Wound Care

T0093561

made Incredibly Easy!

Fourth Edition

Clinical Editor

Patricia Albano Slachta, PhD, RN, APRN, ACNS-BC, CWOCN
President, Nursing Educational Programs and Services
State College, Pennsylvania

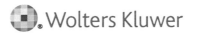 Wolters Kluwer

Philadelphia · Baltimore · New York · London
Buenos Aires · Hong Kong · Sydney · Tokyo

Vice President and Publisher: Julie K. Stegman
Director of Nursing Education and Practice Content: Jamie Blum
Acquisitions Editor: Joyce Berendes
Manager of Content Editing: Staci Wolfson
Editorial Coordinator: Priyanka Alagar
Editorial Assistant: Devika Kishore
Marketing Manager: Amy Whitaker
Production Project Manager: Catherine Ott
Design Coordinator: Stephen Druding
Art Director, Illustration: Jennifer Clements
Manufacturing Coordinator: Bernard Tomboc
Prepress Vendor: S4Carlisle Publishing Services

Fourth Edition

Library of Congress Cataloging-in-Publication Data

ISBN-13: 978-1-975209-21-6

Cataloging in Publication data available on request from publisher.

shop.lww.com

Dedication

To my children, grandchildren, and my husband Greg who have supported me in my professional pursuits over the years, thank you and I love you all. And to my parents, Corable and Angelo Albano, who were always there for me with love and support. I miss you every day.

Patricia Albano Slachta, PhD, RN, APRN, ACNS-BC, CWOCN

Contributors

Michele (Shelly) Burdette-Taylor, PhD, MSN, RN, CWCN, CFCN, NPD-BC, LTC
Associate Professor
Nursing Program
St Martin University
Lacey, Washington

Denise C. Connelly, RN, BSN, CWCN
Dermatology Wound Care Nurse
VA Medical Center
Cherry Hill, New Jersey

Jill Cox, PhD, RN, APN-c, CWOCN, FAAN
Clinical Professor
Division of Nursing Science
Rutgers University
Newark, New Jersey
Wound Ostomy Continence Advanced
  Practice Nurse
Englewood Health
Englewood, New Jersey

Arturo Gonzalez, DNP, APRN, ANP-BC, CWCN-AP
Clinical Associate Professor
Graduate Nursing Department
Nicole Wertheim College of Nursing &
  Health Sciences
Florida International University
Miami, Florida

Joan Junkin, RN, MSN
Wound Consultant and Educator
The Healing Touch, Inc.
Lincoln, Nebraska

Kathleen McLaughlin, DNP, RN, CWOCN
Manager, Wound and Ostomy Care
Wound Care
Texas Health Resources Fort Worth
Fort Worth, Texas

Jody Scardillo, DNP, RN, ANP-BC, CWOCN
Nurse Practitioner
Department of Surgery
Albany Medical College
Albany, New York
Graduate Nursing Program Director
Russell Sage College
Troy, New York

Charleen Singh, PhD, MBA, MSN/ED, FNP-BC, CWOCN, RN
Assistant Program Director MEPN
Betty Irene Moore School of Nursing
University of California Davis
Sacramento, California

Previous Edition Contributors and Consultants

Carol Calianno, MSN, RN, CWOCN

Erin Fazzari, MPT, CLT, CWS, DWC

Joan Junkin, MSN, APRN-CNS

Michelle Marineau, PhD, APRN-Rx

Kathleen McLaughlin, MSN, RN, CWOCN

Jody Scardillo, MS, RN, CWOCN

Tracey Siegel, EdD, MSN, RN, CNE, CWCN

Karen Zulkowski, DNS, RN

Preface

From the first edition in 2003 when I wrote the foreword for this book to now, much has changed in the wound care world. "Pressure ulcers" are "pressure injuries," wet-to-dry dressings are not our first choice, and there are many negative-pressure therapy options available, not to mention different types of dressings.

This edition of *Wound Care Made Incredibly Easy!* combines the best of the third edition with *Wound Care Made Incredibly Visual.* As before, *Wound Care Made Incredibly Easy!* begins at the beginning by reviewing the basics: the integumentary system and wound healing as well as assessing and monitoring wounds. Our previous editions included procedures and products as chapters, but these are now in appendices with the chapters focusing on the larger concepts of wound bed preparation and wound management.

Two new chapters have been added with content on external threats to skin integrity and pediatric skin and wound care. Atypical and malignant wounds content from *Visual* has been incorporated into this *Easy* fourth edition.

Throughout the book, there are key points identified in the "Get wise to wounds," "Handle with care," and "Memory jogger" boxes. Diagrams and photos are provided to enhance understanding of selected concepts and wounds. Charts are used to highlight specific information in a categorized manner. Quizzes are still at the end of each chapter to assist you in your self-evaluation. In the appendices, wound assessment, basic procedures, nutritional guidelines, pressure injury prevention and documentation, and dressing decision tools are available.

Wounds are all around us, regardless of our practice setting. If you are providing care for people with wounds, this book provides well-organized and evidence-based content presented by experts in the field to assist you in your wound care decision-making. We can change a person's life by helping them to manage their wound effectively with minimal pain and cost. Open your mind to new ways of caring for wounds by reviewing the evidence discussed. We have continued with references at the end of each chapter to provide you with the resources to support your wound care decisions.

Acknowledgments

In appreciation to:

Carolyn Cuttino, BSN, RN, CWCN who shared her knowledge when I was discovering the wound and ostomy specialty, and Patty Burns, MSN, RN who generously spent her own time distributing and collecting my dissertation surveys! You have both been amazing colleagues throughout the years.

I would be remiss in not thanking Miss Catherine Zeller, Miss Thelma Taylor, and Miss Lily Martin from Donegal High School, my English and mathematics teachers, and my guidance counselor. The excellent education and guidance I received from these women prepared me for success in my profession.

Contents

Appendices and index

Chapter 1

Skin anatomy and physiology and wound healing

Just the facts

In this chapter, you'll learn about:

♦ layers and functions of the skin

♦ types of wounds

♦ phases of wound healing

♦ factors that affect the skin's ability to heal

♦ complications of wound healing

A look at the skin

The skin, or integumentary system, is the largest organ in the body. It accounts for about 6 to 8 lb (2.5 to 3.5 kg) of a person's body weight and has a surface area of more than 20 sq ft. The thickest epidermal skin is located on the hands and on the soles of the feet; the thinnest skin is located around the eyes and over the tympanic membranes in the ears. The thickest dermal skin is on the back, where it can be 30 to 40 times thicker than the overlying epidermis.

Beauty's only skin deep

Skin protects the body by acting as a barrier between internal structures and the external world. Because skin also stands between each of us and the social world around us, we're also affected by its appearance. Healthy, unblemished skin with good tone (firmness) and color is valued in our society and can therefore contribute to positive self-image. Skin also reflects the body's general physical health. For example, skin may look bluish if blood oxygen levels are low, and it may appear flushed or red if a fever is present.

A wound by any other name

Any damage to the skin is considered a wound. Wounds to the skin can result from planned events (such as surgery), accidents (such as a fall from a bike), or exposure to the environment (such as the damage caused by ultraviolet [UV] rays in sunlight).

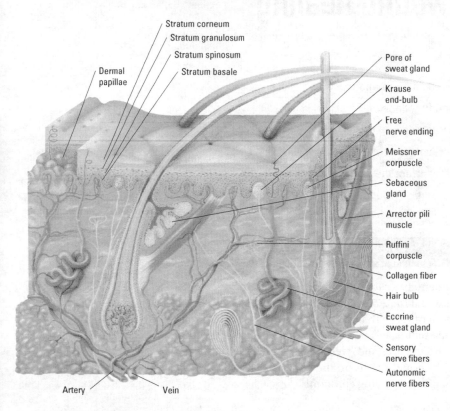

Stratum corneum
Stratum granulosum
Stratum spinosum
Stratum basale
Dermal papillae
Pore of sweat gland
Krause end-bulb
Free nerve ending
Meissner corpuscle
Sebaceous gland
Arrector pili muscle
Ruffini corpuscle
Collagen fiber
Hair bulb
Eccrine sweat gland
Sensory nerve fibers
Autonomic nerve fibers
Artery
Vein

Collaboration is key. The skin is made up of two separate layers, which consist of unique sublayers that function as a single unit. A third layer, the subcutaneous tissue or hypodermis, sits just below the dermis.

Anatomy and physiology

Skin is composed of two main layers that function as a single unit: the epidermis and the dermis. The *epidermis* (outermost layer) is made up of distinct layers. Covering the epidermis is the *keratinized epithelium*, a layer of cells that migrate up from the underlying dermis and die upon reaching the surface. These cells are continuously generated and replaced. The *dermis* (innermost layer) is made up of living cells that receive oxygen and nutrients through an extensive network of small blood vessels. In fact, every square inch of skin contains more than 15 ft of blood vessels! A layer of subcutaneous fatty connective tissue, sometimes called the *hypodermis*, lies beneath these layers.

The outer limits: Our epidermis

When intact with skin oil (sebum) to seal it, the epidermis protects the body from the outside world successfully and prevents excessive fluid and heat loss. Let's take a closer look at some fun and useful facts about the outer limits—the epidermal layers of skin.

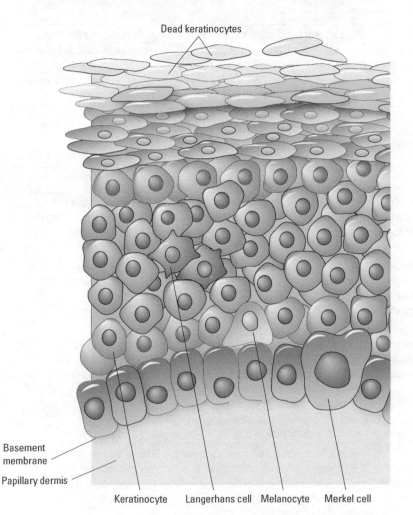

Dead keratinocytes

Basement membrane

Papillary dermis

Keratinocyte   Langerhans cell   Melanocyte   Merkel cell

We live in an "acid mantle," meaning the pH of the skin is naturally acidic when healthy—around 4.5 to 6.2. This creates a hostile environment for bacteria, fungi, and other pathogens. While many bacteria are present on the skin, they don't normally cause infection because the acidic environment of the skin keeps them from multiplying enough to cause infection.

Each of the layers of the epidermis has a name that reflects either its structure or its function. Let's look at them from the outside in:

What's in the epidermis?

Component	Function	Did you know?
Top layer (stratum corneum): A superficial layer of dead skin cells (keratinized epithelium) that's in contact with the environment; sealed with lipids and proteins	Has an acid mantle that helps protect the body from some fungi and bacteria. Cells in this layer continuously migrate through epidermal layers below and die upon reaching the surface. These dead cells are shed daily and are completely replaced every 4–6 weeks. This outer layer regulates the amount and rate of percutaneous absorption of chemicals and organisms unless it is damaged (too dry, too wet, or trauma).	With conditions like eczema and psoriasis, the stratum corneum may become abnormally thick and irritate skin structures and peripheral nerves.
Stratum lucidum: A single layer of cells. Most evident in areas where skin is thick, such as the palms and soles.	Is designed to help these areas withstand friction	This layer appears to be absent where skin is especially thin, such as the eyelids.
Stratum granulosum: Granular layer that is one to five cells thick and is characterized by flat cells with active nuclei. This layer has proteins, lamellar granules, and lipids.	Aids in keratin formation and helps to strengthen the skin	This layer acts as a waterproof barrier to prevent fluid loss from the body.
Stratum spinosum: Composed of keratinocytes and keratin that create intercellular bridges between the keratinocytes	Contains involucrin, a soluble protein that stabilizes the epidermal layers and increases resistance to invading organisms. This layer also contains Langerhans cells that originate in bone marrow and are essential as the first immunologic line of defense.	Langerhans cells can be damaged by UV B rays. Cells begin to flatten as they migrate to the surface.
Stratum basale (stratum germinativum): Just one cell thick and is the only layer of the epidermis in which cells undergo mitosis to form new cells	Forms the dermoepidermal junction—the area where the epidermis and dermis are connected. Protrusions of this layer (called *rete pegs* or *epidermal ridges*) extend down into the dermis where they're surrounded by vascularized dermal papillae.	This unique structure supports the epidermis and facilitates the exchange of fluids and cells between the skin layers.
Melanocytes: Present in the stratum basale layer, and the hypothalamus regulates melanin production by secreting melanocyte-stimulating hormone.	Generate melanin that gives skin and hair its unique color and protects from UV ray damage.	There are two kinds of melanin—eumelanin (black or brown pigment) and pheomelanin (red or yellow pigment). Gray or white hair occurs when melanocytes no longer produce melanin.

What's in the epidermis?

Component	Function	Did you know?
Keratinocytes	Tough guys! These proliferate in the basal layer of epidermis. As they work their way upward to the outer layers, they produce keratin (fibrous protein) and growth factors. They form a tight barrier when healthy.	These cells also have a role as immunomodulators should a wound occur. They are grown in labs to create wound healing tissue products.
Langerhans cells	Sentinels! These take antigens from bacteria and other foreign substances and present them to T-helper lymphocytes in the blood to activate an active immune response if needed.	They are also found in the dermis around blood vessels, mucosa of the mouth, the foreskin, and the vagina. When skin is inflamed, blood monocytes can change into replacement Langerhans cells.
Merkel cells: These cells are in the stratum basale layer.	Touchy! Associated with terminal filaments of cutaneous nerves and have a role in light touch sensation	We have the most Merkel cells in our lips and fingertips.

Sebaceous and sweat glands

Although these glands appear to originate in the dermis, they're actually appendages of the epidermis that extend downward into the dermis. These saclike glands produce sebum, a fatty substance that lubricates and softens the skin. These glands are under androgen control and are very small in infants before beginning to enlarge in preadolescence. For some adolescents, inflammation and infection of the sebaceous glands result in hard-to-manage acne.

Sweat glands: Tightly coiled and tubular; the average person has roughly 2.6 million sweat glands. The secreting portion of the sweat gland originates in the dermis with its outlet on the surface of the skin.	Help regulate body temperature and provide moisture to skin and hair follicles. The sympathetic nervous system regulates sweat production, which in turn helps control body temperature.	There are no sweat glands in the borders of the lips, external ear canals, nail beds, and the glans penis.
Sebaceous glands	Secretes oily/waxy matter (sebum) that lubricates the hair and skin	There are no sebaceous glands on the palms of the hands or soles of the feet. Sebaceous lipids supply vitamin E, a natural antioxidant, to the skin.

What lies beneath: The dermal layers of our skin

The dermis includes all the living structures in the skin, including about 1 million nerves. When healthy, these nerves facilitate sensations such as itching, heat, cold, sharpness of pain, dullness of pain, and the soothing touch of loved ones. There are lots of tiny blood vessels and important connective tissue that keep the skin healthy and intact. The sublayers of connective tissue are:

• The papillary dermis, the outer layer composed of collagen and reticular fibers. Capillaries in the papillary dermis carry the nourishment needed for metabolic activity in this layer.

- The reticular dermis, the inner layer formed by thick networks of collagen bundles. These bundles anchor onto subcutaneous tissue and underlying support structures, such as fasciae, muscle, and bone.
    The dermal layer is thicker in comparison to the epidermal layer and contributes to skin turgor. See the following box for more information on collagen and elastin.

Structural supports: Collagen and elastin

After you pull on the skin, it normally returns to its original position. This is because of the actions of the connective tissues collagen and elastin—two key components of skin.

Understanding the components
Collagen and elastin work together to support the dermis and give skin its physical characteristics.

Collagen
Collagen fibers form tightly woven networks in the papillary layer of the dermis—thick bundles that run parallel to the skin's surface. These fibers are relatively inextensible and nonelastic; therefore, they give the dermis high tensile strength. In addition, collagen constitutes about 70% of the skin's dry weight and is its principal structural body protein.

Elastin
Elastin is made up of wavy fibers that intertwine with collagen in horizontal arrangements at the lower dermis and vertical arrangements at the epidermal margin. Elastin makes skin pliable and is the structural protein that enables extensibility in the dermis.

Seeing the effects of age
As a person ages, collagen and elastin fibers break down, and the fine lines and wrinkles that are associated with aging develop. Extensive exposure to sunlight accelerates this breakdown process. Deep wrinkles are caused by changes in facial muscles. Over time, laughing, crying, smiling, and frowning cause facial muscles to thicken and eventually cause wrinkles in the overlying skin.

Let's take a look at some of these structures.

What's in the dermis?

Component	Function	Did you know?
Fibroblast cells	Produce collagen, elastin, and viscous gel	Collagen makes up 70% of the dermis and gives skin its structure and durability.
Blood and lymph vessels	Provide oxygen and nutrients and carry off waste	The superficial plexus is made of tiny arterioles and venules lying close to the epidermis. The deep plexus is made of vessels that are larger and connect vertically to the superficial plexus. The lymphatic drainage conserves plasma proteins and scavenges foreign material, antigenic substances, and bacteria.

What's in the dermis?

Component	Function	Did you know?
Nerve fibers, pressure and vibration sensors (Pacinian corpuscles), and touch receptors (Meissner corpuscles)	Sensation for safety, information, and pleasure	Autonomic nerves in the skin cause: • blood vessels to dilate in response to excess heat or constrict in response to cold. • sweat glands to secrete moisture to help cool body temperature. • arrector pili muscles to alert us to danger (a hair-raising experience!) but mainly meant to trap air between the erect hairs, helping hairier mammals retain heat.
Hair follicles	The sebaceous glands near every follicle keep hair and surrounding skin healthy.	The bulb in the dermis grows the hair, which follows a tunnel out through the epidermis.
Cholesterol	Converted into cholecalciferol from which the liver makes calcitriol (an active form of vitamin D)	Vitamin D is essential for normal absorption of calcium and phosphorous for bone health; it has many other functions as well.

The layered look

Subcutaneous tissue, or the hypodermis, is the subdermal (below the skin) layer of loose connective tissue that contains major blood vessels, lymph vessels, and nerves. Did you know that medications administered to the hypodermis are absorbed more slowly because it is mostly made up of fat with few blood vessels? This layer is also useful as padding and insulation, and it connects the skin to the muscles and bones beneath it. With aging, the hypodermis shrinks, and the skin tends to sag. Let's take a look at what makes up the hypodermis.

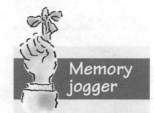

Memory jogger

Keep the skin layers straight by remembering that the prefix **epi-** means "upon." Therefore, the **epi**dermis is upon, or on top of, the dermis.

Two types of sweat glands

- *Eccrine* glands are active at birth and are found throughout the body. They're densest on the palms, soles, and forehead. These glands connect to the skin's surface through pores and produce sweat that lacks proteins and fatty acids. Eccrine glands are smaller than apocrine glands.
- *Apocrine* glands begin to function at puberty. These glands open into hair follicles; therefore, most are found in areas where hair typically grows, such as the scalp, groin, and axillary region. The coiled secreting portion of each gland lies deep in the dermis (deeper than eccrine glands), and a duct connects it to the upper portion of the hair follicle. The sweat produced by apocrine glands

contains water, sodium, chloride, proteins, and fatty acids. It's thicker than the sweat produced by eccrine glands and has a milky white or yellowish tinge. (See *Bacteria make the odor!*)

Blood supply

The skin receives its blood supply through vessels that originate in underlying muscle tissue. Here, arteries branch into smaller vessels, which then branch into the network of capillaries that permeate the dermis and subcutaneous tissue.

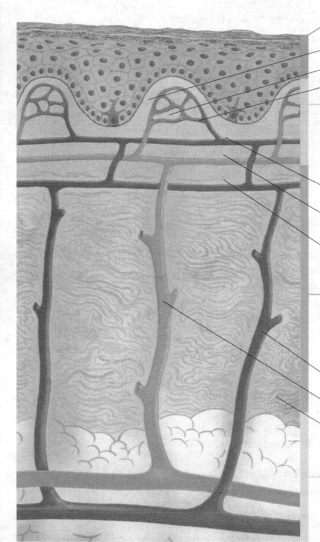

Epidermis

Terminal arteriole

Capillary

Postcapillary venule

Papillary dermis
superficial layer composed of loose connective tissue and capillaries; extends up into the epidermis through the dermal papillae

Upper superficial venular plexus

Superficial arterial plexus

Deep superficial venular plexus

Reticular dermis
deeper layer composed of irregular connective tissue with collagen, collagen bundles, and elastin

Descending venule

Ascending arteriole

Elastic fibers

Subcutaneous tissue

What's in the hypodermis?

Component	Function	Did you know?
Adipose tissue	Fatty tissue (mostly adipocytes) that provides insulation and acts as a shock absorber to protect organs, muscles, and bones from harm; also stores energy	Individuals with more testosterone tend to have thicker adipose tissue in the abdomen, upper arms, shoulders, and lower back. Individuals with more estrogen tend to have thicker adipose tissue at the buttocks, hips, and thighs.
Connective tissue	Includes collagen and elastin, which help keep the skin connected to underlying tissue	With aging, the hypodermis thins and with less connective tissue, skin begins to sag and tears more easily.
Blood and lymph vessels	Provide oxygen and nutrients and carry off waste	Blood flow to the skin is reduced by 40% between the ages of 20 and 70 years. The vasoconstriction associated with smoking can be reversed within 4 weeks after cessation.

Just passing through

Within the vascular system, only capillaries have walls thin enough (typically only a single layer of endothelial cells) to let solutes pass through. These thin walls allow nutrients and oxygen to pass from the bloodstream into the interstitial space around skin cells. At the same time, waste products pass into the capillaries and are carried away. The pressure of arterial blood entering the capillaries is about 30 mm Hg. The pressure of venous blood leaving the capillaries is about 10 mm Hg. This 20-mm Hg difference in pressure within the capillaries is quite low when compared with the pressure found in the larger arteries in the body (85 to 100 mm Hg), which is known as *blood pressure*. (See *Fluid movement through capillaries*.)

Fluid movement through capillaries

The movement of fluids through capillaries—a process called *capillary filtration*—results from blood pushing against the walls of the capillary. That pressure, called *hydrostatic pressure*, forces fluids and solutes through the capillary wall.

When the hydrostatic pressure inside a capillary is greater than the pressure in the surrounding interstitial space, fluids and solutes inside the capillary are forced out into the interstitial space, as shown on the following page. When the pressure inside the capillary is less than the pressure outside, fluids and solutes move back into it.

(continued)

Fluid movement through capillaries *(continued)*

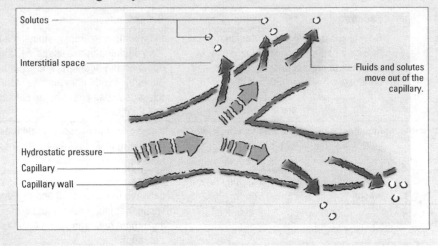

Solutes

Interstitial space

Fluids and solutes move out of the capillary.

Hydrostatic pressure

Capillary

Capillary wall

Lymphatic system

The skin's lymphatic system helps remove waste products, including excess proteins and fluids, from the dermis.

Go with the flow

Lymphatic vessels, or *lymphatics* for short, are similar to capillaries in that they are thin-walled, permeable vessels; however, lymphatics aren't part of the blood circulatory system. Instead, lymphatics belong to a separate system that removes proteins, large waste products, and excess fluids from the interstitial spaces in skin and then transports them to the venous circulation. The lymphatic vessels merge into two main trunks—the thoracic duct and the right lymphatic duct—that empty into the junction of the subclavian and internal jugular veins.

Functions of the skin

Skin performs or participates in a host of vital functions, including:
- protection of internal structures
- sensory perception
- thermoregulation
- excretion
- metabolism
- absorption
- social communication

Damage to skin impairs its ability to carry out these important functions. Let's take a closer look at each.

	Function	Description
	Protection	• Acts as a physical barrier to microorganisms and foreign matter • Two kinds of flora exist on the skin: *resident* (live on the skin) and *transient* (not normally found on the skin). • Most people carry over 20 strains of resident bacteria and fungi on their skin. • Transient bacteria are acquired by contact with others or the environment and are typically removed by hand washing and bathing. • Bathing patients who are hospitalized with pH-balanced chlorhexidine gluconate 4% (CHG 4%) significantly reduces transient flora, which are responsible for central line– and catheter-associated urinary tract infections. • Protects the body against infection from the environment with Langerhans cells, which trigger the immune system • Protects underlying tissue and structures from mechanical injury (Consider the feet: As a person walks or runs, the soles of the feet withstand a tremendous amount of force, yet the underlying tissue and bone structures remain unharmed.) • Protecting the heel from constant pressure prevents deep tissue injury over the heel, which is not accustomed to constant direct pressure. • Maintains a stable environment inside the body by preventing the loss of water, electrolytes, proteins, and other substances. Any damage jeopardizes this protection. When it is damaged, the skin goes into repair mode to restore full protection by increasing the normal process of cell replacement. • Damage or breaks in the skin allow for transient bacteria to enter into the bloodstream, resulting in infections or sepsis.
	Sensory perception	• Contains nerve endings and sensory receptors (Merkel cells) • Sensory nerve fibers originate in the nerve roots along the spine and supply specific areas of the skin known as *dermatomes*. Dermatomes are used to transmit sensory function. This same network helps a person avoid injury by making them aware of pain, pressure, heat, and cold. • Although sensory nerves exist throughout the skin, some areas are more sensitive than others—for example, the fingertips are more sensitive than the back. Any loss or reduction of sensation (local or general) increases the chance of injury.
	Thermoregulation	• Contains nerves, blood vessels, and eccrine glands in the dermis to control body temperature • Causes blood vessels to constrict (reducing blood flow and conserving heat) when exposed to cold or drops in internal body temperature • Causes small arteries in the skin to dilate and increases sweat production to promote cooling when skin becomes hot or internal body temperature rises • Facilitating heat flow and moisture within skin folds using moisture-wicking fabric helps regulate the patient's microclimate.

(continued)

(continued)

	Function	Description
	Excretion	• Transmits trace amounts of water and body wastes to the environment through its more than 2 million pores • Thermoregulation and electrolyte and hydration balances are maintained as sweat carries water and salt to the skin surface, where it evaporates (the healthy adult loses approximately 500 mL of water this way). • Prevents dehydration by ensuring that the body doesn't lose too much water while lipids in the skin help prevent unwanted or dangerous fluids from entering the body • Sebum excretion helps maintain the skin's integrity and suppleness. • Maintaining adequate airflow around a patient's skin is an essential component to maintaining skin integrity.
	Metabolism	• Synthesizes vitamin D via a photochemical reaction in the skin (which is crucial to the metabolism of calcium and phosphate) when exposed to the UV spectrum in sunlight. (Overexposure to UV light causes damage that reduces the skin's ability to function properly.) • Helps maintain the mineralization of bones and teeth
	Absorption	• Allows for some drugs and toxic substances (e.g., pesticides) to be absorbed directly through the skin and into the bloodstream • Areas such as the face and forearms are extremely vulnerable to absorption. • Infants and small children are especially at risk for absorption of chemicals through the skin. Even sunscreen is not recommended until 6 months of age. • The skin's ability to absorb substances can be used to treat certain disorders through topical medications and via skin patch systems. One example is the transdermal drug delivery method used in some nicotine withdrawal programs. This technology is also used to administer some forms of contraception, hormone replacement therapy, nitroglycerin, and pain medications.

Social communication

A commonly overlooked but important function of the skin is its role in self-esteem development and social communication. Every time a person looks in the mirror, they decide whether they like what they see. Although bone structure, body type, teeth, and hair all have an impact, the condition and characteristics of the skin sometimes have the greatest impact on a person's self-esteem. If a person likes what they see, self-esteem rises; if they don't, it sags.

You should have seen your face

Every interpersonal exchange includes the nonverbal languages of facial expression and body posture. A person's level of self-esteem and skin characteristics—which are visible at all times—have an impact on how they communicate, both verbally and nonverbally, and how they are received by a listener.

Because the physical characteristics of skin are so closely linked to self-perception, a proliferation of skin care products and surgical techniques are available to keep skin looking healthy.

Aging and skin function

Over time, skin loses its ability to function as efficiently or as effectively as it once did. (See *How skin ages.*) As a result, advanced age places a person at greater risk for injuries, such as pressure injuries as well as various other skin conditions.

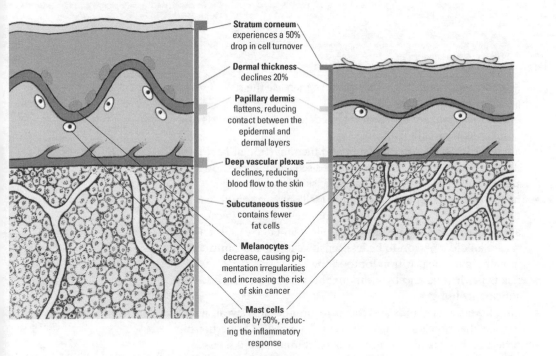

Stratum corneum experiences a 50% drop in cell turnover

Dermal thickness declines 20%

Papillary dermis flattens, reducing contact between the epidermal and dermal layers

Deep vascular plexus declines, reducing blood flow to the skin

Subcutaneous tissue contains fewer fat cells

Melanocytes decrease, causing pigmentation irregularities and increasing the risk of skin cancer

Mast cells decline by 50%, reducing the inflammatory response

How skin ages

Change	Findings in older adult patients
Pigmentation	Paler color than when younger
Thickness	• Wrinkling, especially on the face, arms, and legs • Parchment-like appearance, especially over bony prominences and on the dorsal surfaces of the hands, feet, arms, and legs

(continued)

How skin ages *(continued)*

Change	Findings in older adult patients
Moisture	Dry, flaky, and rough
Turgor	"Tents" and stands alone
Texture	Numerous creases and lines
Papillary dermis	Flattening of papillae in the dermoepidermal junction (meeting of the epidermis and dermis), which reduces adhesion between layers
Subcutaneous tissue	Redistribution of this tissue to the stomach and thighs
Mast cells, fibroblasts, and Langerhans cells	Decline, reducing the inflammatory response

Injury alert

As a person ages, physiologic changes also increase the risk of various injuries. For example, older adults:

- bruise easily and are more prone to edema around wounds due to reduced skin vascularization.
- are more likely to suffer pressure and thermal (hot and cold) damage to the skin due to diminished sensation even though the same number of nerve endings in the skin is retained.
- have a higher incidence of ischemia (cell damage resulting from too little oxygen reaching cells) in compressed tissue because bony areas have less subcutaneous cushioning, and decreased sensation causes an older person to be less sensitive to the discomfort of remaining in one position for too long.
- risk hyperthermia and hypothermia because of decreased subcutaneous tissue.
- have fewer sweat glands and therefore produce less sweat, which hinders thermoregulation and increases the risk of hyperthermia.
- have a higher risk of infection because thinner skin is a less effective barrier to germs and allergens and because the skin contains fewer Langerhans cells to fight infection and fewer mast cells to mediate the inflammatory response.
- are slower to exhibit a sensitization response (redness, heat, discomfort) due to the reduction in Langerhans cells, resulting in overuse of topical medications and more severe allergic reactions (because signs aren't evident early on).
- risk overdose of transdermal medications when poor absorption prompts them to reapply the medication too often.
- have a much higher incidence of shear and tear injuries due to compromised skin layer adhesion and less flexible collagen.

A look at wounds

Any injury to the skin is considered a wound. Tissue damage in wounds varies widely, from a superficial break in the epithelium to deep trauma that involves the muscle and bone. A "clean" wound is a wound produced by surgery. A wound is described as "dirty" if it contains bacteria or other debris. Trauma typically produces dirty wounds. The rate of wound recovery varies according to the extent and type of damage incurred and other intrinsic factors, such as the patient's circulation, nutrition, and hydration. Although the recovery rate varies, the healing process is much the same in all cases.

Types of wound healing

A wound is classified by the way it closes. A wound can close by primary, secondary, or tertiary intention.

Primary intention

Primary intention is the process by which a surgical wound is closed. The skin edges are approximated to each other and secured with suture, staples, or skin glue. These wounds usually heal in 4 to 14 days and result in minimal scarring. A palpable healing ridge begins to develop at 48 hours. Utilizing an antimicrobial dressing immediately following closure reduces the impact of transient flora and facilitates formation of the healing ridge.

Clean incision

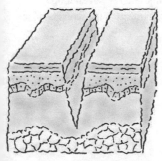

Wound has well-approximated edges.

Early suture

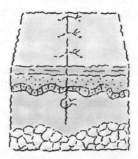

Clean edges can be pulled together neatly.

Hairline scar

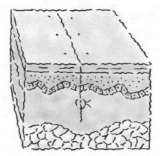

Because there's no loss of tissue and little risk of infection, these wounds usually heal in 4 to 14 days and result in minimal scarring.

Secondary intention

Infected wounds or wounds that involve some degree of tissue loss with edges that can't be easily approximated heal by secondary intention. Depending on a wound's depth, it can be described as partial thickness or full thickness:

- Partial-thickness wounds extend through the epidermis and into but not through the dermis. These are superficial wounds that usually close in 7 to 14 days, typically with little or no scarring.
- Full-thickness wounds extend through the epidermis and dermis and may involve subcutaneous tissue, muscle, and possibly bone.

During healing, full-thickness wounds that heal by secondary intention fill with granulation tissue; then a scar forms, and reepithelialization occurs, primarily from the wound edges. Pressure injuries, burns, dehisced surgical wounds, and traumatic injuries are examples of this type of wound. These wounds also take longer to heal, result in scarring, and have a higher rate of complications than wounds that heal by primary intention.

Occasionally, the delayed healing in this type of wound can lead to hypergranular tissue. Hypergranular tissue is frequently raised above the level of intact skin; is very red, "beefy," and bleeds easily (friable); and typically is a response to chronic inflammation and heavy bacterial burden or excessive moisture.

Gaping irregular wound

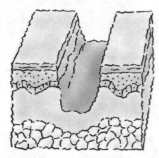

Edges can't be easily approximated.

Granulation

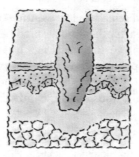

Wound fills with granulation tissue.

Epithelium growth over scar

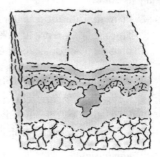

A scar forms, and reepithelialization occurs, primarily from the wound edges.

Tertiary intention

Wounds that are intentionally kept open to allow edema or infection to resolve or to permit removal of exudate heal by tertiary intention (also called "delayed primary intention"). These wounds are later closed with sutures, staples, or adhesive skin closures. Wounds that heal by tertiary intention result in more scarring than wounds that heal by primary intention but less than wounds that heal by secondary intention.

Phases of wound healing

The healing process is the same for all wounds, whether the cause is mechanical, chemical, or thermal. Health care professionals discuss the process of wound healing in four specific phases: hemostasis, inflammation, proliferation, and maturation (remodeling).

Open wound

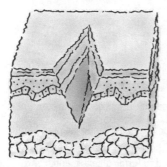

Wound is intentionally kept open (typically for 3 to 5 days) to allow edema or infection to resolve or to permit removal of exudate.

Increased granulation

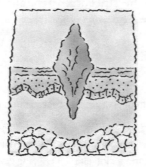

Wound fills with granulation tissue.

Late suturing with wide scar

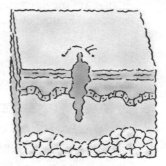

Wound is sutured late, and a wide scar results.

Wound healing process

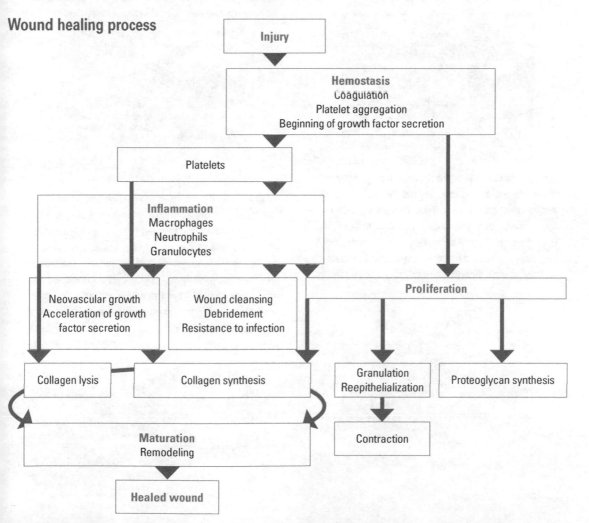

Injury

Hemostasis
Coagulation
Platelet aggregation
Beginning of growth factor secretion

Platelets

Inflammation
Macrophages
Neutrophils
Granulocytes

Neovascular growth
Acceleration of growth
factor secretion

Wound cleansing
Debridement
Resistance to infection

Proliferation

Collagen lysis

Collagen synthesis

Granulation
Reepithelialization

Proteoglycan synthesis

Maturation
Remodeling

Contraction

Healed wound

Although this categorization is useful, it is important to remember that healing rarely occurs in this strict order. Typically, the phases of wound healing overlap. (See *How wounds heal*.)

How wounds heal

The healing process begins at the instant of injury and proceeds through a repair "cascade," as outlined here.

1. Hemostasis: When tissue is damaged, serotonin, histamine, prostaglandins, and blood from the injured vessels fill the area. Blood platelets form a clot, and fibrin in the clot binds the wound edges together. The inflammation stage is initiated during hemostasis, and this process may last a few days.

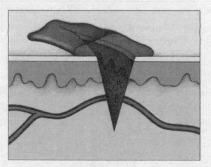

2. Inflammation: Lymphocytes initiate the inflammatory response, increasing capillary permeability. Wound edges swell, and white blood cells from surrounding vessels move in and ingest bacteria and cellular debris, demolishing the clot. Redness, warmth, swelling, pain, and loss of function may occur. Platelets heavily secrete growth factors during this phase.

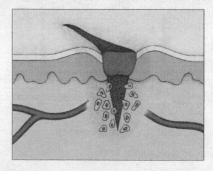

3. Proliferation: Adjacent healthy tissue supplies blood, nutrients, fibroblasts, proteins, and other building materials needed to form soft, pink, and highly vascular granulation tissue, which begins to bridge the area. Inflammation may decrease, or signs and symptoms of infection (increased swelling, increased pain, fever, and pus-filled discharge) may develop.

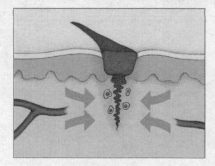

4. Maturation: Fibroblasts in the granulation tissue secrete collagen, a gluelike substance. Collagen fibers criss-cross the area, forming scar tissue. Meanwhile, epithelial cells at the wound edge multiply and migrate toward the wound center. This epithelial tissue will create a light pink "halo" that grows around the edge of the wound until it fills the whole wound with a scar. As it heals, color deposited into the wound will be the same color as the skin.

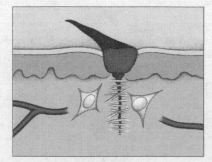

How wounds heal

5. Over months or years, damaged tissue (including lymphatics, blood vessels, and stromal matrices) regenerates. Collagen fibers shorten, and the scar diminishes in size. Scar size may decrease and normal function may return or the scar may hypertrophy, leading to the formation of a keloid and the development of contractures.

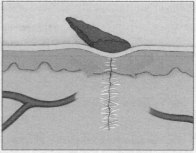

Hemostasis

Immediately after an injury, the body releases chemical mediators and intercellular messengers called *growth factors* that begin the process of cleaning and healing the wound.

Slow that flow!

When blood vessels are damaged, the small muscles in the walls of the vessels contract (vasoconstriction), reducing the flow of blood to the injury and minimizing blood loss. Vasoconstriction can last as long as 30 minutes. Next, blood leaking from the inflamed, dilated, or broken vessels begins to coagulate. Collagen fibers in the wall of the damaged blood vessels activate the platelets in the blood that's in the wound. Aided by the action of prostaglandins, the platelets enlarge and stick together to form a temporary plug in the blood vessel, which helps prevent further bleeding. The platelets also release additional vasoconstrictors, such as serotonin, which help prevent further blood loss. Thrombin forms in a cascade of events stimulated by the platelets, and a clot forms to close the small vessels and stop bleeding.

This initial phase of wound healing occurs almost immediately after the injury occurs and works within minutes in small wounds. Hemostasis is less effective at stopping the bleeding when larger vessels are involved.

Inflammation

The inflammatory phase is both a defense mechanism and a crucial component of the healing process in which the wound is cleaned and rebuilding begins. (See *Understanding the inflammatory response*.)

Understanding the inflammatory response

This flowchart outlines the sequence of events in the inflammatory process.

Microorganisms invade damaged tissue.

▼

Basophils release heparin, and histamine and kinin production occurs.

▼

Vasodilation occurs along with increased capillary permeability.

▼

Blood flow increases to the affected tissues and fluid collects within them.

▼

Neutrophils flock to the invasion site to engulf and destroy microorganisms from dying cells.

▼

This sets the stage for the next phase: proliferation.

During the inflammatory phase, vascular permeability increases, permitting serous fluid carrying small amounts of cells and plasma proteins to accumulate in the tissue around the wound (edema). The accumulation of fluid causes the damaged tissue to appear swollen, red, and warm to the touch.

Search and destroy

During the early phase of the inflammatory process, neutrophils (one type of white blood cell) enter the wound. The primary role of neutrophils is phagocytosis (removal and destruction of bacteria and other contaminants).

As neutrophil infiltration slows, monocytes appear. Monocytes are converted into activated macrophages and continue the job of cleaning the wound. The macrophages play a key role early in the process of granulation and reepithelialization by producing growth factors and by attracting the cells needed for the formation of new blood vessels and collagen.

Telling time

The inflammatory phase of healing is important for preventing wound infection. The process is negatively influenced if the patient has a systemic condition that suppresses their immune system or if they are undergoing immunosuppressive therapy. In clean wounds, the inflammatory response lasts about 36 hours. In dirty, infected wounds or wounds in individuals with impaired immune systems, the response can last much longer.

Proliferation

During the proliferation phase of the healing process, the body:
- fills the wound with connective tissue (granulation).
- contracts the wound edges (contraction).
- covers the wound with epithelium (epithelialization).

Presto change-o!

All wounds go through the proliferation phase, but it takes much longer in wounds with extensive tissue loss. Although phases overlap, wound granulation generally starts when the inflammatory response is complete. As the inflammatory phase subsides, wound exudate (drainage) begins to decrease.

The proliferation phase involves regeneration of blood vessels (angiogenesis) and the formation of connective or granulation tissue. The development of granulation tissue requires an adequate supply of blood and nutrients. Endothelial cells in the blood vessels of the surrounding tissue reconstruct damaged or destroyed vessels by first migrating and then proliferating to form new capillary beds. As the beds form, this area of the wound takes on a red, "beefy," granular appearance. This tissue is a good defense against contaminants, but it is also quite fragile, can bleed easily, and become reinfected.

Let the rebuilding begin

During the proliferation phase, growth factors prompt fibroblasts to migrate to the wound. Fibroblasts are the most common cell in connective tissue. They are responsible for making the fibers and ground substance (also known as *extracellular matrix*) that provide support to cells. At first, fibroblasts populate just the margins of the wound; they later spread over the entire wound surface.

Fibroblasts have the important task of synthesizing collagen fibers that in turn produce keratinocyte, a growth factor needed for reepithelialization. This process necessitates a delicate balance of collagen synthesis and lysis (making new and removing old collagen). If the process yields too much collagen, increased scarring results. If the process yields too little collagen, scar tissue is weak and easily ruptured. Because fibroblasts require a supply of oxygen to perform their important role, capillary bed regeneration is crucial to the process.

Pulling it all together

As healing progresses, myofibroblasts and the newly formed collagen fibers contract, pulling the wound edges toward each other. Contraction reduces the amount of granulation tissue needed to fill the wound, which speeds the healing process. (See *Contraction versus contracture.*) The right dressing can facilitate the process and the wrong dressing can inhibit it.

Contraction versus contracture

Contraction and contracture occur during the wound healing process. While they have mechanisms in common, it is important to understand how contraction and contracture differ:

• Contraction, a desirable process that occurs during healing, is the process by which the edges of a wound pull toward the center of the wound to close it. Contraction continues to close the wound until tension in the surrounding skin causes it to slow and then stop.

• Contracture is an undesirable process and a common complication of burn scarring. Typically, contracture occurs after healing is complete. Contracture involves an inordinate amount of pulling or shortening of tissue, resulting in an area of tissue with only limited ability to move. It is especially problematic over joints, which may be pulled to a flexed position, limiting normal use. Stretching and maintaining mobility during the healing is the only way to mitigate contracture. Patients typically require physical therapy and encouragement to use the extremity.

Complete healing occurs only after epithelial cells have completely covered the surface of the wound. When this occurs, keratinocytes switch from a migratory mode to a differentiation mode. The epidermis thickens and becomes differentiated, and the wound is closed. Any remaining scab comes off and the new epidermis is toughened by the production of keratin, which also returns the skin to its original color.

Maturation

The final phase of wound healing is maturation, which is marked by the shrinking and strengthening of the scar. This is a gradual, transitional phase of healing that can continue for months or even years after the wound has closed. Massaging over the maturing wound can minimize scaring.

Movin' on

During maturation, fibroblasts leave the site of the wound, vascularization is reduced, the scar shrinks and becomes pale, and the mature scar forms. If the wound involved extensive tissue destruction, the scar won't contain hair, sweat, or sebaceous glands.

The wound gradually gains tensile strength. In wounds that heal by primary intention, tissues will achieve about 30% to 50% of their original strength between days 1 and 14. When fully healed, tissue will at best achieve about 80% of its original strength. Scar tissue will always be less elastic than the surrounding skin.

Wound healing: Partial- versus full-thickness wounds

Partial-thickness wounds involve the top layers of skin, specifically the epidermal and dermal layers. Partial-thickness wounds heal by epithelialization only. In contrast, full-thickness wounds extend through the dermis and into the subdermal structures. The more damage done to the tissues, the more mechanisms of healing are required. Full-thickness wounds will have evidence of healing in the form of scars.

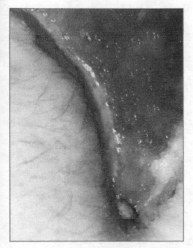

Full-thickness wound with epithelial "halo." Epithelial tissue migrating from intact skin over granulation tissue.

Full-thickness wound around a colostomy

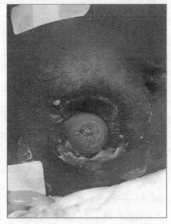

Note the wound is beginning to fill in with granulation tissue and has an epithelial halo starting.

Wound healing: Acute versus chronic wounds

Simply put, acute wounds progress along the healing phases in an orderly, predictable fashion. The mechanism of injury is easily identifiable in acute wounds, for example, those from surgery or trauma. Delays in wound healing are typically minimal and easily addressed.

Chronic wounds do not follow the healing process in an orderly, timely manner. Sometimes they "fall off" the healing cascade. Due to various factors, these wounds stall in one of the phases and require long-term follow-up.

Debridement may be used to convert a wound from a chronic to an acute one. The debridement activates the healing cascade, and normal healing may commence. All systemic factors must be addressed, or the wound will not continue to heal along the cascade.

Factors that affect healing

The healing process is affected by many factors. The most important influences include:
- nutrition
- oxygenation

- infection
- age
- chronic health conditions
- medications
- smoking
- environment

Nutrition

Proper nutrition is arguably one of the most important factors in wound healing; however, malnutrition is a common finding among patients with wounds. It is estimated that between 20% and 50% of all hospitalized persons are malnourished, and the problem is more pervasive for older adults (Cass & Charlton, 2022). Malnutrition has been reported in over half of all hospitalized patients aged 65 years and older (Cass & Charlton, 2022).

Poor nutrition prolongs hospitalization and increases the risk of medical complications. The severity of complications is directly related to the severity of the malnutrition. In older patients, malnutrition is known to increase the risk of pressure injuries and delay wound healing. It may also contribute to poor tensile strength in healing wounds with an associated increase in the risk of wound dehiscence. (See *Tips for detecting nutritional problems.*)

Tips for detecting nutritional problems

Nutritional problems may stem from physical conditions, drugs, diet, or lifestyle factors. The list that follows can help you identify risk factors that make your patient particularly susceptible to nutritional problems.

Physical condition
- Chronic illnesses (such as diabetes) and neurologic, cardiac, or thyroid problems
- Draining wounds or fistulas
- Weight issues—weight loss of 5% of normal body weight, weight less than 90% of ideal body weight, weight gain or loss of 10 lb (4.5 kg) or more in last 6 months, obesity, or weight gain of 20% above normal body weight
- History of gastrointestinal (GI) disturbances
- Anorexia or bulimia
- Depression or anxiety
- Severe trauma
- Recent chemotherapy or radiation therapy
- Physical limitations, such as paresis or paralysis
- Recent major surgery
- Pregnancy, especially during adolescence or with multiple births

Drugs and diet
- Fad diets
- Steroid, diuretic, or antacid use
- Mouth, tooth, or denture problems
- Excessive alcohol intake
- Liquid diet or nothing by mouth for more than 3 days without supplementation

Lifestyle factors
- Lack of support from family or friends
- Lack of resources for obtaining healthy foods

Protein power

Protein is crucial for wounds to heal properly. In fact, a person needs to double the recommended dietary allowance of protein (from 0.8 to 1.5 g/kg/day) before tissue even begins to heal. If a significant amount of body weight has been lost in connection with the injury, as much as 50% of the lost weight must be regained before healing will begin. A patient with low protein reserves heals slowly, if at all, and a patient who is borderline malnourished can easily become malnourished under this demand.

The body needs protein to form collagen during the proliferation phase. Without adequate protein, collagen formation is reduced or delayed and the healing process slows. Studies of malnourished patients indicate that they have lower levels of serum albumin, which results in slower oxygen diffusion and in turn a reduction in the ability of neutrophils to kill bacteria. Wound exudate alone can contain up to 100 g of protein per day.

Nifty nutrients

Fatty acids (lipids) are used in cell structures and play a role in the inflammatory process. Also, vitamins C, B complex, A, and E and the minerals iron, copper, zinc, and calcium are important in the healing process. A zinc deficiency adversely affects the proliferation phase by slowing the rate of epithelialization and decreasing the strength of collagen produced and thus the strength of the healing skin.

In addition to protein and zinc, collagen synthesis requires supplies of carbohydrates and fat. Collagen cross-linking requires adequate amounts of vitamins A and C, iron, and copper. Vitamin C, iron, and zinc are important to developing tensile strength during the maturation phase of wound healing.

Oxygenation

Wound healing depends on a regular supply of oxygen. For example, oxygen is critical for leukocytes to destroy bacteria and for fibroblasts to stimulate collagen synthesis. If the supply is hindered by poor blood flow to the area of the wound or if the patient's ability to take in adequate oxygen is impaired, the result is the same—impaired healing.

Possible causes of inadequate blood flow to the area of the wound include pressure, arterial occlusion, or prolonged vasoconstriction, possibly associated with such medical conditions as peripheral vascular disease and atherosclerosis. Possible causes of a lower than necessary systemic blood oxygenation include:

- hypothermia or hyperthermia
- anemia
- alkalemia
- medical conditions such as chronic obstructive pulmonary disease that limit oxygen intake

Infection

An infection can be systemic or localized in the wound. A systemic infection, such as pneumonia or tuberculosis, increases the patient's metabolism and thus consumes the fluids, nutrients, and oxygen that the body needs for healing. Treatment of infections takes 48 hours to reach the wound bed.

Damaging developments

A localized infection in the wound itself is more common. Remember, any break in the skin allows bacteria to enter. The infection may occur as part of the injury or may develop later in the healing process. For example, when the inflammatory phase lingers, wound healing is delayed and metabolic byproducts of bacterial ingestion accumulate in the wound. This buildup interferes with the formation of new blood vessels and the synthesis of collagen. Infection can also occur in a wound that has been healing normally. This is especially true for larger wounds involving extensive tissue damage. New or increased pain, redness, heat, and drainage are signs of a new infection. In any case, healing can't progress until the cause of infection is addressed.

Age

Skin changes that occur with aging can prolong healing time in older adult patients. Although delayed healing is partially due to physiologic changes, it is usually complicated by other problems associated with aging, such as poor nutrition and hydration, the presence of a chronic condition, and the use of multiple medications. (See *Effects of aging on wound healing.*)

Effects of aging on wound healing

In older adults, factors that impede wound healing include:
* slower turnover rate in epidermal cells
* poorer oxygenation at the wound due to increasingly fragile capillaries and a reduction in skin vascularization
* altered nutrition and fluid intake resulting from physical changes that can accompany aging, such as reduced saliva production, a declining sense of smell and taste, or decreased stomach motility
* altered nutrition and fluid intake attributable to personal or social disturbances, such as loose-fitting dentures, financial concerns, eating alone after the death of a partner, or problems preparing or obtaining food
* impaired function of the respiratory or immune systems
* reduced dermal and subcutaneous mass leading to an increased risk of chronic pressure injuries
* healed wounds that lack tensile strength and are prone to reinjury

Chronic health conditions

Respiratory problems, atherosclerosis, diabetes, autoimmune diseases, and malignancies can increase the risk for wounds and interfere with wound healing. These conditions can interfere with systemic and peripheral oxygenation and nutrition, which affect healing.

Getting complicated

Impaired circulation, a common problem for patients with diabetes and other disorders, can cause tissue hypoxia (lack of oxygen). Neuropathy associated with diabetes reduces a person's ability to sense pressure. As a result, a patient with diabetes may experience trauma, especially to the feet, without realizing it. Insulin dependency can impair leukocyte function, which adversely affects cell proliferation.

Hemiplegia and quadriplegia involve the breakdown of muscle tissue and a reduction in the padding around the large bones of the lower body. Because a patient with one of these conditions lacks sensation, they are at risk for developing chronic pressure injuries. The impaired nerve conduction slows down the wound healing time.

Other conditions that can delay healing include dehydration, end-stage kidney disease, thyroid disease, heart failure, peripheral vascular disease, vasculitis, collagen vascular disorders, and other chronic infections such as hepatitis or human immunodeficiency virus (HIV).

Day and night shifts

Normally, a healthy person shifts position every 15 minutes or so, even during sleep. This prevents tissue damage from ischemia. Anything that impairs the ability to sense pressure, including the use of pain medications, spinal cord lesions, or cognitive impairment, puts the patient at risk for trauma because the patient can't feel the growing discomfort of pressure and respond to it.

Medications

Any medications that reduce a patient's movement, circulation, or metabolic function, such as sedatives and tranquilizers, have the potential to inhibit the ability to sense and respond to pressure. Also, because movement promotes adequate oxygenation, lack of motion means that peripheral blood delivers less oxygen to the extremities than it should. This is especially problematic for older adults. Remember, oxygen is important; without it, the healing process slows and the potential for complications rises.

At a turtle's pace

Some medications, such as steroids and chemotherapeutic agents, reduce the body's ability to mount an appropriate inflammatory response. This interrupts the inflammatory phase of healing and can dramatically lengthen healing time, especially in patients with compromised immune systems.

Smoking

Carbon monoxide, a component of cigarette smoke, binds to the hemoglobin in blood in the place of oxygen. This significantly reduces the amount of oxygen circulating in the bloodstream, which can impede wound healing. To some extent, this reaction also occurs in people regularly exposed to secondhand smoke.

Complications of wound healing

The most common complications associated with wound healing are hemorrhage, dehiscence and evisceration, and infection. Fistulas, tunneling, and undermining can also occur as complications of wound healing.

Hemorrhage

Internal hemorrhage (bleeding) can result in the formation of a hematoma—a blood clot that solidifies to form a hard lump under the skin. Hematomas are commonly found under bruised skin.

External hemorrhage is visible bleeding from the wound. External bleeding during healing isn't unusual because the newly developed blood vessels are fragile and rupture easily. This is one reason that a wound needs to be protected by a dressing. However, each time the new blood vessels suffer damage, healing is delayed while repairs are made.

Dehiscence and evisceration

Dehiscence is a separation of the skin and underlying tissue layers. It is most likely to occur 1 to 2 weeks after the injury is sustained and may follow surgery. Evisceration is similar but involves the protrusion of underlying visceral organs as well. (See *Recognizing dehiscence and evisceration.*)

Dehiscence may constitute a surgical emergency, especially if the wound is large. Evisceration usually involves an abdominal wound and is always a surgical emergency. A dehisced wound will need to heal by secondary intention. Poor nutrition and advanced age are two factors that increase a patient's risk of dehiscence and evisceration. Obesity also increases the risk of these complications. (See *Wound healing and obesity.*)

Recognizing dehiscence and evisceration

In wound dehiscence, the layers of a wound separate. In evisceration, the viscera (in this case, a bowel loop) protrude through the wound.

**Dehisced abdominal wound
(with a colostomy)**

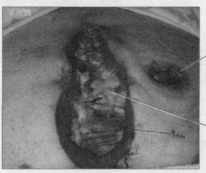

Colostomy

Red granulation tissue

Necrotic tissue

**Healing dehisced abdominal wound
by secondary intention**

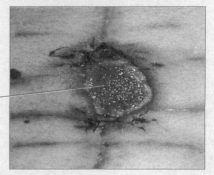

Wound dehiscence   **Evisceration of bowel loop**

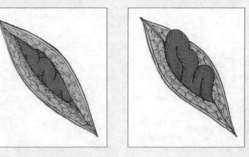

Wound healing and obesity

A patient with obesity is at risk for delayed wound healing due to:

• reduced tissue perfusion in adipose tissue and increased tension at the suture line caused by the weight of excess body fat.

• excess skin folds (especially if the wound is within one of the folds or if the folds of excess tissue cover a suture line, which may keep the wound moist and allow bacteria to accumulate).

• comorbid medical conditions such as type 2 diabetes mellitus.

• protein depletion (can be missed due to weight; assess protein levels).

   The patient with obesity is also at increased risk for dehiscence and evisceration because the diet may not include essential minerals and vitamins necessary for proper wound healing.

Infection

Infection is a relatively common complication of wound healing that should be addressed promptly. Infection can lead to cellulitis or a bacterial infection that spreads to surrounding tissue. Keep in mind that the signs and symptoms of infection can be different in acute and chronic wounds. (See *Signs and symptoms of infection.*)

Signs and symptoms of infection

Acute wounds	Chronic wounds
• Pain	• Serous drainage with inflammation
• Purulent drainage	• Delayed healing
• Odor	• Discolored granulation tissue
• Edema	• Friable granulation tissue
• Erythema	• Pocketing
• Induration	• Foul odor
• Fever	• Wound breakdown
• Lethargy	• Increasing pain
• Elevated white blood cell count	• Tenderness surrounding tissue or underlying joint
• Tachycardia	
• Changes in blood pressure	
• Confusion	

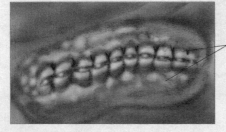

Redness and swelling along the incision line and in surrounding tissue

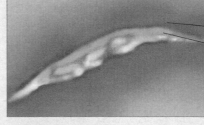

Redness

Pus

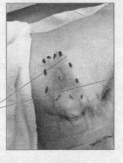

Dotted area outlines erythema for this infected wound. Compare to noninfected wound.

Fistulas and sinus tracts

A fistula is an abnormal passage between an organ or a vessel and another organ, vessel, or area of the skin. A sinus tract, also known as *tunneling*, is a channel that extends through part of a wound and into adjacent tissue. These complications can result in dead space and infection.

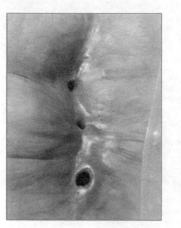
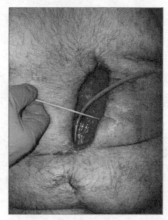

Tunnel measures 4 cm at 4 o'clock.

Undermining

Undermining is tissue destruction that occurs around a wound's edges, causing the skin to come away from the base of the wound (even though it may appear intact). This injury may be the result of friction and shear. It can develop into sinus tracts to nearby tissue.

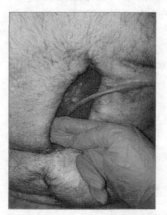

The wound demonstrates 2 cm undermining from 7 to 9 o'clock.

Quick quiz

1. Which layer of the epidermis contains pigment-producing cells?
    A. Stratum corneum
    B. Basal layer
    C. Stratum spinosum
    D. Papillary dermis

Answer: B. Melanocytes, the pigment-producing cells, are in the basal layer of the epidermis.

2. The layer of skin that contains apocrine sweat glands is the:
    A. stratum corneum.
    B. dermis.
    C. subcutaneous tissue.
    D. stratum basale.

Answer: B. Apocrine glands are situated in the dermis and have ducts that empty into hair follicles.

3. In aging skin, which factor causes a decrease in cellular immunity?
    A. Decreased synthesis of vitamin D
    B. Slower cell turnover in the stratum corneum
    C. Decreased numbers of fibroblasts and mast cells
    D. Decreased Langerhans cells

Answer: D. Langerhans cells originate in the bone marrow and are essential for the skin's cellular immunity.

4. The main functions of the skin include:
    A. support, nourishment, and sensation.
    B. protection, sensory perception, and temperature regulation.
    C. fluid transport, sensory perception, and aging regulation.
    D. support, protection, and communication.

Answer: B. The skin's main functions involve protection from injury, noxious chemicals, and bacterial invasion; sensory perception of touch, temperature, and pain; and regulation of body heat.

5. Which type of wound can be closed by primary intention?
    A. Second-degree burn
    B. Pressure injury
    C. Deep cut by a kitchen knife
    D. Dog bite

Answer: C. A clean cut in which there is no deep tissue loss and the wound edges are well approximated can be closed by primary intention.

6. Which phase of the wound healing process is responsible for cleaning the wound and starting the rebuilding process?
   A. Hemostasis
   B. Inflammation
   C. Proliferation
   D. Maturation

Answer: B. The inflammatory phase is both a defense mechanism that is vital to preventing infection of the wound and a crucial component of the healing process.

7. Identify the five layers of epidermis indicated in this illustration.

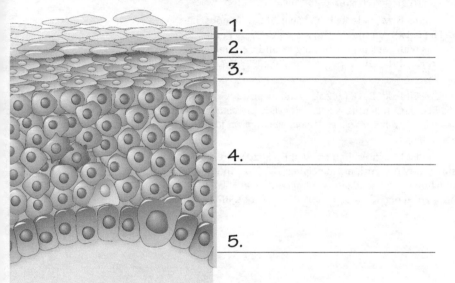

1. _____
2. _____
3. _____

4. _____

5. _____

Answer: 1. Stratum corneum; 2. Stratum lucidum; 3. Stratum granulosum; 4. Stratum spinosum; 5. Stratum germinativum

Scoring

★★★ If you answered all seven questions correctly, congrats! It looks like the information in this chapter has gotten under your skin.

★★ If you answered five or six questions correctly, good job! It's our sensory perception that you're well-healed.

★ If you answered fewer than five questions correctly, don't sweat it! After a quick review, this topic won't "phase" you at all.

Select references

Beitz, J. (2022). Wound healing. In L. L. McNichol, C. R. Ratliff, & S. S. Yates (Eds.), *Wound, Ostomy, and Continence Nurses Society core curriculum: Wound management* (2nd ed., pp. 38–54). Wolters Kluwer.

Cass, A. R., & Charlton, K. E. (2022). Prevalence of hospital-acquired malnutrition and modifiable determinants of nutritional deterioration during inpatient admissions: A systematic review of the evidence. *Journal of Human Nutrition and Dietetics, 35*(6), 1043–1058. https://doi.org/10.1111/jhn.13009

Friedrich, E., Posthauer, M., & Dorner, B. (2022). Nutritional strategies for wound management. In L. L. McNichol, C. R. Ratliff, & S. S. Yates (Eds.), *Wound, Ostomy, and Continence Nurses Society core curriculum: Wound management* (2nd ed., pp. 115–134). Wolters Kluwer.

Haines, J., LeVan, D., & Roth-Kauffman, M. (2020). Malnutrition in the elderly: Underrecognized and increasing in prevalence. *Clinical Advisor.* https://www.clinicaladvisor.com/home/topics/geriatrics-information-center/malnutrition-in-the-elderly-underrecognized-and-increasing-in-prevalence/

Howell, R. S., Gorenstein, S., Gillette, B. M., Criscitelli, T., Davitz, M. S., Woods, J. S., Acerra, M., & Brem, H. (2018). A framework to assist providers in the management of patients with chronic, nonhealing wounds. *Advances in Skin & Wound Care, 31*(11), 491–501. https://doi.org/10.1097/01.ASW.0000546117.86938.75

Mufti, A., Maliyar, K., Ayello, E., & Sibbald, R. G. (2022). Anatomy and physiology of the skin. In L. L. McNichol, C. R. Ratliff, & S. S. Yates (Eds.), *Wound, Ostomy, and Continence Nurses Society core curriculum: Wound management* (2nd ed., pp. 13–37). Wolters Kluwer.

Munoz, N., Posthauer, M. E., Cereda, E., Schols, J., & Haesler, E. (2020). The role of nutrition for pressure injury prevention and healing: The 2019 international clinical practice guideline recommendations. *Advances in Skin & Wound Care, 33*(3), 123–136. https://doi.org/10.1097/01.ASW.0000653144.90739.ad

Chapter 2

Wound assessment and monitoring

Just the facts

In this chapter, you'll learn about:

♦ assessment methods

♦ ways to classify wounds according to type, age, and depth

♦ accurate documentation of wound progress

♦ tools to track wound healing

Holistic patient assessment

Each time you assess a wound, remember that you're assessing a patient with a wound—not simply the wound itself. This will help keep you focused on the big picture as you perform your initial assessment and will set the stage for effective monitoring and successful healing.

The words used to describe a wound must communicate the same thing to members of the health care team, insurance companies, regulators, the patient's family, and, ultimately, the patient. When you gather information about a wound, use all your senses. Be sure to cover the key assessment considerations discussed in the next section as well as assessing the wound itself. As you perform your assessment, remember that it doesn't matter what tool you use to record your observations as long as you're consistent.

Key assessment considerations

Several factors influence the body's ability to heal itself, regardless of the type of injury sustained. You should consider these elements in your assessment:

• immune status
• blood glucose levels, especially glycosylated hemoglobin (HbA1c)
• hydration
• nutrition

- blood albumin and prealbumin levels
- oxygen and vascular supply
- pain
- wound etiology
- patient's age

Immune status

The immune system plays a central role in wound healing. If the patient's immune system is impaired due to chronic diseases, infections such as human immunodeficiency virus (HIV), or as a result of chemotherapy or radiation, you should monitor the wound for impaired healing. There is a wide array of medications on the market that are used to treat cancer and chronic inflammatory diseases such as arthritis and to prevent organ rejection in people who have received transplants.

Many people today are on tumor necrosis factor (TNF) medications or corticosteroids to treat skin and systemic disorders. Keep in mind these medications depress immune system function.

Blood glucose levels

Blood glucose levels should be below 100 mg/dL when fasting and below 140 mg/dL after eating for satisfactory healing, regardless of the wound's cause. Levels of 140 mg/dL or more can impair the function of white blood cells (WBCs), which are important in wound healing because they help prevent infection.

HbA1c is also an indication of glucose control and the efficacy of diabetes therapy. This test reflects blood glucose levels over the past 12 weeks. An elevated HbA1c level has the same consequences as an elevated blood glucose level: impaired wound healing and reduced ability to fight infection.

Hydration

Be sure to closely monitor and optimize the patient's hydration status—successful healing depends on it. Skin and subcutaneous tissues need to be well-hydrated from the inside. Dehydration impairs the healing process by slowing the body's metabolism. Dehydration also reduces skin turgor, or fullness, leaving skin vulnerable to new wounds.

Nutrition

Nutritional status helps you determine the patient's vulnerability to skin breakdown as well as the body's overall ability to heal. A comprehensive assessment of the patient's nutritional status also helps you plan effective care.

Body mass index is the calculation of an individual's body mass divided by the square of their height; the value is stated in units of kilogram per square meter (kg/m^2). This calculation is helpful in determining if your patient's weight is classified as underweight, normal weight, overweight, or obese. It is an assessment of body weight in relationship to height that is helpful in determining general health and nutritional status. Keep in mind, however, that people of any weight can have nutritional deficiencies.

Nutrition is complex. If your assessment leads you to believe that the patient's nutritional status places them at risk for skin damage or for delayed wound healing, collaborate with a health care provider and a dietitian to develop the best possible treatment plan.

Blood albumin and prealbumin levels

Blood albumin and prealbumin levels are essential factors in wound assessment for two important reasons:

- Skin is primarily constructed of protein, and albumin is a protein. If albumin levels are low, the body lacks an important building block for skin repair.
- Albumin is the blood component that provides colloid osmotic pressure, the force that prevents fluid from leaking out of blood vessels into nearby tissues. Albumin has a half-life of approximately 20 days and reflects your patient's serum protein status for the past month. (See *A closer look at albumin*.) If albumin levels fall below 3.5 g/dL, the patient can develop edema (fluid leakage into tissues), which compromises wound healing. The patient also risks developing hypotension (low blood pressure) as fluid leaks out of the bloodstream into tissues. If blood pressure falls to the point at which adequate blood flow is no longer maintained through the capillaries near the wound, healing slows or stops. Prealbumin is a protein with a half-life of approximately 2 days.

A closer look at albumin

Albumin, a large protein molecule, acts like a magnet to attract water and hold it inside the blood vessel.

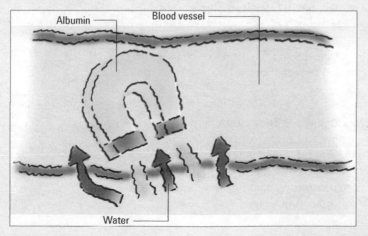

Albumin — Blood vessel —

Water —

A patient's prealbumin level is a better indication of their nutritional status because a normal level (16 to 35 mg/dL) is less affected by liver and kidney disease and hydration status than other serum proteins. This test can be used to identify early protein malnutrition, and because of its short half-life, it can also be used to monitor improving protein status in patients on a nutritional recovery program. However, prealbumin is affected by inflammation, infection, and recent trauma. Use the patient's prealbumin level as a rapid screening test to determine if a patient needs a more in-depth nutritional assessment.

Oxygen and vascular supply

Healing requires oxygen—it's that simple. Therefore, anything that impedes full oxygenation also impedes healing. During your assessment, you should consider factors that may reduce the amount of oxygen available for healing. Possible problems include:
- impaired gas exchange, causing decreased oxygen levels in the blood
- hemoglobin levels too low to transport adequate oxygen
- low blood pressure that fails to drive oxygenated blood through capillaries
- insufficient arterial and capillary supply in the wound area
  Any of these problems on their own or in combination can deprive the wound of the oxygen needed for successful healing.

Smoke bomb

Smoking is a modifiable factor that impedes oxygenation of the wound. If the patient smokes, explain the ways in which smoking affects wound healing:
- Nicotine is a powerful vasoconstrictor that narrows peripheral blood vessels, thereby compromising blood flow to the skin.
- Because it is easier for hemoglobin to bind to the carbon monoxide present in cigarette smoke than it is for it to bind to oxygen, the blood that does squeeze through carries far less oxygen than it should.
- Lung tissue damaged by smoke doesn't function as well as it should, resulting in decreased oxygenation.

Pain

Pain control also has a practical purpose. In response to pain, the body releases epinephrine, a powerful vasoconstrictor. Vasoconstriction reduces blood flow to the wound. When you relieve pain, vasoconstriction subsides, blood vessels dilate, and blood flow to the wound improves. In addition, controlling pain promotes patient comfort and allows the patient to focus on healing.

Pain assessment is an important part of wound assessment. Note pain associated with the injury itself along with pain associated with healing and therapies employed to promote healing. Use one of the approved scales to begin the pain conversation, and then independently watch to see how the patient responds to pain and the therapies provided. As always, remember to record your findings. (See *How to assess pain*.)

How to assess pain

To properly assess your patient's pain, consider the patient's descriptions and your own observations of their reactions to pain and treatments.

Talk to your patient

Begin your pain assessment by asking your patient the following questions:
• Where is the pain located? How long does it last? How often does it occur?
• What does the pain feel like? (Let your patient describe it; don't prompt them.)
• What relieves the pain? What makes it worse?
• How do you usually get relief?
• How would you rate your pain on a scale of 0 to 10, with 0 representing no pain and 10 representing the worst pain?

Talking with your patient about pain in this manner helps define the pain for both you and the patient, and it helps you evaluate the effectiveness of therapies used to relieve it.

Monitor and observe your patient

As you work with your patient, observe their responses to pain and to interventions intended to relieve it.

Behavioral responses to watch for include:
• altered body position
• moaning
• sighing
• grimacing
• withdrawing from painful stimuli
• crying
• restlessness
• muscle twitching
• immobility

Sympathetic responses, normally associated with mild to moderate pain, include:
• pallor
• elevated blood pressure
• dilated pupils
• tension in the skeletal muscles
• dyspnea (shortness of breath)
• tachycardia (rapid heartbeat)
• diaphoresis (sweating)

Parasympathetic responses, which are more common in cases of severe, deep pain, include:
• pallor
• lower-than-normal blood pressure
• bradycardia (slower-than-normal heartbeat)
• nausea and vomiting
• weakness
• dizziness
• loss of consciousness

Listen and learn

If the patient is conscious and can communicate, have them rate the pain before and during each dressing change. If your notes reveal that the pain is higher before the dressing change, it may indicate an impending infection, even before any other signs appear. Remember that the patient may also experience apprehension prior to the dressing change, which may increase their pain level. This can be managed in part by explaining what the patient can expect.

If the patient says the dressing change itself is painful, consider administering pain medication before the procedure or changing the dressing technique itself. For example, if treatment calls for a debridement technique, you can anticipate that the patient will experience pain and administer preprocedural pain medication accordingly. Remember to document this pain and report it to the health care provider. Keep in mind that wet-to-dry dressings are no longer a recommended standard of care. There are many more effective and less painful methods of removing dead tissue. If there is an order for wet-to-dry dressings, be sure to request a reevaluation of treatment plan and document the patient's pain. If it is not documented and communicated, the wet-to-dry dressing orders may stand and the patient may suffer unnecessary discomfort.

Easy does it
In general, when removing adherent dressings, it's less painful for the patient if you soak the dressing. Over intact skin, you can also use an adhesive remover. Remember to keep the skin taut. Press down on the skin to release the dressing rather than just pulling it off. If the patient still says that dressing removal is painful, the team may wish to choose a less adherent dressing type.

Etiology

Focus on the etiology of the wound to help ensure that you consider all factors that can influence healing. For instance, if you're assessing a patient with an ulcer related to a chronic venous disorder, you should not only measure the wound, but you should also measure calf circumference regularly to determine if efforts to reduce edema are succeeding. The best interventions for a venous insufficiency ulcer won't heal the wound if edema is left unchecked.

Diabetes details
Similarly, if you're assessing the wound of a patient with diabetes, check to make sure that the blood glucose is well-controlled and that the calluses around a neuropathic foot ulcer are removed regularly. Otherwise, healing will be impeded.

In other words, as you focus on specific wound characteristics and track the healing process, never lose sight of the big picture.

Patient's age
Remember, the older your patient, the slower the healing time. This is especially true for those over the age of 65 years and for lower extremity wounds. Aging decreases the skin's tensile strength and elasticity and can limit mobility and place your patient at increased risk for

multiple wounds. Your older adult patient's medications, nutritional status, and hydration are especially important to monitor because they cannot return to a normal baseline as quickly as in a younger patient.

Wound classification

One way to classify wounds is to use a basic system that focuses on three categories of fundamental characteristics:
- type
- age
- depth

Type

Wounds are often classified by the mechanism of injury. For instance, a surgical wound is caused by a surgical procedure. A nonsurgical wound can be caused by a disease process and/or trauma, such as a pressure injury, neuropathic ulcer, or lower extremity ulcer due to venous or arterial disease.

Age

When determining wound age, you need to first determine if the wound is acute or chronic. However, this determination can present a problem if you adhere solely to a timeline. For instance, just how long is it before an acute wound becomes a chronic wound?

Chronic wounds are defined as wounds that have failed to proceed through an orderly and timely reparative process to produce anatomic and functional integrity over a period of 3 months or a wound that does not decrease in size by 30% in 3 weeks or by 50% in 4 to 5 weeks. If a wound does not decrease in size by 50% in 4 weeks, there is a 91% chance it will not be healed within 12 weeks.

Chronic wounds have a decreased ability to mount an acute inflammatory response in the presence of infections. Consequently, patients with older wounds can have muted or subacute signs and symptoms of infection.

Chronic wounds don't heal as easily as acute wounds. The drainage in chronic wounds contains a greater amount of destructive enzymes and fibroblasts (i.e., the cells that function as the architects in wound healing). They are less effective at producing collagen, divide less often, and send fewer signals to other cells telling them to divide and fill the wound. They also typically have biofilms on the surface. Biofilms are colonies of bacteria that have adapted the wound environment to promote their proliferation on the host.

Depth

Depth is another fundamental characteristic used to classify wounds. In your assessment, record wound depth as partial thickness or full thickness (you will describe extent of tissue loss in more detail in your wound assessment). (See *Classifying wound depth.*)

Get wise to wounds

Classifying wound depth

Partial-thickness wounds involve the epidermis and extend partially into the dermis but not through it. Full-thickness wounds extend through the dermis into tissues beneath and may expose adipose tissue, muscle, or bone.

Focused wound assessment

The 10 points of wound assessment include:
1. Extent of tissue loss
2. Wound type
3. Anatomic location
4. Size and shape
5. Wound bed characteristics
6. Exudate
7. Tracts and tunnels
8. Undermining
9. Edges
10. Periwound skin

Extent of tissue loss

Remember, depth of wound is one of the ways to classify a wound, but identifying the extent of tissue loss is also important for determining wound management. Partial-thickness wounds normally heal quickly because they involve the epidermal and partial dermal layers of the skin. The dermis remains at least partially intact to generate the new epidermis needed to close the wound. Partial-thickness wounds are also less susceptible to infection because part of the body's first level of defense (the partial dermis) is still intact. These wounds tend to be painful and need protection to reduce pain and minimize risk of localized infection.

Full-thickness wounds penetrate completely through the skin into underlying tissues. The wound may expose adipose tissue (fat), muscle, tendon, or bone. In the abdomen, you may see adipose tissue or omentum (the covering of the bowel). If the omentum is penetrated, the bowel may protrude through the wound (evisceration). Granulation tissue may be visible if the wound has started to heal.

Staging

Pressure injury staging (see Chapter 6) or categories for staging neuropathic foot ulcers (see Chapter 7) provide information on the amount of tissue loss in a wound. Arterial and venous ulcers also have staging systems, so remember to check if your agency uses these classification systems.

Wound type

The comprehensive assessment as well as the wound assessment will help you determine the etiology of the wound. The most common wound types are:
- Pressure injury
- Skin tear
- Moisture-associated skin damage (MASD)
- Medical adhesive-related skin injury (MARSI)
- Venous ulcer
- Arterial ulcer
- Neuropathic ulcer
- Acute wounds such as surgical or trauma wounds

Anatomic location

The location of a wound often helps us determine etiology. For instance, a neuropathic ulcer is on the plantar surface of the foot and is unlikely to be a venous ulcer.

Size and shape

Assess the wound bed and the surrounding skin only after they have been cleansed. Shape is evaluated by looking at the wound perimeter and may assist with identifying the etiology of the wound. In general:
- Round and "punched out" suggest an arterial wound.
- A butterfly or mirror image shape, especially over the sacrum, suggests deep-tissue pressure injury (DTPI), terminal pressure injury, or skin failure.
- A linear wound in the gluteal cleft or matching wounds on bilateral buttocks suggest MASD.
- Oval, irregularly shaped wounds are often venous.

The most common method of measuring wound dimensions is to use a disposable, single-use, measuring guide. Record the length of the wound as the longest overall distance across the wound with a head-to-toe orientation, and record the width as the longest measurement perpendicular (at a right angle) to your length measurement. Consistency in measuring is the key factor, and selecting a head-to-toe direction for length and a side-to-side direction for width is the most consistent way to measure. Suggest staff use the clock face to identify 12, 6, 3, and 9 o'clock for reference points for length and width. Record all measurements in centimeters.

Measuring the longest and widest dimensions overestimates the total wound area approximately 70% of the time (Haesler, 2019; Langemo et al., 2008).

Just a trace

Another way to measure the wound is to use wound tracing (wound margins are traced on a sheet of clear plastic with a grid printed on it). You can use the tracing to calculate an approximate wound surface area. This method provides only a rough estimate and is less accurate for very irregularly shaped wounds, but it is simple and fairly quick. Unless you are using a disposable tracing material, this method can pose an infection control hazard.

How deep

To measure wound depth, you'll need a flexible foam- or cotton-tipped device. Gently insert the device into the deepest portion of the wound, and then carefully mark the stick where it meets the edge of the skin. Remove the device and measure the distance from your mark to the end to determine depth. This method can also be used to measure undermining and tunneling. Remember, never probe surgical wounds because they are full-thickness wounds and organs or vessels may be injured.

Because accurately recording wound dimensions is important, many health care facilities use photography as a tool in wound assessment. If photography is available in your facility, it should be included in your assessment of wound characteristics. Some photographic techniques produce a picture with a grid overlay that's useful for measuring. Remember, however, that there are qualities of the wound that a camera simply can't record. (See *What's missing?*) The Health Insurance Portability and Accountability Act (HIPAA, 1996) and the Health Information Technology for Economic and Clinical Health Act (HITECH Act, part of the 2009 American Recovery and Reinvestment Act) apply to wound photography, and the patient needs to sign a consent to be photographed. Check with your facility for the wound photography policy. Photography must be done properly to ensure adequate documentation of a wound. Remember that poor documentation, including photography, can be construed negatively in the event of litigation.

Get wise to wounds

What's missing?

If wound photography is a routine part of your wound documentation system, remember that a picture may be worth a thousand words, but your assessment skills and personal observations are still essential. Many wound characteristics can't be recorded accurately—or at all—on film. These include:

* location
* depth
* measurements of tunnels or undermined areas
* odor
* feel of surrounding tissue
* pain

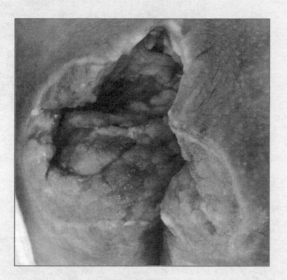

All of this information is needed if the health care team is to make sound treatment decisions.

Wound bed characteristics

Characteristics of the wound bed provide important information about the wound and how it's healing. Tissue may be viable (healthy) or nonviable (necrotic). Noting the percent of the different tissue types and their location in the wound is part of the assessment.

Viable (healthy)	Nonviable (necrotic)

Granulation

- Pink or red
- Shiny
- Moist
- Appears granular (cobblestone appearance)

Slough

- Yellow, tan, gray, black, or brown
- Stringy
- Moist or dry and adherent

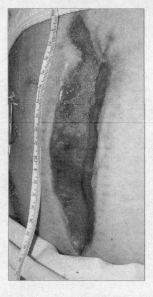

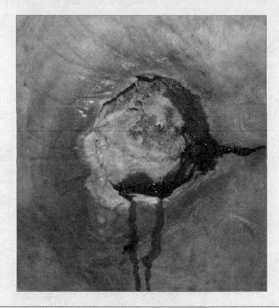

Epithelial tissue

- Silver to light pink
- Growing in from the edges or on the wound surface

Eschar

- Usually the hard (knock, knock) tissue
- Black or brown

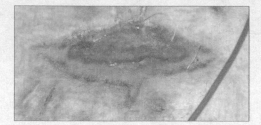

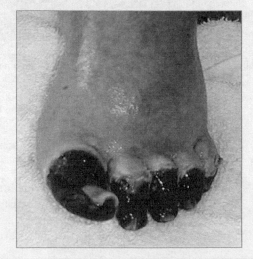

What do you see?

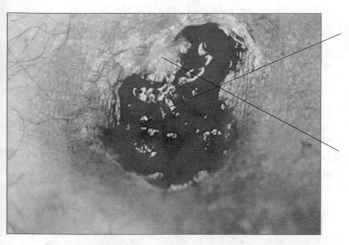

Red, bumpy, shiny tissue in the base of an ulcer
- This indicates **granulation tissue**.
- As a wound heals, it develops more and more granulation tissue.
- Beware, beefy red tissue that is friable (bleeds easily) may indicate excessive bio-burden in the wound. This colonized wound needs to be treated topically.

Pale or pearly pink skin
- This indicates **epithelial tissue**.
- Epithelial tissue first appears at ulcer borders in full-thickness wounds and as islands around hair follicles in partial-thickness wounds.

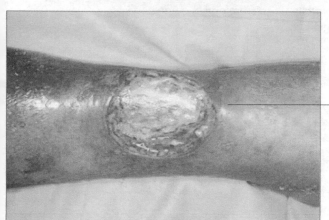

Moist yellow, tan, or gray area of tissue that's separating from viable tissue
- This is **slough** and indicates soft, necrotic tissue.
- Slough provides an ideal medium for bacterial growth.

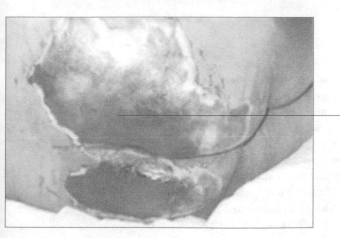

Thick, hard, leathery black tissue
- This is **eschar** and indicates dry, necrotic tissue.
- For healing to occur, necrotic tissue, drainage, and metabolic wastes must be removed.

Exudate

The wound bed should be moist—but not overly moist. Moisture allows the cells and chemicals needed for healing to move about the wound surface.

Desert storm

In dry wound beds, cells involved in healing, which normally exist in a fluid environment, can't move. WBCs can't fight infection, enzymes such as collagenase can't break down dead material, and macrophages can't carry away debris. The wound edges curl up to preserve the moisture that remains in the edge, and epithelial cells (new skin cells) fail to grow over and cover the wound. Healing grinds to a halt, and necrotic tissue builds up.

Flood watch

Too much moisture poses a different problem. It floods the wound and spills out onto the skin, where the constant moisture causes damage to intact skin cells at the wound edge.

Documenting exudate

Amount	Consistency	Color	Odor
• None	• Thin	• Pink	• None
• Scant	• Thick	• Red	• Mild
• Small	• N/A	• Brown	• Moderate
• Moderate		• Yellow	• Strong
• Heavy		• Green	
		• N/A	

Also consider the consistency of the drainage. If the drainage has a thick, creamy texture, the wound contains excessive amounts of bacteria; however, this doesn't necessarily mean a clinically significant infection is present. Document the characteristics of the drainage. Drainage might be creamy because it contains WBCs that have killed bacteria. The drainage is also contaminated with surface bacteria that naturally live in moist environments on the human body. Because of this bacterial colonization, guidelines recommend against using swab cultures to identify wound infections. However, some practitioners still order swab cultures because they are easy to collect and inexpensive. See Chapter 3,

"Wound Bed Preparation," for more information on obtaining a wound culture.

If kept clean, a noninfected wound usually produces little if any odor. (One exception is the odor normally present under an occlusive dressing, such as a hydrocolloid, that develops as a byproduct of the degradation process.) A newly detected odor might be a sign of infection. When documenting wound odor, it's important to include when you noted the odor and whether it was still present after wound cleansing. Think about where you are physically when you smell the wound—entering the home or unit (strong) or after you remove the dressing (mild).

If an odor is present, it can present an embarrassing or otherwise uncomfortable situation for the patient as well as their family, guests, and/or roommate. If you notice an odor or the patient says they notice one, after fully assessing the wound for changes, you can use dressings that reduce odor and, if needed, a spray odor eliminator. Odor eliminators differ from air fresheners because they aren't scents that mask odors but rather compounds that bind with and neutralize the molecules responsible for the odor.

Tracts, tunnels, and undermining

It's also important to measure tunnels (extensions of the wound bed into adjacent tissue) and undermining (areas of the wound bed that extend under the skin). Measure tunneling and undermining just as you would wound depth. These measurements should be recorded and identified in relation to a clock face and are a consideration for filling "dead space" when determining the dressing to be used.

Carefully insert the device to the bottom of the tunnel, then mark the stick and measure the distance from your mark to the end of the device. If a tunnel is large, palpate it with a gloved finger rather than a foam- or cotton-tipped device because you can sense the end of the tunnel better with your finger. This also avoids damaging the tissue. Sinus tracts are very small tunnels that cannot be intubated (i.e., you cannot insert a measuring device). You may see a small opening and note drainage from it, but do not attempt to measure depth as this may widen the tract. Often, sinus tracts are pathways from an organ or a body cavity. Record what you see and communicate your findings to the patient's health care provider.

Probing the issue

- Put on clean or sterile gloves based on your facility policy. Gently probe the wound bed and edges with a sterile applicator to assess for wound undermining or tunneling.
- Gently insert the applicator around the wound edges for undermining or into the wound in the direction where the deepest tunneling occurs. Below is an illustration of undermining measurement.

Marking progress

- Grasp the applicator where it meets the wound edge.
- Remove the applicator, keeping your hand in place, and place it next to the measuring guide to determine the measurement of the undermining in centimeters, as shown below.

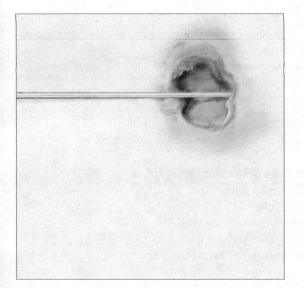

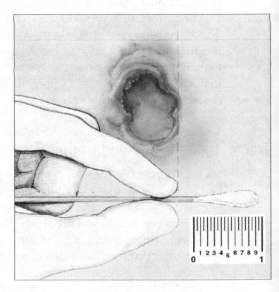

Undermined tissue is destruction of tissue extending under the skin edges (margins) so the wound is larger at its base than at the skin surface.

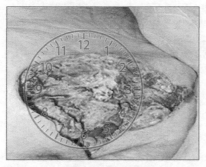

Undermining from 6 to 10 o'clock.

Edges

When assessing wound edges, note that they should be open and at-tached, clear and distinct, and even or flush with the wound base to enhance epithelialization. You'll want to see skin that's smooth—not rolled—and tightly adherent to the wound bed.

Rolled skin may indicate that the wound bed is too dry (epibole). Loose skin at the edges may indicate additional shearing injury (sepa-ration of skin layers), possibly due to a rough transfer or reposition-ing. In this case, improve transfer and repositioning techniques to prevent recurrence. Callus or hyperkeratosis especially around a foot wound indicates pressure. Debride the callus and offload the area to allow healing.

Periwound skin

When assessing the periwound skin, you'll assess at least 4 cm beyond the wound margins.

Rainbow connections

The color of the skin around the wound can alert you to impending problems that can impede healing. Also note if the periwound skin is intact.

- Denuded skin is excoriated or eroded, and the area may be painful though superficial.

- White skin indicates maceration, or too much moisture, and signals the need for a skin protector or a protective barrier around the wound, a dressing that remains in the wound, and a more absorbent dressing.
- Erythema, or red skin, can indicate inflammation, injury (e.g., tape burn, excessive pressure, chemical exposure), or infection. (Remember that inflammation is healthy only during the inflammatory phase of healing.) Generally, erythema of 2 to 3 cm from the wound's edge is an indication of local infection. Be aware though that darker skin may obscure erythema, so you will have to be on the lookout for other signs.

Let your fingers do the talking

During your assessment of the area around the wound, use your fingers to gain valuable information. For example, gently probe the periwound tissue (i.e., the skin immediately around the wound bed) to determine if edema is present or if the tissue is soft or hard (indurated). Indurated tissue, even in the absence of erythema (redness), is one indication of infection. Similarly, if the patient has dark skin, it may be difficult to see some color cues. Again, your fingers can help. Probe the area around the wound bed and compare the feel to surrounding healthy skin. A tender area of skin that appears shiny and feels hard may indicate inflammation. Be sure to record the size of the area of induration around the open wound.

During periwound palpation, a wavy feeling under the tissue may indicate fluctuance because of trapped fluid. Crepitus is identified as a crackling or popping sensation. It signifies an accumulation of gas or air in the tissues and may be indicative of anaerobic infection.

As you palpate, also identify if there is pain in the periwound area, and have the patient rate the pain on the scale used by the facility or agency.

Wound monitoring

Monitor the patient throughout the healing process, periodically reassessing their status and documenting progress of the wound toward full healing. Wound monitoring is a requirement for some regulatory agencies, including the Centers for Medicare & Medicaid Services (CMS).

Paint a picture

Your initial assessment sets the benchmark for subsequent monitoring and reassessment activities. One assessment is a static report; a series of assessments, however, can illustrate the dynamic aspect of the healing process. In this way, all members of the health care team can see the patient's progress toward healing (or failure to heal), the development of complications, or the relative success of interventions. This will depend on the accuracy, quality, and consistency of your documentation.

In the course of a wound assessment, you amass quite a bit of useful information about the patient, their environment, the characteristics of the wound, and the current status in the healing process. When documenting your assessment, be sure to include the date and time of your observations. Also strive to obtain accurate measurements, using appropriate units of measurement. Make sure that the entire health care team is using the same tool to measure the patient's wound. Remember to document only the facts, not your opinions, about the wound.

The prospect of monitoring, reassessing, and documenting over time may seem daunting; however, there is a research-based documentation tool available—or your facility may have its own tool—to help you manage the task.

Bates–Jensen Wound Assessment Tool

The Bates–Jensen Wound Assessment Tool (BWAT) is a validated wound assessment tool that measures wound status on a continuum. See the BWAT in Appendix 1.

Recognizing complications

It is important to monitor and track, or reassess, wound status to identify signs and symptoms of complications or failure to heal as early in the process as possible. Early intervention improves the likelihood of resolving complications successfully and getting the healing process back on track.

You'll conduct your reassessments using the same criteria as that in the initial assessment with one added advantage—perspective. Careful monitoring can help you catch failure to heal early so you can intervene appropriately. (See *Recognizing failure to heal*.)

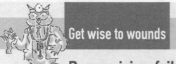

Recognizing failure to heal

This chart presents the most common signs of failure to heal as well as associated probable causes and appropriate interventions.

Sign	Causes	Interventions
Wound bed		
Too dry	• Exposure of tissue and cells normally in a moist environment to air • Inadequate hydration	Use a dressing that maintains moisture, such as a transparent film, hydrocolloid, or hydrogel dressing if possible.
No change in size or depth for 2 weeks	• Pressure or trauma to the area • Poor nutrition, poor circulation, or inadequate hydration • Poor control of disease processes such as diabetes • Biofilm or heavy colonization • Infection	Reassess the patient for local or systemic problems that impair wound healing and intervene as necessary.
Increase in size or depth	• Ischemia due to excess pressure or poor circulation • Infection	• Reassess the patient for local or systemic problems that impair wound healing, and intervene as necessary. • Consult the appropriate health care provider.
Necrosis	Ischemia	Debride if the remaining living tissue has adequate circulation.
Increase in drainage or change of drainage color from clear to purulent	• Autolytic or enzymatic debridement: If caused by autolytic or enzymatic debridement, no intervention is necessary. An increase in drainage or change of drainage color is expected because of the breakdown of dead tissue. • Infection	Assess the wound for infection.
Tunneling	• Pressure over bony prominences • Presence of foreign body • Deep infection • Shearing forces	• Protect the area from pressure and shear. • Irrigate tunnel and lightly fill dead space. If the tunnel doesn't shorten in length each week, thoroughly clean it and obtain a tissue biopsy.
Wound edges		
Red, hot skin; tenderness; and induration	Inflammation due to excess pressure or infection: If pressure redistribution doesn't resolve the inflammation within 24 hours, antimicrobial therapy may be indicated.	Protect the area from pressure.

Recognizing failure to heal

Sign	Causes	Interventions
Maceration (white skin)	Excess moisture in wound	Protect the skin with a skin protectant or protectant dressing.
Rolled skin edges	Too dry wound bed	Use moisture-retentive dressings. If rolling isn't resolved in 1 week, debridement of the edges may be necessary.
Undermining or ecchymosis of surrounding skin (loose or bruised skin edges)	Excess shearing force to the area	Initiate measures to protect the area, especially during patient transfers.

The sooner, the better

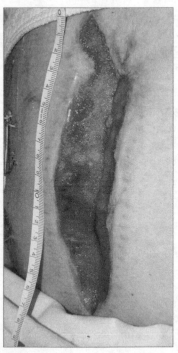

Granulation tissue in an abdominal wound

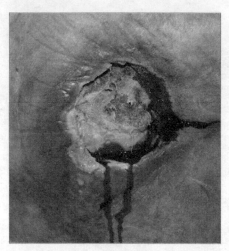

Sacral pressure injury with 75% of the surface area covered in yellow necrotic slough

Success or failure of the healing process has a tremendous impact on the patient's quality of life as well as their family's quality of life. Early intervention can mean that a patient with a neuropathic foot ulcer can avoid amputation or a patient who is paraplegic with an ischial pressure injury can once again sit up and lead an active life.

Chronic wounds pose a particularly difficult problem not only for individual practitioners but also for the health care industry as a whole. Treating chronic wounds is expensive because they're difficult to heal and often reoccur. Consequently, the people responsible for the largest portion of the bill—government and private insurers—are placing increased emphasis on early intervention and prevention.

Winning in wound healing

Now that you know what to look for when things *aren't* going well, let's take a look at what you can expect to see when healing is progressing smoothly.

In this case, the patient:
- is well-hydrated, well-nourished, comfortable, and warm.
- is well-managed for associated or contributing diseases, such as diabetes, heart failure, or kidney failure.
- exhibits normal immune system response.

In addition, the wound itself:
- receives the oxygen and nutrients it needs (adequate vascular supply).

- is moist and protected from the environment.
- is free from necrotic tissue.

These conditions optimize wound healing. By using the assessment techniques presented in this chapter, you'll be a part of this success.

Wound healing isn't a simple matter to coordinate. Through vigilance and consistent assessment and documentation, success is much more likely. By using your senses, you can have a tremendous influence on whether a wound heals or becomes chronic and harder to manage. Recognizing red flags that warn of failure to heal and knowing the appropriate interventions make you a part of the winning wound healing team!

Quick quiz

1. A wound that extends through the epidermis and partway into the dermis is classified as a:
    A. chronic wound.
    B. acute wound.
    C. partial-thickness wound.
    D. full-thickness wound.

Answer: C. Partial-thickness wounds extend into but not through the dermis, which retains function that helps the healing process.

2. Which characteristics indicate normal, healthy granulation tissue?
    A. Red with a bumpy or pebble appearance
    B. Red with a shiny gel-like surface
    C. Thin, yellow-tan fibers easily removed
    D. Thick, black, dry surface

Answer: A. Red tissue with a bumpy or pebble appearance indicates healthy granulation tissue.

3. Which management techniques would be appropriate for a wound bed covered in 80% fibrin slough?
    A. Cover the wound to keep it clean and protect it using a transparent film, hydrocolloid, or hydrogel dressing.
    B. Consider sharp or enzymatic debridement to degrade the fibrinous material.
    C. Apply topical antimicrobials.
    D. Keep clean and dry.

Answer: B. Consider sharp or enzymatic debridement to degrade the fibrinous material.

4. If you see multiple colors in a wound bed, the best way to describe the wound is to describe the:

    A. percentage of tissue types.
    B. least healthy color you see.
    C. color most visible.
    D. number of colors present.

Answer: A. Describe a wound with multiple colors according to the percentage of tissue types in the wound bed.

5. Which term could be used to accurately describe drainage that is thin and bright red?

    A. Serous
    B. Sanguineous
    C. Serosanguineous
    D. Purulent

Answer: B. Sanguineous drainage is red, usually due to the presence of fresh blood.

6. Which is an appropriate intervention for a wound that has tunneling?

    A. Provide warmth to the area.
    B. Perform conservative sharp debridement.
    C. Protect the area from shear and pressure.
    D. No intervention is necessary.

Answer: C. Because tunneling may be caused by shear and pressure over bony prominences, the wound should be protected from pressure.

7. What would your assessment of a nonhealing wound show if the cause was a too dry wound bed?

    A. Rolled skin edges
    B. Maceration
    C. Red, hot skin
    D. Undermining

Answer: A. A wound bed that's too dry exhibits rolled skin edges and requires moisture-retentive dressings or debridement.

Scoring

✮✮✮   If you answered all seven questions correctly, stand up and bow! You're a wound care all-star.

✮✮   If you answered five to six questions correctly, great job! You're a cut above the rest.

✮   If you answered fewer than four questions correctly, don't worry! You've just skimmed the surface of wound care; there are eight more chapters to go.

Select references

Goto, T., & Saligan, L. N. (2020). Wound pain and wound healing biomarkers from wound exudate: A scoping review. *Journal of Wound, Ostomy and Continence Nursing, 47*(6), 559–568. https://doi.org/10.1097/WON.0000000000000703

Haesler, E. (Ed.). (2019). *European Pressure Ulcer Advisory Panel, National Pressure Injury Advisory Panel and Pan Pacific Pressure Injury Alliance. Prevention and treatment of pressure ulcers/injuries: Clinical practice guideline.* European Pressure Ulcer Advisory Panel, National Pressure Injury Advisory Panel and Pan Pacific Pressure Injury Alliance. Cambridge Media.

Langemo, D. K., Anderson, J., Hanson, D., Hunter, S., & Thompson, P. (2008). Measuring wound length, width, and area: Which technique? *Advances in Skin & Wound Care, 21*(1), 42–45. https://doi.org/10.1097/01.ASW.0000284967.69863.2f

Smollock, W., Montenegro, P., Czenis, A., & He, Y. (2018). Hypoperfusion and wound healing: Another dimension of wound assessment. *Advances in Skin & Wound Care, 31*(2), 72–77. https://doi.org/10.1097/01.ASW.0000527964.87741.a7

WOCN Board of Directors Task Force. (2020). Recommendations for wound assessment and photodocumentation in isolation. *Journal of Wound, Ostomy and Continence Nursing, 47*(4), 319–320. https://doi.org/10.1097/WON.0000000000000672

Chapter 3

Wound bed preparation

Just the facts

In this chapter, you'll learn about:

♦ components of wound bed preparation

♦ wound cleaning and irrigation techniques

♦ debridement techniques

♦ specimen collection techniques

TIMERS

In 2000, Sibbald et al. first identified the concept of preparing the wound bed (as cited in Sibbald et al., 2011). One framework used in this paradigm of wound bed preparation (WBP) was the "TIME" acronym first introduced in 2003. While TIME focused on only the wound, in 2019, a consensus panel identified a new acronym, TIMERS, to include repair of tissue and social factors:

- T—Tissue: nonviable or deficient
- I—Inflammation/infection
- M—Moisture
- E—Edge: not advancing or undermining
- R—Regeneration/repair of tissue
- S—Social factors

Because your observation of the wound is important for the wound care decisions you make, you can go about assessment in a uniform manner, using the TIMERS acronym.

Tissue	Is there devitalized tissue in the wound?
	Is debridement needed?
	How should the wound be cleansed?
Inflammation/infection	Is the wound red?
	Is the wound bed tissue friable (bleed easily)?
	Is there drainage or odor?

Moisture	Is there excess moisture in or around the wound?
Edge	Are the wound edges flat, rounded, or connected to other tissues?
Regeneration/repair	Do the wound orders support healing (advanced wound therapies)?
Social factors	Consider the environment the patient lives in, cost, and availability of treatment. Does the patient understand the plan? Does the patient have a goal of wound healing?

Let's investigate TIMERS letter by letter.

Tissue

Clean machine

Cleansing the wound is the first step and should be done before assessment. Because open wounds are colonized with bacteria, observe clean technique using clean, nonsterile gloves during wound care unless sterile dressing changes are specified. Always follow standard precautions.

Cleaning techniques

To clean a linear-shaped wound, such as an incision, gently wipe from top to bottom in one motion, starting directly over the wound and moving outward, as shown below.

For an open wound, such as a pressure injury, gently wipe in concentric circles, starting directly over the wound and moving outward, as shown below.

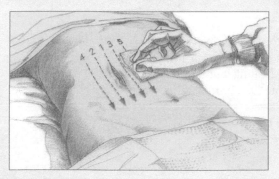

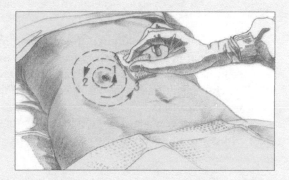

The goal of wound cleaning is to remove debris and contaminants from the wound without damaging healthy tissue. The wound should be cleaned initially; repeat cleaning as needed or with each dressing change. See *Wound cleansing solutions* and Appendix 2 for wound cleansing procedure.

Wound cleansing solutions

Normal saline	Hydrogen peroxide	Acetic acid	Sodium hypochlorite (Dakin's solution)	Povidone-iodine	Chlorhexidine	Polyhexamethylene biguanide
• Not cytotoxic to new cells • May be used in wound irrigations	• Commonly used at half strength • Used to irrigate the wound and aid in mechanical debridement • Foaming action warms the wound, promoting vasodilation and reducing inflammation • Do not use this solution in surgical wounds.	• Used to treat *Pseudomonas* infection • Verify active infection by culture before use. • 0.5%–5% strength depending on order	• Used to kill Gram-negative bacteria per culture • Slightly dissolves necrotic tissue • Must be freshly prepared every 48 hours and kept away from sunlight	• Used to kill broad spectrum of bacteria • May dry and stain the surrounding skin; protect from contact • Toxic with prolonged use or over large areas • Avoid use in patients with thyroid disease	• Used to kill Gram-positive and Gram-negative bacteria • Must be diluted • Do not use on face or mucous membranes.	• Effective against a broad spectrum of microbes • No evidence of resistance • Preservative free • Surfactant quality (aids cleaning)

Normal saline solution is the most commonly used cleansing solution, but antiseptic solutions may also be used. Note that antiseptic solutions may damage tissue and delay healing, but infected or newly contaminated wounds may require more than normal saline or wound cleansers.

For deeper wounds, wound irrigation may be needed. See Appendix 2 for wound irrigation procedures.

Debridement

Debridement of nonviable tissue is an important factor in WBP. Wound healing can't take place until necrotic tissue is removed. Necrotic tissue may present as moist, yellow or gray tissue that is separating from viable tissue. If this moist, necrotic tissue becomes dry, it presents as thick, hard, leathery black eschar. Areas of necrotic tissue may mask underlying fluid collections or abscesses. Although debridement can be painful (especially with burns), it is necessary to prevent infection and promote healing.

Understanding debridement methods

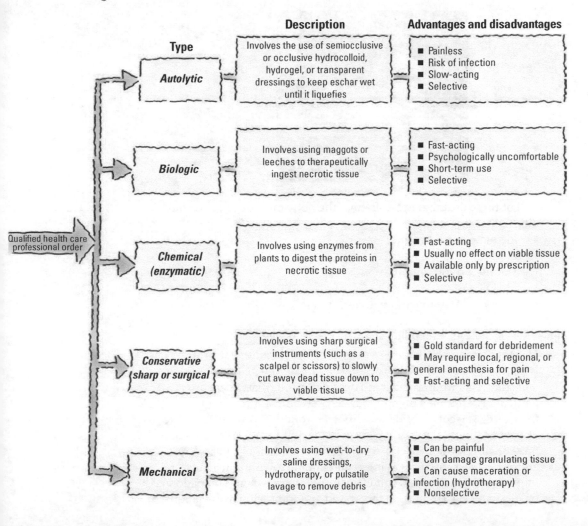

Type	Description	Advantages and disadvantages
Autolytic	Involves the use of semiocclusive or occlusive hydrocolloid, hydrogel, or transparent dressings to keep eschar wet until it liquefies	▪ Painless ▪ Risk of infection ▪ Slow-acting ▪ Selective
Biologic	Involves using maggots or leeches to therapeutically ingest necrotic tissue	▪ Fast-acting ▪ Psychologically uncomfortable ▪ Short-term use ▪ Selective
Chemical (enzymatic)	Involves using enzymes from plants to digest the proteins in necrotic tissue	▪ Fast-acting ▪ Usually no effect on viable tissue ▪ Available only by prescription ▪ Selective
Conservative sharp or surgical	Involves using sharp surgical instruments (such as a scalpel or scissors) to slowly cut away dead tissue down to viable tissue	▪ Gold standard for debridement ▪ May require local, regional, or general anesthesia for pain ▪ Fast-acting and selective
Mechanical	Involves using wet-to-dry saline dressings, hydrotherapy, or pulsatile lavage to remove debris	▪ Can be painful ▪ Can damage granulating tissue ▪ Can cause maceration or infection (hydrotherapy) ▪ Nonselective

Qualified health care professional order

Autolytic debridement

Autolytic debridement involves the use of moisture-retentive dressings to cover the wound bed. Necrotic tissue is then dissolved through self-digestion of enzymes in the wound fluid.

Polyurethane films	Hydrocolloids	Gels	Alginates	Honey
Tegaderm Opsite	DuoDERM Tegasorb	Requires a secondary dressing	Requires a secondary dressing	Requires a secondary dressing

For more information on these dressings, see Chapter 9.

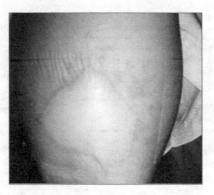

For these dressings to be effective, the body must be in good condition, meaning it has:

- adequate nourishment.
- an intact immune system.

And the wound must have:

- adequate WBP.
- no urgent need to remove necrotic tissue.

Biologic or larval therapy (everything that's old is new again)

Maggot therapy, also known as maggot debridement therapy (MDT), is the use of medical-grade maggots (larvae) for the treatment of skin and soft-tissue wounds that need debridement. Fly larvae are not particularly appealing to most, but they serve an admirable role in the world. Maggots debride and disinfect wounds as well as stimulate wound healing. They dissolve any proteins that have died by secreting proteolytic enzymes, ingest necrotic tissue with their mouths, secrete antibiotic-like substances to ingest and kill microbes in their guts, and improve oxygenation and stimulate fibroblast growth and migration by mechanically stimulating the wound and improving oxygenation.

They are pretty awesome little helpers as it turns out, but don't count on the ones that may be found in the garbage. MDT requires a specific species of larvae because some varieties eat live tissue also. They are ordered from a lab that grows them in an aseptic environment and will ship them overnight to clean up wounds full of slough or eschar. Medicare codes them as a "device," which may seem disrespectful, but they do reimburse for them. Dressings need to be inspected at least daily; any escaped maggots are disposed of and not reapplied to the wound.

When they're used
Medicinal maggots are used to debride necrotic materials in a wound bed. They are discontinued when there is no more slough or eschar.

What's the advantage?
- Maggots are nature's solution to dead flesh.
- They may be less expensive than other methods of debridement.
- The only side effect is the *ick* factor, though some patients may experience pain as the maggots begin to eat the dead tissue. Over-the-counter acetaminophen often helps.

What to consider
If MDT is ordered, properly prepare the patient, their loved ones, and the staff prior to using them.
- Education of the patient and family is crucial.
- People who can feel MDT may report a slight *crawling* sensation, but most are able to accept this as a part of the healing.
- Explain the importance of avoiding pressure on the wound area because pressure can squash the maggots and kill them.
- Ensure that the patient and family know that the dressing shouldn't get saturated during bathing because the maggots can drown in water.
- A mesh dressing is cemented to a hydrocolloid frame around the wound in order to let the maggots breathe while they work without letting them roam from the wound bed.
  Be sure to have storage, dressing, and maggot removal protocols in place prior to applying medical maggots. Protocols are available from the distributors.

Chemical debridement
Effectiveness is achieved by carefully following each manufacturer's guidelines, as certain cleansers, iodine products, silver products, and Dakin's solution may render the enzyme ineffective in chemical debridement. Consider stopping the enzymes when the wound is clean with granulation tissue, choosing another method to continue moist wound healing.

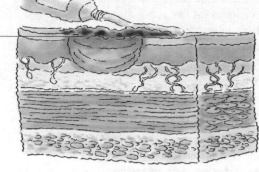

Necrotic
tissue

1

First, apply the debriding agent to the surface of the wound after crosshatching any eschar (scoring it with a scalpel in a meshlike pattern), taking care to apply to entire wound bed per manufacturer recommendations.

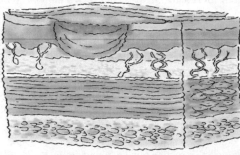

2

Apply damp NSS dressing over ointment and then cover with dry dressing.

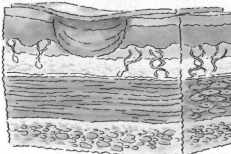

3

Once daily, remove the dressing and irrigate the wound to remove the liquefied necrotic material. Afterward, apply more debriding agent and a clean dressing.

When applied directly to moist necrotic or devitalized tissue, an enzyme debriding agent can break the collagen bonds holding the dead tissue, allowing it to be removed. Consider an enzyme debriding agent for wounds with moderate to large amounts of necrotic tissue, especially in cases for which surgical debridement isn't an option. Dead tissue in a wound has to be broken down so it can be washed away during dressing changes. This happens only when two requirements are met: the wound bed is moist and there is adequate enzyme to break down the dead tissue. Some people with minimal or compromised circulation to a wound do not generate enough natural enzyme to accomplish autolytic debridement, natural breakdown of dead tissue. For these wounds, adding an enzyme may be useful. An enzyme debriding agent augments the collagenase in one's own bloodstream for wounds that do not have optimal microcirculation to bring one's natural enzymes to the wound bed.

What to consider

Debriding agents add cost to wound care, so it is best to utilize natural autolytic debridement when possible. In addition, they:

- may contain known allergens.
- require secondary dressings. It is essential to keep the wound moist at all times for effective debridement to occur, whether adding an enzyme or using autolytic debridement.
- may cause irritation if they come in contact with surrounding skin.
- may cause a burning sensation in the wound during application, though this is rare.

Use the acronym "MEND" to remember application technique:

- M—Moist wound bed (use normal saline solution dressing over enzyme)
- E—Edge-to-edge application of enzyme ointment
- N—Nickel-thick (2 mm)
- D—Daily dressing change

Surgical debridement

Follow your institution's policy regarding informed consent and time-out procedures. Caution should be used when performing surgical sharp debridement on patients who have low platelet counts or who are taking anticoagulants. Surgical debridement is often done in an operating room with the use of anesthesia.

Mechanical debridement

Mechanical debridement includes conservative sharp debridement, wet-to-dry dressings, and pulsatile lavage.

Eschar-go

Conservative sharp debridement involves the removal of necrotic tissue only. It is usually performed by a qualified health care professional. During conservative sharp debridement, loosened eschar is carefully lifted and cut with forceps and scissors to separate it from viable tissue beneath. As one of the most painful types of debridement, it may require either topical or systemic analgesic administration. This may also require informed consent and a time-out procedure per your facility's guidelines.

Sticky situation

Wet-to-dry dressings, typically used for wounds with extensive necrotic tissue and minimal drainage, require an appropriate technique, and the dressing materials used are critical to the outcome. The practitioner places a moist dressing in contact with the lesion and covers it with an outer layer of bandaging. As the dressing dries, it sticks to the wound. When the dried dressing is removed, the necrotic tissue comes off with it. Unfortunately, this is a non-selective form of debridement and should not be the method of choice as healthy tissue may be removed too. The gauze *cannot* differentiate healthy tissue from necrotic tissue. It can also cause pain for the patient.

Finger on the pulse

Pulsatile lavage involves the use of a pressurized antiseptic solution or normal saline, which cleans tissue and removes wound debris and excess drainage.

Pulsatile lavage can be used with almost any wound type: acute or chronic, large or small, infected or noninfected, and clean or necrotic. It is a modality used by physical therapists with health care provider orders.

Indications for pulsatile lavage include:
- clean wounds—to increase granulation tissue formation.
- slow-healing wounds—to increase granulation tissue formation.
- infected or heavily contaminated wounds—to decrease bioburden levels.
- WBP—for grafting with either skin grafts or cellular tissue products (CTPs).
- removal of necrotic tissue or other particulate.

Puttin' on the spritz

Sterile normal saline solution at room temperature is typically used for pulsatile lavage. It is applied by spray gun using a plastic, disposable fan tip. A tunneling tip is used for deep wounds with tunnels or extensive undermining.

The solution is delivered under pressure to the wound bed and concurrently aspirated by negative pressure through a separate plastic tube in the spray gun. The therapist can control both the delivery or impact pressure of the sterile normal saline solution and the suction pressure for aspiration of the contaminated fluid. (See *Pressures for pulsatile lavage.*)

Pressures for pulsatile lavage

The amount of pressure used for pulsatile lavage depends on the patient's wound type:
- High-impact and suction pressures are used for contaminated, necrotic wounds.
- Intermediate pressures are used for infected wounds.
- Low pressures are used for clean, granulating wounds.

Specific impact, or delivery pressures, and suction pressures are listed below.

Wound type	Impact pressure (psi)	Suction pressure (mm Hg)
Clean or granulating	4–8	60–80
Infected	8–10	80–100
Necrotic	10–12	100–120

Note: Impact pressures of less than 15 psi are recommended for wound management in order to prevent bacteria from being driven into the deeper tissues of the wound.

Pulsatile precautions

Currently, no contraindications for pulsatile lavage are recognized; however, you should consider premedicating the patient with analgesia for comfort during the procedure. Suggested precautions include:
- using personal protective equipment when delivering therapy.
- having the patient in a private room as particles can become airborne.
- using lower-impact and suction pressures on fragile tissue.
- avoiding direct pressure over exposed nerves and blood vessels.
- avoiding high-impact pressure over malignant tissue.
- avoiding high-impact and suction pressures and static delivery in areas where excess suction may draw tissue into the tip as well as over grafts and exposed organs and body cavities.

Inflammation and infection

The evolution of a wound from contamination to infection is difficult for the naked eye to evaluate. Consider the following points:
- The length of time a wound remains unhealed is significant as the amount of bacteria acquired begin to multiply.
- When wound colonization has taken place, bacteria have multiplied but the wound tissue is not damaged.

- When surface and deeper tissue damage occurs, bacteria have invaded this wound tissue, and local or systemic infection may occur. This is the point at which a wound culture should be done.
- Critical colonization, now referred to as local infection, is often described quantitatively as a bacterial burden of *greater than 10^5 colony-forming units per gram of tissue*. If critical colonization is not treated, the wound will progress to an infection, and microbes will damage the deeper tissues.

Remember that proteases (enzymes that digest protein) are activated to help with wound debridement by:

- facilitating bacteria removal.
- stimulating migration of cells needed for wound healing.
- activating growth factors.
- remodeling scar tissue.

In wound healing, a balance between the activation and inhibition of matrix metalloproteinases (MMPs) occurs during the first days. Chronic wounds have an imbalance and activation of the protease that continues and prolongs the inflammatory phase. In addition, bacteria are producing their own proteases and disrupting the MMP activation/inhibition balance.

When should you take a culture?

In order to identify potential chronic wound infection, consider these early clinical signs:

- Pain
- Delayed healing
- Presence of necrotic tissue
- Wound deterioration
- Classic signs of infection

The mnemonics "NERDS" and "STONEES" were developed to assist with clinically assessing bacterial levels and damage in chronic wounds. As you can see, there are a few characteristics that are the same.

Superficial (NERDS)	Deep (STONEES)
N—Nonhealing	S—Size increasing
E—Exudate increasing	T—Temperature elevation
R—Red, friable granulation tissue	O—Os (probes to bone)
D—Debris or discoloration	N—New breakdown
S—Smell	E—Erythema, edema
	E—Exudate increasing
	S—Smell

Because most wounds are colonized with surface bacteria, the swab specimen technique is limited in that it only obtains surface cultures. Needle aspiration of fluid or punch tissue biopsy is recommended for accurate wound culturing. All cultures are done after the wound has been cleansed as all chronic wounds are contaminated and colonized.

Wound biopsy

Biopsies are in the scopes of practice for medical doctors, physician assistants, and advanced practice registered nurses. A tissue biopsy contains the organisms invading the wound, not just the surface bacteria, and it is done with a punch tool or a scalpel.

To perform a punch biopsy:
- Cleanse wound with normal saline solution, and pat it dry with gauze.
- Select tissue that is not necrotic and at edge of wound if possible (a 2- to 10-mm, full-thickness plug is captured).
- Send the specimen to the lab.

Moisture

In the 1960s, scientists found that cells migrate at their maximal rate across a moist wound bed, but the wound bed must:
- be clean and free of debris.
- have adequate blood supply.
- have adequate nutrition.

Over the years, randomized controlled trials have demonstrated that with moisture, wound healing is achieved at the wound's optimal rate.

Moisture-retentive dressings have many attributes, which overall lead to more cost-effective wound management as they:
- protect the wound.
- increase the capacity for autolysis.
- decrease pain.
- decrease infection.
- decrease dressing changes.

Because of these attributes, wounds with moist wound healing heal:
- at their fastest rate.
- less painfully.
- with less scarring.
- with fewer infections.
- more cost-effectively.

Edge

The edge of the wound should be flush with the wound bed and attached. If there is considerable undermining, callus, or the edges are rolled under (known as epibole), the edge needs attention.

If there is considerable undermining, the wound may need the excess tissue cut away to the "edge" of the wound. To prevent further undermining, lightly fill the wound dead space, keep the wound bed moist, and protect the wound from pressure and shearing forces.

If callus is present, sharp debridement of this dead, hard tissue to expose the flat edge of the wound is necessary. To prevent further callus, offload the wound area to remove pressure.

Epibole indicates that the wound is dry, has been traumatized by a dressing, is infected, or is hypoxic. In epibole, the upper epidermal cells roll down over the lower epidermal cells and then proceed down the sides of the wound instead of across the wound. When the two sets of epithelial cells come into contact, the body thinks the wound is healed and the epithelial migration across the wound stops. Opening this closed edge occurs with conservative or surgical sharp debridement or sometimes with silver nitrate. To prevent further epibole, lightly fill wound dead space, keep the wound bed moist, and protect the wound from pressure.

Regeneration/repair

Wound healing addresses how the wound will be repaired or closed. Wounds may be closed by supporting the body's natural processes with the appropriate cleansing and dressing techniques. It may be necessary to use advanced wound care techniques (e.g., negative pressure wound therapy, hyperbaric oxygen therapy, stem cell therapy) in order to accomplish this goal. Remember to address risk factors as well.

Social factors

Patient care, including wound care, must be conducted with a holistic focus. Consider the following factors when developing a care plan:
1. The patient's social situation and environment must be considered for a safe, effective plan of care. Where is the patient's environment? Their home, long-term care, acute care, or rehabilitation? Identify the patient's goals with environment in mind. Engage the patient in the plan to enhance understanding and adherence.
2. Cost and availability of supplies are essential to consider.
3. The education of the patient and caregivers must be done in a clear and concise manner. Ensure that the patient understands the plan of care by using the teach-back technique in which the patient "teaches" the nurse the information they have learned.

Quick quiz

1. Because conservative sharp debridement may be painful, the procedure should be limited to:
   A. 5 minutes.
   B. 10 minutes.
   C. 20 minutes.
   D. 25 minutes.

Answer: C. Debridement should be performed for no more than 20 minutes. If needed, the procedure can be repeated to completely remove the necrotic tissue.

2. To irrigate a wound, direct the flow of irrigant:
   A. toward the wound.
   B. away from the wound.
   C. toward the center of the wound.
   D. to pool inside of the wound.

Answer: B. Direct the flow away from the wound to prevent contamination.

3. The most commonly used cleaning agent is:
   A. normal saline solution.
   B. hydrogen peroxide.
   C. povidone-iodine solution.
   D. sodium hypochlorite.

Answer: A. Sterile normal saline solution is most commonly used because it provides a moist environment, promotes granulation tissue formation, and causes minimal fluid shifts in healthy adults.

4. Which type of dressing wouldn't be appropriate for a wound with excessive drainage?
   A. Gauze dressing
   B. Transparent film dressing
   C. Alginate dressing
   D. Hydrocolloid dressing

Answer: B. Because a transparent film dressing can't absorb drainage, it should be used only for wounds with minimal drainage.

5. Which methods of wound culturing are most accurate for determining infection?
   A. Swab technique and needle aspiration
   B. Swab technique and punch tissue biopsy
   C. Needle aspiration and punch tissue biopsy
   D. Aerobic and anaerobic swab techniques

Answer: C. Because the surface of most wounds is normally colonized with bacteria, swab cultures may not be accurate. Needle aspiration and punch tissue biopsy provide the most reliable information.

Scoring

☆☆☆   If you answered all five questions correctly, yippee! You're quite a
fine specimen.

☆☆   If you answered four questions correctly, great job! You really
cleaned up in the area of basic wound care procedures.

☆   If you answered fewer than four questions correctly, don't despair!
Irrigate your system and then review the chapter again.

Select references

Bowers, S., & Franco, E. (2020). Chronic wounds: Evaluation and management. *American Family Physician, 101*(3), 159–166. https://www.aafp.org/pubs/afp/issues/2020/0201/p159.html

Brindle, T., & Farmer, P. (2019). Undisturbed wound healing: A narrative review of the literature and clinical considerations. *Wounds International, 10*(2), 40–48. https://www.woundsinternational.com/journals/issue/577/article-details/undisturbed-wound-healing-narrative-review-literature-and-clinical-considerations

Coleman, K., & Neilsen, G. (2019). *Wound care: A practical guide for maintaining skin integrity*. Elsevier Health Sciences.

Goto, T., & Saligan, L. N. (2020). Wound pain and wound healing biomarkers from wound exudate: A scoping review. *Journal of Wound, Ostomy and Continence Nursing, 47*(6), 559–568. https://doi.org/10.1097/WON.0000000000000703

Jaszarowski, K., & Murphree, R. (2021). Wound cleansing and dressing selection. In L. L. McNichol, C. R. Ratliff, & S. S. Yates (Eds.), *Wound, Ostomy, and Continence Nurses Society core curriculum: Wound management* (2nd ed., pp. 156–170). Wolters Kluwer.

Ramundo, J. (2021). Principles and guidelines for wound debridement. In L. L. McNichol, C. R. Ratliff, & S. S. Yates (Eds.), *Wound, Ostomy, and Continence Nurses Society core curriculum: Wound management* (2nd ed., pp. 171–185). Wolters Kluwer.

Rosenbaum, A. J., Banerjee, S., Rezak, K. M., & Uhl, R. L. (2018). Advances in wound management. *Journal of the American Academy of Orthopaedic Surgeons, 26*(23), 833–843. https://doi.org/10.5435/JAAOS-D-17-00024

Sibbald, R. G., Goodman, L., Woo, K. Y., Krasner, D. L., Smart, H., Tariq, G., Ayello, E. A., Burrell, R. E., Keast, D. H., Mayer, D., Norton, L., & Salcido, R. (2011). Special considerations in wound bed preparation 2011: An update. *Advances in Skin & Wound Care, 24*(9), 415–436. https://doi.org/10.1097/01.ASW.0000405216.27050.97

Sibbald, R. G., Woo, K., & Ayello, E. A. (2006). Increased bacterial burden and infection: The story of NERDS and STONES. *Advances in Skin and Wound Care, 19*(8), 447–461. https://doi.org/10.1097/00129334-200610000-00012

Chapter 4

External threats to skin integrity

Just the facts

In this chapter you'll learn about:

♦ Factors that compromise skin integrity
♦ Effects of friction, adhesive, and trauma on the skin
♦ Effects of excessive moisture exposure on skin

Seriously?

Why take skin injuries from external factors seriously? The top three reasons are:

1. First of all, they hurt! For anyone with normal sensation, abrasions and moisture-related injuries are painful.
2. Secondly, they are a break in the body's first line of immune defense, and there are some nasty organisms out there waiting to invade and cause trouble!
3. Thirdly, anything that compromises skin health puts the person at higher risk for more serious skin injuries such as pressure injuries.

So let's get to it!

Trouble in paradise

Many factors can make the skin more susceptible to injury from external forces. With aging, for example, the body produces less sebum and natural moisturizing factor (NMF), and the skin gets drier and thinner. Add to this the natural decline in microcirculation, and we see the effects manifest in wrinkling and thinner, more fragile skin. We also see accelerated skin compromise caused by disease complications, such as microcirculatory changes from diabetic neuropathy and peripheral arterial disease. Nurses can counsel patients to make healthy lifestyle choices that improve skin health and can review the use of medications that affect skin.

Modifiable factors that can compromise skin

Factor	Common effect on skin	Interventions
Long-term systemic steroid use	Skin atrophy (thinning) most commonly in the skin folds; purpura; fragility; telangiectasia; acne; susceptibility to bacterial, fungal, and viral skin infections; slow wound healing	The key is using the lowest-potency steroid and lowest dose effective for the condition being treated. Vitamin A supplementation may increase collagen content (Krasner et al., 2007, p. 132), and use of vitamin A analogs such as retinol sometimes reverses steroid effects on wound healing (Krasner et al., 2007, p. 293).
Long-term (longer than 4 weeks) topical steroid use in the potent, very potent, and extremely potent classes	Permanent stretch marks with severe pruritus; localized atrophy with resulting fragility	Atrophy may be permanent, but the sooner the steroid is discontinued the better. Topical tretinoin may encourage collagen production to prevent or reverse atrophy.
Overexposure to sunlight	Ultraviolet (UV) light damages collagen and elastin fibers, which give skin its toughness and elasticity, and results in wrinkles and more fragile skin as well as an increased risk of skin cancer.	For longer than 15 minutes of sun exposure, apply sun protection factor 30 or higher to exposed skin.
Cigarette smoking	Nicotine narrows capillaries, damages collagen and elastin.	Smoking cessation if possible or decreased use with support systems
Air pollution	Induces oxidative stress	Avoid longer outdoor exposure on days when air quality is listed as unhealthy.

Cleanup without compromise

How can we keep skin as healthy as possible with gentle cleansing when it is fragile? Traditional soap, such as bars for cleansing, have an alkaline pH that can destroy the natural "acid mantle" function. Healthy skin has a pH of 4.5 to 5.5, which is hostile to pathogens and therefore beneficial to us. Most soaps also contain surfactants, which dissolve the natural lipids that protect the epidermis. Newer cleansers such as synthetic detergents (also called syndets) provide cleansing at a natural skin pH level and avoid harsh surfactants, leaving high-risk skin in better condition. It is also helpful to avoid hot water for showering or bathing and to bathe only as often as necessary for good hygiene.

Picky, picky, picky!

Our skin has multiple mechanisms to maintain moisture balance, keeping excess moisture from causing damage and protecting it from excess dryness. However, there is a delicate balance that can be disturbed in many ways. The keratin produced in the dermis is a waxy substance that helps keep excess outside moisture from causing trouble and prevents excess evaporation from the dermis too. NMF occurs in the epidermis and includes urea, lactate, amino acids, pyrrolidone carboxylic acid (PCA), and salts. NMF holds moisture to keep skin from becoming overly dry, but it decreases with aging (especially the amino acids) and can be overwhelmed by excessive washing or excess UV light exposure. This leaves our skin vulnerable to excess dryness and damage from external wetness.

Xerosis: Overly dry skin

When skin is too dry with less sebum and NMF, it becomes flaky and rough, sometimes scaly. This increases the chances of abrasions, fissures, and skin tears.

Skin care ingredients to improve dry skin

Ingredient type	Purpose	Tips
Humectants (urea, lactate, hyaluronic acid, aloe vera, glycerin)	Bind and hold water in the epidermis	Look for these ingredients to help dry skin, but avoid using them in high amounts to protect skin that is overexposed to wetness.
Occlusives (petrolatum, lanolin, emu oil, shea butter, cocoa butter, jojoba oil, castor oil, safflower oil, argan oil, olive oil)	Barriers that prevent transepidermal water loss	These reduce evaporation and act as emollients to smooth rough skin. Be aware that they also reduce the absorbency of incontinence products such as briefs and underpads. In some situations, such as incontinence, they further reduce evaporation, which is not helpful if skin is already overhydrated.
Emollients (include above occlusives plus dimethicone, triglycerides, squalene, colloidal oatmeal)	Soften, smooth, and protect skin	Dimethicone is an emollient but is nonocclusive, so it is often used in barrier products to protect skin from incontinence when protection is needed and overhydration is common.

Different forms of skin products

Lotions

Lotions are dissolved powder crystals held in suspension by surfactants. They have the highest water content, which is why lotions feel cool as they're applied. They also evaporate faster than any other type of moisturizer; consequently, they must be applied more often. Keep in mind that evaporation is drying, so lotion may not be the best choice for xerosis (super dry skin).

Creams

Creams are preparations of oil and water that are a bit more occlusive than lotions. They don't have to be applied as often as lotions. Usually, three or four applications per day should be sufficient. Creams are better for preventing moisture loss due to evaporation than for replenishing skin moisture.

Ointments

Ointments are preparations of water in oil (typically lanolin or petroleum). They're the most occlusive and longest-lasting form of moisturizer. For dry skin, they are most effective if applied while skin is still moist following a shower or bath. Because they are occlusive, oils are not preferred for areas that are exposed to too much moisture, such as in the skin folds, between toes, and areas often exposed to wetness as with incontinence. If using ointments on the feet, put socks on before walking to avoid slipping. Socks and gloves can prevent the ointment from rubbing off too quickly from feet and hands and make nighttime application very effective.

Does this rub you the wrong way?

Friction is a physical force that occurs when two surfaces rub against each other. When healthy skin rubs lightly against a surface, like sheets on a bed, this can cause a bit of warmth but will not cause damage. It is a different story when fragile, rough, flaky skin or overly moist skin rubs on a surface, increasing friction that can result in exfoliation of layers of epidermis (an abrasion), or even into the dermis, depending on the weight and whether the area being rubbed is a flat surface of skin (forearm) or curved (buttocks and heels). Friction itself cannot cause a pressure injury, but any compromise of the skin increases risk. An abrasion occurs when skin cells are removed due to friction; depending on the amount of damage and the health of the skin, blisters may form. Fissures, or linear cracks in the skin, and skin tears can occur due to friction or blunt trauma when xerosis is present. This is most common in compromised or very thin skin and in seriously dry skin (xerosis), often found on the heels and lower legs of older adults.

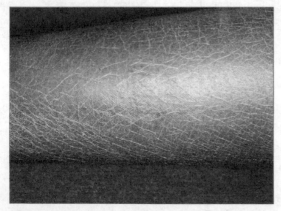

Craft. N., & Fox, L. P. (2010). *VisualDx: Essential adult dermatology.* Wolters Kluwer Health/Lippincott Williams & Wilkins.

Health care providers and others who must wash their hands frequently also may experience painful fissures in fingertips and hands. Try your own experiment! Tonight at bedtime, apply your favorite lotion to one hand and apply an ointment (dimethicone or petrolatum based) to the other hand. Put a glove on each hand. In the morning, check to see how soft your hands are and how the cracks in your fingertips have responded. Usually, the ointment heals them faster! Try it on your heels with socks too!

Keys to protecting skin from friction damage include preventing or treating xerosis and preventing overhydration. One method to reduce skin tears and abrasions is to cover any high-risk areas. Skin prone to dryness on the lower legs can be protected with pant legs or knee-high socks; don't forget to keep the long socks on the patient during transfers, especially while in a wheelchair. Skin tears on the shins can even occur during a short trip for a bath! Forearms are also especially vulnerable to abrasions and skin tears and can be protected with long sleeves or separate sleeves meant for this protection.

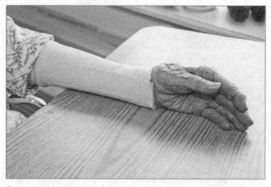

Goldschmidt, W. M., & Carter, P. J. (2009). *Lippincott's textbook for long-term care nursing assistants: A humanistic approach to caregiving.* Lippincott Williams & Wilkins.

A trial of protective socks made with Kevlar fibers (used in stab-proof vests and motorcycle protective clothing) showed these products can decrease skin tears in lower extremities (Powell et al., 2017). There is also a special type of linen meant to reduce friction and abrasions. This might be considered when frequent friction injuries occur, but keep in mind when friction is reduced, extra caution must be taken to prevent falls, such as slipping out of bed.

Skin tears

Accidental separation of a flap of skin occurs frequently in people who have fragile, overly dry, or overly moist skin. Especially vulnerable are those who depend on others for care and those who become restless or agitated and have poor coordination or safety awareness. These are most often minor injuries and for the most part heal without complications. However, they can be unsightly, painful, and may trigger more severe skin injuries. For example, a patient with chronic lower extremity edema who sustained a small bump to the shin with a small skin tear may end up with a chronic wound. The constant weeping from the edema does not allow the wound to close (without adequate compression) and the subcutaneous tissue may be compromised due to the chronic injury from poor edema control. Chapter 7 includes methods to control such edema and allow the skin tear to heal.

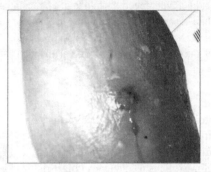

This bump and small skin tear occurred on the way to a shower. Because of the chronic lymphedema (unhealthy subcutaneous tissue), this injury took 7 months to heal and required Unna wraps for compression, changed weekly. Remember to keep legs covered until after transferring into a shower chair!

Risk factors and prevention

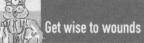

Get wise to wounds

A 6-month prospective cohort study in two Japanese long-term care hospitals reported a 13% incidence of skin tears (Minematsu et al., 2021). They noted predictive factors such as dry skin and actinic purpura (mild bruises that occur without known trauma to fragile capillaries usually due to aging). In another study, an Australian hospital reported a prevalence of skin tears of 8.9%, most often happening in patients over age 70 and most often due to falls or collisions with equipment (Miles et al., 2022). A 4-week study of a long-term care population in Ontario, Canada, showed a prevalence of 20.8% and incidence of 18.9% (LeBlanc et al., 2020). A report from six U.S. long-term care facilities showed a 9% prevalence rate with an average age of 83 among those sustaining wounds (Hawk & Shannon, 2018). The majority had mobility limitations, supporting mobility as a risk factor, and a third of the skin tears were due to falls.

What can be done to reduce the occurrence of skin tears? Certainly, preventing falls is essential, but simple nursing interventions such as encouraging good nutrition and hydration and twice-daily moisturizer for at-risk skin are also helpful. A review of literature showed that a comprehensive skin tear bundle, or a standardized way to prevent and treat skin tears, can decrease incidence and prevent complications (Al Khaleefa et al., 2022).

Classification of skin tears

In order to standardize treatments for skin tears, it is helpful to speak the same language about the severity of the injury. The International Skin Tear Advisory Panel (ISTAP) Classification System is one tool for categorizing skin tears.

Skin Tear Classification

Type 1: No Skin Loss   Type 2: Partial Flap Loss   Type 3: Total Flap Loss

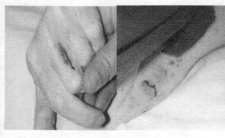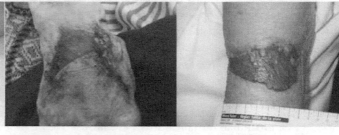

Linear or Flap* Tear which can
be repositioned to cover the
wound bed

Partial Flap Loss which
cannot be repositioned
to cover the wound bed

Total Flap Loss exposing
entire wound bed

*A flap in skin tears is defined as a portion of the skin (epidermis/dermis) that is unintentionally separated from
its original place due to shear, friction, and/or blunt force. This concept is not to be confused with tissue that is
intentionally detached from its place of origin for therapeutic use e.g. surgical skin grafting.*

International Skin Tear Classification System. https://www.skintears.org/

According to ISTAP, this is a type 2 skin
tear. The partial flap remaining was repositioned to serve as a skin graft and speed healing. No adhesive fixation strips were used to
secure the flap due to the fragile nature of the
skin. A long nonadherent pad was covered
in petrolatum-based ointment and secured
over the area using tubular dressing retention
netting.

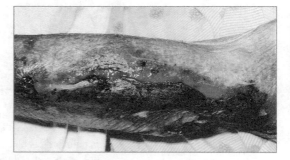

Medical adhesive–related skin injuries

A medical adhesive is any product meant to help a medical device
stick to the skin: adhesive tape, ostomy skin barriers, dressings
with adhesive edges, and electrodes. Many may think the "rip the
Band-Aid off quickly" technique makes removal hurt less, but this
approach can be harmful to anyone with compromised skin. This
includes very young children, older adults, and anyone with fragile
skin. This method can lead to medical adhesive–related skin injuries (MARSIs).

Handle with care

A university hospital in China reported their intensive care unit (ICU) MARSI incidence rate of 11.86% including epidermal stripping and skin tears (Gao et al., 2020). It makes sense since there are many medical devices in the ICU and many patients in the ICU are those with fragile skin. This group noted independent risk factors included moderate-to-severe edema, hyperthermia, and use of medications such as immunosuppressants and anticoagulants.

Unfortunately, "tape burns," as they used to be called, are common and often occur near wounds, surgical incisions, or where medical devices penetrate the body.

Preventing MARSIs

Twice-daily moisturizing of dry skin is helpful, but this is not an option under adhesive devices or dressings. There are some alternative methods to consider.

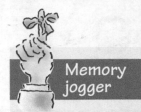

Memory jogger

A unique way to think about any superficial break in skin is as if it is a Petri dish in a lab—full of nutrients to grow germs. Imagine that as soon as the first line of defense is broken (skin), the bacteria that is always present on the surface sees a neon "OPEN" sign. If this is near a wound or entry point for a device like an intravenous line, it can be a recipe for disaster!

Method	How it works	Did you know?
Liquid skin barrier application prior to adhesive application	Provides an extra layer of protection of breathable "plastic" film if applied prior to tape or clear film protective dressings; can reduce trauma during removal	The nonalcohol versions prevent stinging of nearby open wounds or previously damaged skin and also tend to be more durable.
Remove clear polymer film dressings by stretching the film parallel to the skin, not pulling up away from the skin level. Put pressure on the edge you are pulling away from to prevent it from stripping skin.	Staying parallel to skin level reduces the amount of force needed to detach the adhesive, lessening the chance of MARSI. Anchoring the dressing as you stretch it prevents it from tearing off the skin.	Clear film dressings can be removed by loosening opposite edges with adhesive remover or oil then grasping both edges and pulling them apart parallel to the skin. This breaks the adhesive in the center easily.

Method	How it works	Did you know?
Use medical adhesive remover while removing tape or other adhesive.	Dissolves the adhesive rather than tearing it off the skin	No medical adhesive remover handy? Any skin product such as lotion or a skin barrier with oil in it can also help prevent skin damage during clear film dressing, tape, or ostomy barrier removal. Prior to applying new tape or an ostomy barrier, the adhesive remover or oil must be cleansed from skin. Do not use these products close to any incision closed in surgery with a medical adhesive rather than sutures or stitches; it will dissolve it, and the incision may dehisce.
Use silicone tape rather than adhesive tape.	Adheres to skin well (except on very moist skin) but does not strip it when removed. Be sure to dry skin well before applying and press it into place.	For persons with fragile skin there is silicone-based clear film for protecting intravenous devices and silicone-based drape available to seal negative pressure wound therapy dressings.

Moisture-associated skin damage

Moisture-associated skin damage (MASD) includes damage to skin related to contact with external moisture and often includes the effects of friction on the overly moist skin. It usually manifests in inflammation of the skin (becoming red, hot, and tender), sometimes with erosion or denudement and possibly weeping of serous fluid causing the skin to glisten. The location often tells the story about which bodily fluid is causing the damage.

Effects of excess moisture on skin health

We've discussed the problems associated with excessively dry skin and what to do about it. Now let's examine the opposite side of the coin—too much moisture. Skin has a delicate balance when it comes to moisture content and the risk of skin damage is high when it is overhydrated. When skin gets "drowned," maceration occurs. The skin becomes lighter in color and often wrinkled (a common example is how skin looks after soaking in a bathtub too long). For people with healthy skin, some layers of epidermis slough off and we're left with intact and still functional skin. Those with less healthy skin may experience additional consequences, often before the maceration becomes apparent. Let's look at what happens to unprotected skin when exposed to external moisture such as sweat or urine.

Effects of external moisture on unprotected skin

Process	How it affects skin health	What may happen if barrier is not restored
The pH becomes alkaline.	The acid mantle function of the skin is impaired.	Bacteria and fungi can proliferate to the point of causing infection because they thrive in an alkaline environment.
The barrier becomes more permeable because lipids are impaired and the tight junctions between cells are loosened.	The permeability allows even more fluid and caustic materials (such as destructive enzymes) to penetrate the skin.	Inflammation (dermatitis) occurs due to the penetration of irritants.
Overly moist skin has an increased friction coefficient.	Skin sticks to linens and clothes.	Skin tears, blisters, and abrasions may occur, especially over heels and fleshy prominences like the buttocks. If skin sticks in place and gravity pulls the skeleton downward kinking blood vessels, shearing injury can occur, causing ischemia and pressure injuries over bony prominences.

Get wise to wounds

In long-term care, MASD is reported to the Centers for Medicare & Medicaid Services (CMS) in the Minimum Data Set (MDS). Data available up to 2017 show that the percentage of residents with MASD in quarter 1 of 2013 was 5.8, 2016 was 6.9, and 2017 was 6.63. Between 2013 and 2016, it is likely that reporting of MASD had improved with education efforts (Ayello, 2017). Hopefully, when newer data become available, the percentages will improve. However, during the COVID-19 pandemic, there was likely an increase in all skin issues due to declining health of long-term care residents and shortage of staff plus fatigue and difficulty working with personal protective equipment.

Nothing new under the sun, except terminology

International Classification of Disease (ICD) codes from the World Health Organization are used by most countries in the world to define causes of mortality and morbidity and for data collection. In the United States, the ICD codes are also how organizations bill insurance companies for reimbursement for health care and supplies. The United States is currently using ICD-10. ICD-11 was released in January 2022, but due to the complexity of changing electronic data collection systems, it will probably not be implemented until at least 2025. In the meantime, in October of 2021, the CMS and the Centers for Disease Control and Prevention (CDC) approved a clinical modification called the ICD-10-CM. The definition from the ICD-10-CM for MASD is "irritant contact dermatitis due to friction, sweating, or contact with body fluids." This is an improvement from "diaper dermatitis" in the ICD-9, reflecting more current science thanks to the work of the Wound, Ostomy, and Continence Nurses Society™ and others who testified to Congress to get more precise terms.

ICD-10-CM codes for MASD conditions

- L24.A0 Irritant contact dermatitis due to friction or contact with body fluids, unspecified
  - L24.A1 Irritant contact dermatitis due to saliva
  - L24.A2 Irritant contact dermatitis due to fecal, urinary, or dual incontinence
  - L24.A9 Irritant contact dermatitis due to friction or contact with other specified body fluids

- L24.B0 Irritant contact dermatitis related to unspecified stoma or fistula
  - L24.B1 Irritant contact dermatitis related to digestive stoma or fistula
  - L24.B2 Irritant contact dermatitis related to respiratory stoma or fistula
  - L24.B3 Irritant contact dermatitis related to fecal or urinary stoma or fistula

If you work in an organization that bills insurance for care and supplies, you have someone (or a team) that determines ICD-10-CM codes for billing purposes. They may get this from a medical diagnosis but quite often, especially for more superficial skin issues, they look at the nurses' documentation. It is more important than ever to be specific when it is moisture that causes damage. When you chart the pattern (diffuse edges rather than distinct edges like a pressure injury) and the location (in the area affected by incontinence or around a wound, stoma, or in a moist skin fold), more appropriate reimbursement occurs because the condition was coded correctly.

Intertriginous dermatitis

Excessive moisture buildup in skin folds can cause intertriginous dermatitis (ITD), also called erythema intertrigo. This type of MASD often appears as a symmetrical shape on the opposing skin surfaces (mirror image). In a deep skin fold, there is little or no opportunity for moisture to evaporate, and the two opposing skin surfaces slide against each other, creating friction in a high-risk environment of overhydrated skin.

The first sign of injury is inflammation. The skin then becomes edematous and likely peels. This sets up an ideal environment for pathogens such as bacteria and fungi to proliferate, especially since overly moist skin develops an alkaline pH over time, which favors the pathogens. Areas most likely to be affected include the inframammary area (under the breasts), under the pannus (fatty abdominal apron), groins, gluteal cleft (between the buttocks), and interdigital areas (especially between toes). It is important to examine other skin fold areas in people that have contractures or other deep folds.

Risk factors for ITD include excessive sweating, deep skin folds, atrophy of skin and decreased sebum (due to aging, medications, or disease), atopy (genetic susceptibility to irritants), diabetes, and immune deficiency.

Get wise to wounds

Over the course of 2 years, Arnold-Long and Johnson (2019) studied inpatients in a U.S. acute care and acute rehabilitation hospital who had been referred for any reason to a wound and ostomy care nurse. The mean prevalence of ITD among these patients was 40%, and the mean incidence of hospital-acquired ITD was 33%. Incidence was higher in those classified as obese, and the most common location was the gluteal cleft.

Treating ITD

Because of the association between deeper skin folds and ITD, one long-term approach to improving the risk is to assist with weight loss when feasible. Most literature on the topic recommends avoiding oil-based ointments ("no grease in the crease") because oil further reduces evaporation. Consider zinc oxide preparations instead because these barriers absorb small amounts of sweat or weeping. When skin fold moisture is likely to be a long-term problem, another strategy is to use a textile woven to wick fluid laterally. Three products available contain silver, which is useful to combat fungal and bacterial skin infections. The products are InterDry Ag from Coloplast, DermaTex Ag from Hartmann, and McKesson Silver Moisture Wicking Fabric. Follow directions and leave at least 2 in of the fabric hanging outside the fold to allow evaporation. When using a wicking textile with silver, it is not necessary to add another antifungal medication as the silver is considered the treatment when used as directed. Medline offers a wicking cloth that slowly releases hydrogen peroxide and is called DriGo-HP Intensive Skin Therapy Barrier Sheet.

Two products help maintain dry skin folds but without antimicrobials, so they can be used long term. Medline offers a Skinfold Dry Sheet that has an absorbent core to wick moisture off the skin. It cannot be cut but can be folded to fit into a crease and holds up to 8 oz. It is also sold under the name UltraSorbs. A similar product from Tranquility is called ThinLiner Moisture Management. These are preferred alternatives to towels and pillowcases often used in skin folds because cloth absorbs moisture and holds it against the skin, and many towels and washcloths are rough.

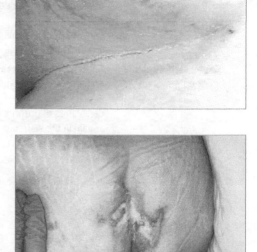

This inframammary (under the breast) example of the effects of ITD shows inflammation and maceration of the deepest crease. Teaching nursing assistants and technicians to recognize this as moisture damage and report it before it worsens is a great way to achieve success in prevention because early treatment saves skin.

This deep ITD occurred in a continent patient who was in a chair constantly due to pain issues. The patient was diaphoretic from pain and did not let nursing staff check the area for over a week. This is not a pressure injury as weight-bearing surfaces for this man who remained upright, not slouched, were ischial tuberosities, not the sacrum. There is a deep gluteal fold, and the buttocks were not separated for care initially. Once care of the area resumed, the ITD healed in a few weeks using zinc oxide applied to an anal leakage pad twice a day along with gentle cleansing with a disposable bathing cloth.

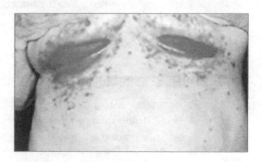

This inframammary ITD shows evidence of skin infection, likely fungal. Skin infections in moist areas that cause itching (pruritus) and have "satellite lesions" (macules and papules around the margins) are likely fungal, though they can sometimes be bacterial. The wicking textile with silver can treat either type, but if you are using an antifungal and having no success after 2 weeks, consider a culture.

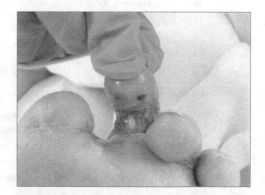

When toes are deformed, be sure to check under and between for ITD, especially dangerous for a patient with diabetes who may lose toes due to infection that is allowed to penetrate the macerated skin. Lamb's wool rope woven between toes wicks moisture away and prevents ITD between the toes.

Area at risk for ITD	Warning signs	Interventions
Inframammary (below the breasts) or below the pannus (fatty abdominal apron)	Any inflammation or rash; superficial peeling; maceration, especially along the deepest crease; foul odor Complaints of pruritus (itching) or pain in the skin fold	If only mild erythema is present, zinc oxide can be applied to both sides of a nonadherent pad and replaced twice daily after gently cleansing with an acidic pH cleanser. For more serious damage or suspected fungal/bacterial infection, consider using a wicking textile with silver; leave 2 in of it outside the fold to allow evaporation to occur.
Gluteal cleft (crease between the buttocks)	Any inflammation or rash; maceration or skin split along the deepest crease Complaints of pruritus (itching) or pain in the skin fold	Consider a zinc oxide paste, ointment, or spray for prevention of mild ITD in this area. Zinc oxide paste can be applied to an anal leakage pad or to both sides of a nonadherent pad. Cleanse gently after each incontinence episode with a pH-balanced cleanser (acidic), and reapply. If there are denuded areas, pastes containing carboxymethylcellulose/pectin applied to the denuded skin may be helpful. These products and zinc oxide barriers should only be removed every few days to bare skin and reapplied. In the interim, cleanse stool and urine off the paste, and apply more paste as needed.
Interdigital Toes, especially with deformities such as hammer toes Fingers, especially with hand contractures	Maceration (whitish appearance of skin) often followed by inflammation and fungal or Gram-negative bacterial infection Complaints of burning or pruritus (itching) if sensation is intact	For toes, weave a rope of lamb's wool between the toes to help wick moisture and prevent surfaces from touching. If fungus is suspected, consider an antifungal spray rather than cream or ointment that holds moisture. For fingers and palms with contractures, use wicking textile with silver, leaving at least 2 in of the cloth out in the air to facilitate evaporation.

Incontinence-associated dermatitis

Incontinence-associated dermatitis (IAD), also called incontinence-associated skin damage and perineal dermatitis, is skin injury due to fecal, urinary, or dual incontinence. IAD has received more attention in the last few decades. Prior to recent years, regardless of the age of the affected person, it was called "diaper rash" and incontinence briefs were called "diapers."

Get wise to wounds

The first IAD prevalence study in acute care showed that a rate of 42.5% of patients with incontinence in two U.S. hospitals had related skin injuries (Junkin & Selekof, 2007). A study in multiple American acute care facilities showed a 45.7% prevalence of IAD among patients with incontinence (Gray & Giuliano, 2018). A later study showed a 36.2% prevalence in acute care in Brazil (Ferreira et al., 2020). Though it seems like IAD prevention is not improving, that may be due to better reporting and lower use of urinary catheters, especially in acute care.

When data become available for the time of the COVID pandemic, it is likely that the rates of IAD and other skin issues will show an increase due to severity of patient condition, staff shortages, and difficulty working with personal protective equipment.

Etiology

According to Wounds International, the factors most closely associated with increased risk of damage due to incontinence include the type of fluid (e.g., liquid stool is more damaging due to moisture exposure and enzymes present to digest food); frequency of stools; the duration of exposure; frequency of cleansing; and being incontinent of both urine and feces (Fletcher et al., 2020). One reason dual incontinence is more damaging is that urea from urine sitting on the skin is changed to ammonia with an alkaline pH, and when skin becomes more alkaline, its effectiveness as a barrier decreases.

In a study using synthetic urine–soaked premium wicking pads for females over 65 with healthy skin, within 15 minutes of lying on the pads, their skin pH went from a normal 5.67 to a higher pH of 6.25 and their skin barrier function was affected, including a significant increase in erythema and self-reported discomfort (Phipps et al., 2019). Whenever skin becomes more alkaline, the enzymes in stool, including lipases and proteases, become active and are more corrosive to skin. Stool that has a pH higher than 7.5 causes inflammation without any additional factors.

Resolving incontinence

Fecal incontinence

It's helpful to have an excellent relationship with your nutrition therapy colleagues when caring for patients with fecal incontinence. They can often recommend dietary changes, nutritional products containing soluble fiber, along with medications prescribed by health care providers, to get patients closer to producing formed stool. When stool is formed, even if an involuntary evacuation occurs, it is less likely to cause any skin damage. For the nonambulatory patient, while working to resolve diarrhea, there are several "invasive" fecal collection devices on the market as well as noninvasive devices available for use.

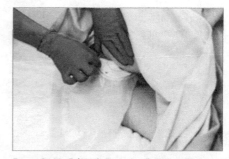

DigniShield™ Stool Management System. Courtesy © Becton, Dickinson and Company.

Evans-Smith, P. (2014). *Taylor's clinical nursing skills.* Lippincott Williams & Wilkins.

Urinary incontinence

Urinary incontinence may be managed temporarily through indwelling catheters, but these carry the risk of urinary tract infection so this intervention is avoided whenever possible. External devices are available, including condom-type catheters for males and padded suction devices to lie between the female labia.

The best option, however, when medically possible, is to correct the cause of urinary incontinence. Sometimes using timed toileting visits or simply making a commode available for quicker access can solve functional incontinence. Appropriate pelvic floor muscle training can also succeed, and incontinence-educated nurses and therapy professionals can offer evaluation and interventions. Dietary changes can help if the patient has triggers for urge incontinence like caffeine, spicy foods, and others. Overflow incontinence from an enlarged prostate may respond to intermittent catheterization. Which approach to take depends on the person's medical status and level of consciousness.

Taking IAD seriously

The pain of contact dermatitis has been described as similar to a thermal burn; stinging and burning are made worse with every touch to the area. However, with IAD, it is impossible to avoid all touch in this region. The person with IAD will be sitting or lying on the painful area, and if skin between the thighs is affected, then ambulation will also be painful. Cleansing the area also causes pain and may be so noxious the patient avoids telling anyone they've experienced incontinence again. No matter what type of product you're using for cleansing, it is important to reduce the amount of friction used because this increases pain and further disrupts the skin barrier.

Let's look at some options for incontinence care that can be less painful and damaging.

Product	Purpose	Comparison	Tips
Synthetic detergent (pH-balanced incontinence cleansers)	Cleansing	Strips less natural skin barrier than soap does Most have an acidic pH closer to the skin's acid mantle	Avoid regular soap, which is usually alkaline and strips natural skin oil away.

Product	Purpose	Comparison	Tips
Microfiber or soft disposable cloth	Used to cleanse soiled skin	Causes less skin stripping than regular washcloths. The nubs on regular washcloths are for the purpose of exfoliation, to remove layers of skin, which is harmful in this situation.	For large stools, consider scooping (not rubbing) the larger portion of stool with the underpad or used brief prior to washing skin. If you need to use toilet paper, add a bit of petrolatum to it to further reduce the friction. The small amount of petrolatum also helps loosen the stool more easily.
Dimethicone-based barrier	Leaves a breathable protective barrier	Allows evaporation so as not to trap excess moisture against skin like oily options do Does not clog up incontinence briefs and underpads like oily options do	The all-in-one products contain a synthetic detergent (gentler), some moisturizer to prevent overdrying, and a dimethicone barrier to protect skin without being occlusive like oily protectants.
Liquid film–forming skin barriers (two types)	Elastomeric terpolymer skin protectant may be applied to intact or superficially eroded skin and is able to adhere to moist areas. It is usually applied every 2–3 days.	Elastomeric terpolymer skin protectants are more expensive, but because they are applied less often than most other barriers, they can be cost-saving in terms of staff time.	If using a liquid film–forming skin barrier, be sure staff knows not to apply any petrolatum barrier of any kind; these will melt away the protective film.
	Nonalcohol cyanoacrylate skin protectant can be used on intact or damaged skin to protect skin.	Check every day and reapply if the clear film is cracked, at least every 3 days.	
Zinc oxide barriers	Protective barrier	Able to absorb weeping or sweating to allow healing even though it is an occlusive barrier	There are a few spray zinc oxide options available. They are not as absorptive but still add protection. If using the thicker types from a tube or a jar, apply the barrier to a pad (nonadherent pad, anal leakage pad, or abdominal pad [ABD]) and apply twice daily and as needed to the injured area. No tape is necessary; just hold it in place with the brief. Do not remove zinc oxide with every stool; just soak the top clean and apply a new pad with zinc oxide. To remove zinc oxide to reassess the skin, apply oil (e.g., petrolatum) to a disposable cloth and wipe it on gently. As the oil mixes with the zinc oxide, it will remove easily with cleanser.

(continued)

(*continued*)

Product	Purpose	Comparison	Tips
Absorptive products	To quickly wick away urine into an inner core and away from the skin	Some types of absorptive briefs and underpads may not be able to trap liquid in the core, so they often include a plastic layer, which further traps moisture and is counterproductive.	It is best to use super-absorbent briefs for ambulation or while up in a chair and use super-absorbent underpads when the patient is in bed to allow airflow to the skin. Some briefs keep the skin more acidic, which maintains a better barrier function. Dignity Compose, Dignity Comfort, and Dignity Complete from Hartmann are briefs with "curly fibers" that help keep the skin's pH acidic.

IAD has a close association with the development of pressure injuries. Anything that damages skin integrity causes an increased risk of pressure-related injuries. An analysis of an international database of 176,689 patients showed that for those who had incontinence (92,889), 16.3% had pressure injuries in the affected areas; those who did not have incontinence had a 4.1% prevalence (Lachenbruch et al., 2016). A data analysis of 5,342 patients published in 2018 showed that the presence of incontinence-related skin damage (odds ratio [OR] 4.56) and immobility (OR 3.56) was associated with significantly increased likelihood of developing full-thickness sacral pressure injury (Gray & Guiliano, 2018). The OR for IAD was even higher than for immobility! This is one area of health care in which an ounce of prevention is worth a pound of cure. It is essential to develop a plan for prevention and treatment and then stick to it.

Classifying IAD

There are several methods of classifying the damage to skin associated with incontinence that range from simple to complex.

One simple method is the Incontinence-Associated Dermatitis Intervention Tool© (IADIT©), meant to give bedside caregivers including family a simple way to match level of risk or skin injury to interventions that may help. This is reprinted here with permission from the author Joan Junkin. It has been translated into several languages to be used in research and education. The German translation (IADIT-D) was used in a long-term care study and was found to have high or very high interrater reliability among 19 assessors of level of severity of IAD due to incontinence (Braunschmidt et al., 2013).

Another simple method to classify IAD is the Ghent Global IAD Categorisation Tool (GLOBIAD). There is a revision of this tool called the GLOBIAD-M that includes daily monitoring tools and more precise marking of areas affected by persistent erythema, skin loss, and signs of infection. The full text of that article including the additional tools is available for free at https://pubmed.ncbi.nlm.nih.gov/29797507/

A more complicated but useful tool to assess severity of IAD due to incontinence is the Incontinence-Associated Skin Damage and Its Severity (IASD.D.2) tool (Bliss et al., 2018). It requires a score from 0 (no damage) to 4 (skin loss) in each of 14 areas where skin is likely to be affected by incontinence. Using the sum of the 14 scores allows tracking over time to quantify improvement and so is useful for research.

Irritant contact dermatitis due to other body fluids

Saliva

The reason long-term exposure to saliva on the skin is damaging is partly due to the moisture exposure. Also, saliva contains digestive enzymes such as alpha-amylase, lysozyme, lactoferrin, and peroxidase, which help begin digestion of food as we chew. Saliva contains immunoglobulins with antibacterial properties that are helpful in the mouth, but not on top of the skin.

One cause of irritation near the mouth from saliva is sialorrhea, excessive drooling. This can be corrected with medication or removal of one or more salivary glands. Another method is salivary gland ablation; injecting the glands with alcohol shrinks them, but they still produce some saliva to prevent dry mouth. Botulism toxin injections have also been used. Using lip protectants is useful for prevention and treatment. Solid versions often contain a wax or other longer-lasting ingredients to help protect perioral skin from the effects of saliva exposure. Other causes of irritant contact dermatitis (ICD) due to saliva are excess licking of the lips, neurologic deficits such as cerebral vascular accident or coma, or a fistula of the oral cavity due to head and neck cancer.

Respiratory secretions from a stoma or fistula

ICD due to respiratory secretions may occur near a related stoma or a fistula. The secretions will be 95% water with a pH around 6.0 but also contain mucus, which holds moisture longer and may be more damaging along with chemokines and cytokines that are known skin irritants. Managing secretions around a respiratory stoma such as a tracheostomy requires a different approach because of the risk of aspiration of many barrier products used to protect skin. Sometimes, a nonalcohol liquid protectant can be utilized successfully. The wicking textiles with silver that can be used in moist skin folds have also been successfully used to wick away copious secretions if they are fairly thin or liquid. Often, woven cotton gauze or foam with a slit cut in it to fit around the tube is used. In some cases, along with regular gentle cleansing and sometimes a nonalcohol liquid skin protectant, this will provide adequate protection if changed every 8 hours. With the sharp rise in tracheostomies needed due to the COVID-19 pandemic, or at any time there is an increase in respiratory illnesses, a less time-intensive method may be useful.

Get wise to wounds

Chuang et al. (2013) found positive results with a pectin-based wafer sometimes used for ostomy care. This barrier could be changed every 4 days with effective results. The device may also help prevent the pressure injuries sometimes associated with any device that must be secured tightly enough to prevent dislodgment, such as a tracheostomy tube.

Karaca and Korkmaz (2018) reported positive results using a durable barrier cream containing dimethicone and acrylate terpolymer once daily after cleansing around the tracheostomy with saline and replacing the gauze as often as necessary based on secretion amount. This cream kept the skin at a more normal acidic pH than the skin in the group using gauze alone. Maintaining the acid mantle of the skin protects it from infection and improves the barrier function.

Digestive or urinary secretions from a stoma or fistula

Just as liquid stools per rectum can be irritating to the skin, so can any digestive system effluent (output) that exits the body through a stoma or fistula, especially if the effluent is liquid. How about a quick review of expected digestive system ostomy output?

Digestive fluid source	Type of effluent	Effects on the skin
Ileostomy or ileal fistula (from the terminal portion of the small intestine)	Liquid with high output, at least at first; as the body adjusts, it can become mushy or pasty.	High in digestive enzymes, which can break down skin as quickly as they do food pH is usually alkaline—around 7.5 and irritating to skin
Jejunostomy or jejunal fistula (from the middle portion of the small intestine)	Liquid with high output; usually remains liquid or mushy	High in digestive enzymes, which can break down skin as quickly as they do food
Colostomy or colon fistula (from the large intestine)	Descending colon—usually formed stool Transverse colon—usually semiformed or pasty stool Ascending colon (less common)—usually mushy or pasty stool	If formed, there is less risk of related dermatitis if there is a leak from ostomy pouching system. If stool is more liquid, there is a mild risk of ICD if skin is exposed often.

The key to preventing dermatitis related to stool or urine effluent due to ostomies or fistulas is consulting a certified ostomy nurse preoperatively. Often an appropriate location for the stoma can be marked to increase the likelihood of success in pouching postoperatively. An ostomy pouching system that fits with fewest leaks is necessary and definitely in the wheelhouse for a nurse certified in ostomy care. Lastly, an education plan for the patient and caregivers regarding the effects on the skin of the various effluents and the containment of these as well as the protection of the skin is essential.

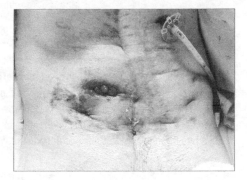

This ileostomy stoma is recessed and with a crease, making leaks more frequent, and ICD is evident. Small bowel fistula below and lateral to the ileostomy and one in the healed midline incision complicate the situation. Patient was on immune suppressant medications due to Crohn disease, making healing of any denudement slower. Also note this gastrostomy tube needs securement or soon there will be corrosive stomach contents leaking too due to enlargement of the opening.

Wound effluent

As discussed, any moisture on the skin for too long can cause ICD, including exudate from a wound. This can cause inflammation and we must determine if the inflammation is due to ICD or another cause. Two other possibilities are local wound infection (or regional if the inflamed area is larger than 2 cm; please refer to Chapter 3 for determination of wound infection) and allergic contact dermatitis. A patch test may be ordered to determine if the person is allergic to one of the dressings, wound cleanser, skin protectant, or tape.

If it is not an infection or allergic contact dermatitis, the likely cause of periwound inflammation is ICD from the wound effluent oozing onto the skin. Refer to Chapter 2 for wound exudate components, which can be very irritating to skin. Chronic wounds such as leg ulcers due to poorly controlled lower extremity edema and neuropathic foot ulcers have been found to be especially high in proteases (which break down proteins including exposed skin), and when the limb is dependent, gravity makes it more likely to increase exudate amount. Therefore, they are the two wounds most likely to result in ICD due to wound exudate.

This leg ulcer in an area of chronic eczema is related to chronic edema changes in the skin and subcutaneous tissue. Maceration around the edges shows that wound exudate (known to be high in proteases) is further compromising the periwound skin. Skin edge injuries were treated with zinc oxide in Unna wrap compression, which also decreased the amount of exudate through compression and allowed healing.

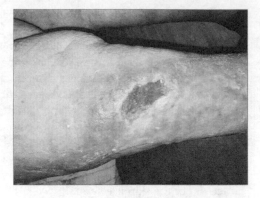

This neuropathic foot ulcer with some callus has maceration at the wound edges, evidence of ICD that impaired wound closure. Paring the callus and replacing the regular foam with a super-absorbent dressing to absorb excess exudate allowed the now healthy wound edges to close.

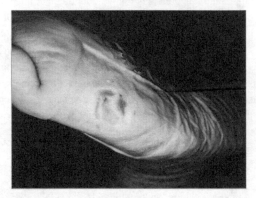

Quick quiz

1. The term "acid mantle" refers to:
   A. wound dressings with an acidic pH.
   B. adult incontinence briefs with curly fibers that are acidic.
   C. function of the skin that protects us from pathogens.
   D. acidic pH of the stomach mucosa that assists in digesting food.

Answer: C. An acidic pH of the skin is a hostile environment to harmful bacteria and fungi.

2. Friction is a physical force that can cause:
   A. pressure injuries.
   B. allergic contact dermatitis.
   C. xerosis.
   D. abrasions.

Answer: D. Any skin injury increases the risk of pressure injuries, but friction cannot cause them. Friction can cause abrasions and skin tears and increase the risk of ITD.

3. An ISTAP skin tear classification type 2 means:
   A. the affected flap of skin has been lost.
   B. there is a partial flap of skin left attached.
   C. the flap of skin is still attached, but it cannot be reposi-
      tioned over the wound.
   D. the entire flap of skin remains attached.

Answer: B. Type 2 means a partial flap of skin remains attached.

4. Medical adhesive–related skin injury can be prevented by:
   A. stretching clear film dressings parallel to skin prior to
      removal.
   B. using gentle, nonionic cleansers rather than soap.
   C. avoiding regular washcloths that have nubs to increase
      friction.
   D. using a dressing with enough absorbency to match the
      amount of wound exudate.

Answer: A. Stretching clear film dressings breaks the adhesive bond
without tearing skin.

5. Urine is especially damaging to skin because:
   A. it contains enzymes that break skin down quickly.
   B. the urea changes to ammonia and makes skin alkaline.
   C. the bacteria cause skin infections.
   D. it is very acidic.

Answer: B. Bacteria on the skin change the urea to ammonia, which
is alkaline and harms the acid mantle function of the skin.

6. A neuropathic foot ulcer exhibits very heavy exudate. Which
dressing type can best help prevent surrounding skin damage?
   A. Alginate
   B. Medical-grade honey
   C. Super-absorbent
   D. Gauze

Answer: C. Super-absorbent dressings can absorb large amounts
of exudate and trap the fluid in the dressing core to prevent it from
oozing back out.

Scoring

✩✩✩ If you answered all six questions correctly, congrats! You have a
"balanced" approach to learning, just like moisture in healthy skin!

✩✩ If you answered four or five questions correctly, good job! Your
learning has not been superficial like the injuries in the chapter.

✩ If you answered fewer than four questions correctly, don't sweat it!
After all, sweat causes skin damage, so instead get some fresh air
and a quick review and you'll be good to go.

Select references

Al Khaleefa, N., Moore, Z., Avsar, P., Connor, T. O., Budri, A., Nugent, L., & Patton, D. (2022). What is the impact of skincare bundles on the development of skin tears in older adults? A systematic review. *International Journal of Older People Nursing, 17*(4), e12455. https://doi.org/10.1111/opn.12455

Alavi, A., Sibbald, R. G., Ladizinski, B., Saraiya, A., Lee, K. C., Skotnicki-Grant, S., & Maibach, H. (2016). Wound-related allergic/irritant contact dermatitis. *Advances in Skin & Wound Care, 29*(6), 278–286. https://doi.org/10.1097/01.ASW.0000482834.94375.1e

Arnold-Long, M., & Johnson, E. (2019). Epidemiology of incontinence-associated dermatitis and intertriginous dermatitis (intertrigo) in an acute care facility. *Journal of Wound, Ostomy, and Continence Nursing, 46*(3), 201–206. https://doi.org/10.1097/WON.0000000000000519

Ayello, E. A. (2017). CMS MDS 3.0 section M skin conditions in long-term care: Pressure ulcers, skin tears, and moisture-associated skin damage data update. *Advances in Skin & Wound Care, 30*(9), 415–429. https://doi.org/10.1097/01.ASW.0000521920.60656.03

Beeckman, D. (2017). A decade of research on incontinence-associated dermatitis (IAD): Evidence, knowledge gaps and next steps. *Journal of Tissue Viability, 26*(1), 47–56. https://doi.org/10.1016/j.jtv.2016.02.004

Bliss, D. Z., Gurvich, O. V., Hurlow, J., Cefalu, J. E., Gannon, A., Wilhems, A., Wiltzen, K. R., Gannon, E., Lee, H., Borchert, K., & Trammel, S. H. (2018). Evaluation of validity and reliability of a revised Incontinence-Associated Skin Damage Severity Instrument (IASD.D.2) by 3 groups of nursing staff. *Journal of Wound, Ostomy, and Continence Nursing, 45*(5), 449–455. https://doi.org/10.1097/WON.0000000000000466

Braunschmidt, B., Müller, G., Jukic-Puntigam, M., & Steininger, A. (2013). The inter-rater reliability of the Incontinence-Associated Dermatitis Intervention Tool-D (IADIT-D) between two independent registered nurses of nursing home residents in long-term care facilities. *Journal of Nursing Measurement, 21*(2), 284–295. https://doi.org/10.1891/1061-3749.21.2.284

Burns, E. S., Pathmarajah, P., & Muralidharan, V. (2021). Physical and psychological impacts of handwashing and personal protective equipment usage in the COVID-19 pandemic: A UK based cross-sectional analysis of healthcare workers. *Dermatologic Therapy, 34*(3), e14885. https://doi.org/10.1111/dth.14885

Chuang, W. L., Huang, W. P., Chen, M. H., Liu, I. P., Yu, W. L., & Chin, C. C. (2013). Gauze versus solid skin barrier for tracheostomy care: A crossover randomized clinical trial. *Journal of Wound, Ostomy, and Continence Nursing, 40*(6), 573–579. https://doi.org/10.1097/01.WON.0000436431.01159.9f

Colwell, J. C., McNichol, L., & Boarini, J. (2017). North America wound, ostomy, and continence and enterostomal therapy nurses' current ostomy care practice related to peristomal skin issues. *Journal of Wound, Ostomy, and Continence Nursing, 44*(3), 257–261. https://doi.org/10.1097/WON.0000000000000324

DeVries, M., Sarbenoff, J., Scott, N., Wickert, M., & Hayes, L. M. (2021). Improving vascular access dressing integrity in the acute care setting: A quality improvement project. *Journal of Wound, Ostomy, and Continence Nursing, 48*(5), 383–388. https://doi.org/10.1097/WON.0000000000000787

Ferreira, M., Abbade, L., Bocchi, S. C. M., Miot, H. A., Boas, P. V., & Guimaraes, H. Q. C. P. (2020). Incontinence-associated dermatitis in elderly patients: Prevalence and risk factors. *Revista Brasileira de Enfermagem, 73*(Suppl 3), e20180475. https://doi.org/10.1590/0034-7167-2018-0475

Fletcher, J., Beeckman, D., Fumarola, S., Boyles, A., Kottner, J. McNichol, L., Moore, Z., Sarkar, N., Stenius, M., & Voegeli, D. (2020). International best practice recommendations: Prevention and management of moisture-associated skin damage (MASD). *Wounds International.* https://www.woundsinternational.com/resources/details/best-practice-recommendations-prevention-and-management-moisture-associated-skin-damage-masd

Gao, C., Yu, C., Lin, X., Wang, H., & Sheng, Y. (2020). Incidence of and risk factors for medical adhesive–related skin injuries among patients: A cross-sectional study. *Journal of Wound, Ostomy, and Continence Nursing, 47*(6), 576–581. https://doi.org/10.1097/WON.0000000000000714

Glass Jr, G. F., Goh, C. C. K., Cheong, R. Q., Ong, Z. L., Khong, P. C. B., & Chan, E. Y. (2021). Effectiveness of skin cleanser and protectant regimen on incontinence-associated dermatitis outcomes in acute care patients: A cluster randomised trial. *International Wound Journal, 18*(6), 862–873. https://doi.org/10.1111/iwj.13588

Gray, M., Bliss, D. Z., & McNichol, L. (2022). Moisture-associated skin damage: Expanding and updating practice based on the newest ICD-10-CM codes. *Journal of Wound, Ostomy, and Continence Nursing, 49*(2), 143–151. https://doi.org/10.1097/WON.0000000000000865

Gray, M., & Giuliano, K. K. (2018). Incontinence-associated dermatitis, characteristics and relationship to pressure injury: A multisite epidemiologic analysis. *Journal of Wound, Ostomy, and Continence Nursing, 45*(1), 63–67. https://doi.org/10.1097/WON.0000000000000390

Hawk, J., & Shannon, M. (2018). Prevalence of skin tears in elderly patients: A retrospective chart review of incidence reports in 6 long-term care facilities. *Ostomy Wound Management, 64*(4), 30–36. https://doi.org/10.25270/owm.2018.4.3036

Junkin, J., & Selekof, J. L. (2007). Prevalence of incontinence and associated skin injury in the acute care inpatient. *Journal of Wound, Ostomy, and Continence Nursing, 34*(3), 260–269. https://doi.org/10.1097/01.WON.0000270820.91694.1f

Karaca, T., & Korkmaz, F. (2018). A quasi-experimental study to explore the effect of barrier cream on the peristomal skin of patients with a tracheostomy. *Ostomy Wound Management, 64*(3), 32–39. https://doi.org/10.25270/owm.2018.3.3239

Kim, S., Ly, B. K., Ha, J. H., Carson, K. A., Hawkins, S., Kang, S., & Chien, A. L. (2022). A consistent skin care regimen leads to objective and subjective improvements in dry human skin: Investigator-blinded randomized clinical trial. *Journal of Dermatological Treatment, 33*(1), 300–305. https://doi.org/10.1080/09546634.2020.1751037

Krasner, D. (Ed.). (2007). *Chronic wound care: A clinical source book for healthcare professionals.* Health Management Publications.

Lachenbruch, C., Ribble, D., Emmons, K., & VanGilder, C. (2016). Pressure ulcer risk in the incontinent patient. *Journal of Wound, Ostomy, and Continence Nursing, 43*(3), 235–241. https://doi.org/10.1097/WON.0000000000000225

Landsperger, J. S., Byram, J. M., Lloyd, B. D., & Rice, T. W. (2019). The effect of adhesive tape versus endotracheal tube fastener in critically ill adults: The endotracheal tube securement (ETTS) randomized controlled trial. *Critical Care, 23*(1), 1–7. https://doi.org/10.1186/s13054-019-2440-7

LeBlanc, K., Whiteley, I., McNichol, L., Salvadalena, G., & Gray, M. (2019). Peristomal medical adhesive-related skin injury: Results of an international consensus meeting. *Journal of Wound, Ostomy, and Continence Nursing, 46*(2), 125–136. https://doi.org/10.1097/WON.0000000000000513

LeBlanc, K., Woo, K. Y., VanDenKerkhof, E., & Woodbury, M. G. (2020). Skin tear prevalence and incidence in the long-term care population: A prospective study. *Journal of Wound Care, 29*(Suppl 7), S16–S22. https://doi.org/10.12968/jowc.2020.29.Sup7.S16

Mijaljica, D., Spada, F., & Harrison, I. P. (2022). Skin cleansing without or with compromise: Soaps and syndets. *Molecules, 27*(6), 2010. https://doi.org/10.3390/molecules27062010

Miles, S. J., Fulbrook, P., & Williams, D. M. (2022). Skin tear prevalence in an Australian acute care hospital: A 10-year analysis. *International Wound Journal, 19*(6), 1418–1427. https://doi.org/10.1111/iwj.13735

Minematsu, T., Dai, M., Tamai, N., Nakagami, G., Urai, T., Nakai, A., Nitta, S., Kataoka, Y., Kuang, W., & Sanada, H. (2021). Risk scoring tool for forearm skin tears in Japanese older adults: A prospective cohort study. *Journal of Tissue Viability, 30*(2), 155–160. https://doi.org/10.1016/j.jtv.2021.02.010

Monari, P., Fusano, M., Moro, R., Baiguini, I., Calzavara-Pinton, P., Vascellaro, A., & Gualdi, G. (2021). Allergic contact versus irritant contact dermatitis in patients with hard-to-heal leg ulcer: Clinical and diagnostic approach. *Journal of Wound Care, 30*(5), 394–398. https://doi.org/10.12968/jowc.2021.30.5.394

Nomoto, T., & Iizaka, S. (2020). Effect of an oral nutrition supplement containing collagen peptides on stratum corneum hydration and skin elasticity in hospitalized older adults: A multicenter open-label randomized controlled study. *Advances in Skin & Wound Care, 33*(4), 186–191. https://doi.org/10.1097/01.ASW.0000655492.40898.55

Parnham, A., Copson, D., & Loban, T. (2020). Moisture-associated skin damage: Causes and an overview of assessment, classification and management. *British Journal of Nursing, 29*(12), S30–S37. https://doi.org/10.12968/bjon.2020.29.12.S30

Phipps, L., Gray, M., & Call, E. (2019). Time of onset to changes in skin condition during exposure to synthetic urine: A prospective study. *Journal of Wound, Ostomy, and Continence Nursing, 46*(4), 315–320. https://doi.org/10.1097/WON.0000000000000549

Powell, R. J., Hayward, C. J., Snelgrove, C. L., Polverino, K., Park, L., Chauhan, R., Evans, P. H., Byford, R., Charman, C., Foy, C. J. W., Pritchard, C., & Kingsley, A. (2017). Pilot parallel randomised controlled trial of protective socks against usual care to reduce skin tears in high risk people: "STOPCUTS." *Pilot and Feasibility Studies, 3*(1), 1–22. https://doi.org/10.1186/s40814-017-0182-3

Røpke, M. A., Alonso, C., Jung, S., Norsgaard, H., Richter, C., Darvin, M. E., Litman, T., Vogt, A., Jurgen, L., Blume-Paytavi, U., & Kottner, J. (2017). Effects of glucocorticoids on stratum corneum lipids and function in human skin—A detailed lipidomic analysis. *Journal of Dermatological Science, 88*(3), 330–338. https://doi.org/10.1016/j.jdermsci.2017.08.009

Stephen-Haynes, J. (2020). The what, who, why and how of skin tears in the community and care homes. *British Journal of Nursing, 29*(20), S14–S17. https://doi.org/10.12968/bjon.2020.29.20.S14

Van Tiggelen, H., LeBlanc, K., Campbell, K., Woo, K., Baranoski, S., Chang, Y. Y., Dunk, A. M., Gloeckner, M., Hevia, H., Holloway, S., Idensohn, P., Karadağ, A., Koren, E., Kottner, J., Langemo, D., Ousey, K., Pokorná, A., Romanelli, M., Santos, V. L. C. G., … Beeckman, D. (2020). Standardizing the classification of skin tears: Validity and reliability testing of the International Skin Tear Advisory Panel Classification System in 44 countries. *British Journal of Dermatology, 183*(1), 146–154. https://doi.org/10.1111/bjd.18604

Voegeli, D. (2020). Intertrigo: Causes, prevention and management. *British Journal of Nursing, 29*(12), S16–S22. https://doi.org/10.12968/bjon.2020.29.12.S16Wound effluent

Chapter 5

Acute wounds

Just the facts

In this chapter, you'll learn about:

◆ types of acute wounds, including those caused by surgery, infection, trauma, and burns

◆ assessment factors for each type of acute wound

◆ nursing interventions and management strategies for different types of acute wounds

A look at acute wounds

Acute wounds proceed through an orderly repair process of hemostasis, proliferation, maturation, and remodeling. This leads to a healed wound with good functional outcome. Acute wounds can be simple or complex, depending on size, location on the body, anatomic structures involved, and bioburden in the wound. Ask these questions when characterizing an acute wound:

• Is the wound new or relatively new?
• Did the wound occur suddenly (as opposed to developing over time)?
• Is the wound healing in a timely, predictable, and measurable manner?

Intent or accident?

Acute wounds can occur by intention or trauma. For example, a surgical incision is an acute wound that's caused intentionally. Traumatic wounds can range from simple to severe. Burns are a category of traumatic wound that have a unique set of causes, potential complications, and treatment options.

Regardless of the cause, when caring for a patient with an acute wound, you'll focus on promoting healing, preventing infection, and restoring normal anatomic structure, physiologic function, and appearance of the wound area (sometimes accomplished by skin grafting).

Surgical wounds

An acute surgical wound is a healthy and uncomplicated break in the skin's continuity resulting from surgery. In an otherwise healthy individual, this type of wound responds well to postoperative care and heals without incident in a predictable period of time.

Factors that affect healing

Several factors can greatly affect the course of postoperative wound healing. These include the patient's age, nutritional status, general health before surgery, presence of infection, oxygenation status, and tobacco use.

Handle with care

Age and wound healing

In infants and older adult patients, surgical wounds may not heal normally.

Infants
In premature infants and infants up to 1 year of age, the immune system and other body systems aren't fully developed, so there's a greater risk for infection before, during, and after surgery. Sterile technique is a critical component of care for very young patients.

Older adult patients
Skin becomes thinner and less elastic with decreased tensile strength as people age. Populations of cells that repair tissues and fight infection decline, and the skin's vascular system is less robust. As a result, surgical wounds in older adult patients heal more slowly, increasing the risk of infection.

Nutrition

Proper nutrition is crucial for the body to heal itself effectively. During your assessment, it is imperative for you to identify nutritional problems early and to develop a plan that addresses deficits. Collaborate with dieticians for assistance.

After surgery, the body quickly depletes its stores of nutrients (especially in the highly exudative wound), and even an otherwise healthy patient can become malnourished if diet is ignored. The care plan must include a diet with adequate nutrients and fluids to maintain homeostasis and create an optimal environment for wound healing. Enteral or parenteral nutrition may be needed in some patients.

Adipose poses problems

A patient with excess adipose has an additional problem because this tissue lacks the extensive vascular supply present in skin. As the amount of adipose tissue increases, blood flow to the skin decreases. This reduces the amount of oxygen and nutrients reaching the wound area, impeding healing and increasing the risk of wound dehiscence.

General health

In most cases, a preexisting illness or infection delays or complicates healing after surgery. Unfortunately, it isn't always possible to delay surgery while an underlying condition resolves itself. In these cases, the care plan must include measures that minimize the impact of the preexisting condition on the healing process. For example:

- Disorders that impede blood flow, such as coronary artery disease, peripheral vascular disease (PVD), and hypertension, can cause problems by reducing the flow of blood reaching the incision site. A patient with one of these conditions requires a care plan that includes interventions to improve circulation.
- Cancer may necessitate more aggressive pain management or a care plan that includes management of such symptoms as nausea and vomiting.
- Diabetes mellitus impedes healing in many ways and increases the patient's risk of infection. Diabetic neuropathy (inflammation and degeneration of peripheral nerves), if present, may interfere with vasodilation and consequently circulation in the area of the incision. Wound healing improves with optimal glucose control.
- Immunosuppression resulting from either a disease or drug therapy (e.g., corticosteroids, chemotherapy) may impair the inflammatory response, delaying wound healing and increasing the patient's risk of infection.

Infection

An infection can also delay or impair healing. Chlorhexidine gluconate (CHG) is commonly used for preoperative bathing and surgical site preparation to decrease the number of pathogens on the skin. Guidelines state that a sterile dressing should be placed in the operating room and remain in place for 48 hours to help prevent infection.

Signs of wound infection include the following:

- increased exudate
- purulent (pus-containing) exudate
- erythema (reddened tissue) around the wound
- warmer skin temperature at or around the wound
- new or increased pain
- general malaise
- fever
- high white blood cell (WBC) count

Although all open wounds are colonized with surface bacteria, infected wounds become overwhelmed with bacteria and are slow to heal. They may have complications such as dehiscence.

Oxygenation status

Adequate oxygenation is critical to the healing process. Any condition that impedes overall oxygenation or the amount of oxygen reaching the wound—atherosclerosis or decreased circulation, for example—slows the healing process.

Assessment and care

Your care should focus on keeping the wound clean and protecting it from trauma. Proper care during healing varies depending on the method of wound closure used, the development of the healing ridge, and the type of dressing ordered. The patient's ability to properly perform wound care after discharge also affects healing.

Assessment and Care

First check the outside...

✔ Is the dressing stained?
- Estimate drainage quantity.
- Note its color, consistency, and odor.

✔ Does the patient have a drainage device?
- Record the amount of drainage.
- Note the color of the drainage.
- Ensure that the device is patent, secure, and free from kinks.

✔ Does the patient have an ostomy (urostomy, colostomy, ileostomy)?
- Describe the output, color, location of the stoma, security of the pouching system, and peristomal skin.

... then go under cover

✔ Is a healing ridge present?
- This is a palpable ridge that forms on the sides of the wound during normal wound healing. It results from a buildup of collagen fibers that begin to form during the inflammatory phase of wound healing and peak during the proliferation phase (~5 to 9 days postoperatively). Ridges typically fail to develop because of mechanical strain on the wound. If you can't feel the ridge, healing isn't progressing as expected, further assessment is required, and you should notify the health care provider. Are there signs and symptoms of infection? Report these to the surgeon.

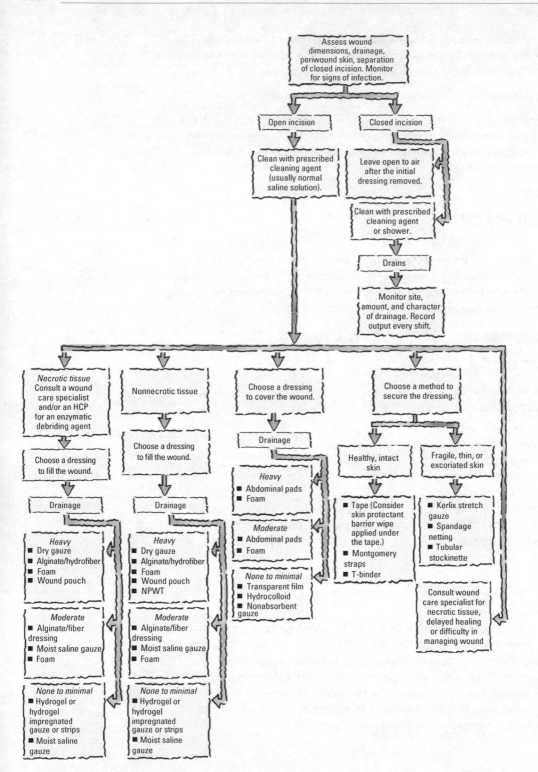

Wound closure

The surgeon determines the appropriate method of wound closure based on the wound's severity and by selecting the least invasive method for closure with the least risk of complications and the best cosmetic result. Wounds that are well-approximated and clean can be closed by primary intention using staples, sutures, skin adhesives, or skin tapes. Negative pressure wound therapy designed for closed wounds may enhance healing. Delayed primary closure is usually performed after 3 to 5 days. Bite wounds and lacerations can be closed with this technique. Wounds that heal by secondary intention heal in by granulation and eventual reepithelialization, so they are not closed. Contaminated wounds, infected wounds, or dehisced surgical wounds can be managed in this way. Negative pressure wound therapy and other advanced wound care products are commonly used for wounds as an adjunct to healing by secondary intention.

Sew ... a needle pulling thread

In suturing, a natural or synthetic thread is used to stitch the wound closed. (See *Suture materials and methods*.)

Suture materials and methods

When closing a surgical wound, the choice of suture material varies according to the suturing method, location, and tissue type.

Materials

Nonabsorbable sutures:
- are used to close the skin surface.
- provide strength and immobility.
- cause minimal tissue irritation.
- are made of silk, cotton, stainless steel, or Dacron.

Absorbable sutures:
- are used when suture removal is undesirable (e.g., sutures are in an underlying tissue layer).
- are made of chromic catgut (a natural catgut treated with chromium trioxide to improve strength and prolong absorption time); plain catgut (a material that's absorbed faster and is more likely to cause irritation than chromic catgut); or synthetic materials (such as polyglycolic acid) that are replacing catgut because they're stronger, more durable, and less irritating.

Methods

The most common suture methods include mattress continuous suture, plain continuous suture, mattress interrupted suture, plain interrupted suture, and blanket continuous suture.

Sutures typically remain in place for 7 to 10 days, depending on the wound's severity, the type of tissue involved, and whether healing is progressing as expected. Factors that affect the timing of suture removal include the patient's overall condition; the shape, size, and location of the incision; and whether inflammation, drainage, or infection develops.

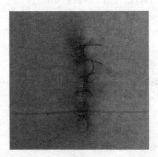

Stainless steel solutions

The surgeon may choose to use skin staples or clips as an alternative to sutures if cosmetic results aren't a concern. These closures secure a wound faster than sutures. Tissue reaction is minimal because they are made of surgical stainless steel. Properly placed staples and clips distribute tension evenly along the suture line, reducing tissue trauma and compression. This promotes healing and minimizes scarring. The surgeon won't use staples or clips if less than 5 mm of tissue exists between the staple and any underlying bone, vessel, or organ. Commonly, Steri-Strips are placed after skin staples are removed to ensure the incision remains secure. (See *Using retention sutures.*)

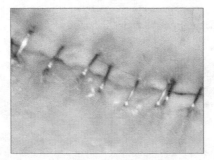

Handle with care

Using retention sutures

Retention sutures can be used to secure wound edges and to support the suture line for patients following bariatric surgery or for high-risk patients, such as someone who has required more than one abdominal surgery in a short time. The use of retention sutures helps support the deep tissues while the more superficial fascia and skin tissues heal. Retention sutures are placed through the abdominal wall before the abdominal layers are closed to reinforce the suture line. These remain in place longer than standard sutures, often several weeks or until a wound left to heal by secondary intention is almost healed.

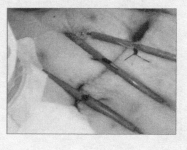

Surgical drains

Surgeons insert closed wound drains during surgery when they expect a large amount of postoperative drainage. These drains suction serosanguineous fluid from the wound site. If a wound produces heavy drainage, the closed wound drain may be left in place for longer than 1 week. Drainage must be frequently emptied and measured to maintain maximum suction and prevent strain on the suture line. Treat the tubing exit site as an additional surgical wound. Be sure to secure the drainage device so it does not pull or become dislodged. When the drain is removed, use a dry gauze dressing or Band-Aid until the area is completely closed. Instruct the patient to change the gauze daily as needed until closed.

Purposes

- Promote healing
- Prevent swelling
- Reduce risk of infection and skin breakdown
- Minimize the need for dressing changes

Closed wound drainage system

A closed wound drain consists of perforated tubing that facilitates drainage and is connected to a portable vacuum unit. (Hemovac and Jackson-Pratt are the most commonly used drainage systems.) The distal end of the tubing lies within the wound and usually leaves the body from a site other than the primary suture line. The drain is usually sutured to the skin. Shown below is a closed wound drainage system in a patient following mastectomy.

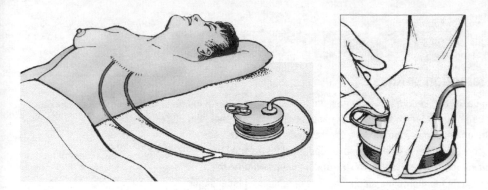

To empty the drainage, remove the plug and empty it into a graduated cylinder. To reestablish suction in a Hemovac unit, compress the drainage unit against a firm surface to expel air, and while holding it down, replace the plug with your other hand as shown.

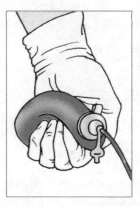

Follow a similar procedure to reestablish suction in a Jackson-Pratt bulb drain shown here.

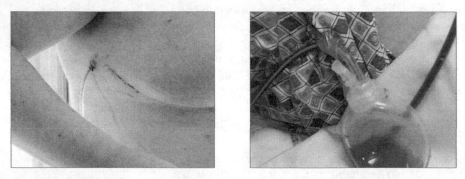

Stick with me!

Smaller wounds with little drainage can be closed with adhesive skin closures, such as Steri-Strips, butterfly closures, or tissue adhesives. As with staples and clips, these closures cause little tissue reaction and are generally used for wounds with little tension. They can be used alone or in combination. Adhesive closures can be used after suture or staple removal to provide ongoing support for a healing incision. (See *Types of adhesive skin closures*.)

Types of adhesive skin closures

The three most common types of adhesive skin closures are Steri-Strips, butterfly closures, and skin adhesives.

Steri-Strips

Steri-Strips (thin strips of sterile, nonwoven tape) are a primary means of holding a wound closed after suture or staple removal.

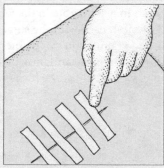

Butterfly closures

Butterfly closures have two sterile, waterproof adhesive strips linked by a narrow, nonadhesive "bridge." They are used to hold small wounds closed to promote healing. They are useful on highly contoured areas of the body.

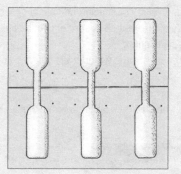

Prior to placing adhesive skin closures, apply a protective barrier film around the area. Steri-Strips and butterfly closures should stay in place for 5 to 7 days and gently removed as they loosen. Apply these one-eighth of an inch apart without tension or pressure to avoid blistering. Skin adhesives are left in place for 5 to 10 days and not removed. The person may shower but should not scrub the wound or put lotions or creams near the adhesive.

Skin adhesives

Skin adhesives usually contain a strong, fast-acting adhesive called *cyanoacrylate*. They can be used for lacerations and surgical wound closure and are often used for laparoscopy incisions. Dermabond is a commonly used product.

Dressings

The incision dressing shields the wound against pathogens and protects the skin surface from irritating drainage. The dressing is the primary aspect of wound management for surgical wounds; therefore, choosing the right type is important. Keeping a surgical dressing in place for 48 hours after surgery is standard practice to prevent surgical site infection (SSI).

Proper dress required

Dressing selection should be guided by the size and depth of the wound and the amount of drainage (see Chapter 9). For complex wounds, biologic or synthetic mesh may be visible in the wound base. Discuss the specific brand of mesh used with the surgeon so that expected progression of healing and granulation can be monitored. Pouching may be used to contain the drainage and protect the surrounding skin of a highly draining wound or fistula. (See *Pouching a wound*.)

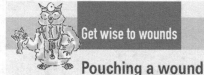

Get wise to wounds

Pouching a wound

If your patient's wound is draining heavily or if drainage may damage surrounding skin, consider applying a pouch. An ostomy pouch or specialized wound collection pouch can be used depending on the size of the wound. Unsure of pouch application? Consult the wound and ostomy care specialty nurse.

• Cleanse the wound and surrounding skin with warm water or pH-balanced no-rinse wound cleanser. Pat dry.
• Apply a skin protectant to the surrounding skin.
• Measure the wound. Cut an opening one-eighth inch larger than the wound in the facing of the collection pouch or wafer.

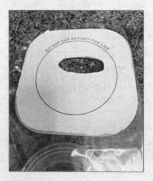

Pouching a wound

• Stoma paste or barrier strips or rings, such as those used in ostomy care, can be used to fill in uneven skin surfaces if needed.

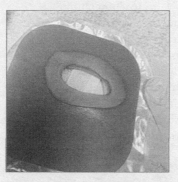

• Be sure to close the drainage port at the bottom of the pouch to prevent leaks. Then gently press the contoured pouch opening or contoured barrier around the wound, starting at the lower edge, to catch any drainage.
• To empty the pouch, put on gloves, a face shield or mask, and eye protection. Insert the lower portion of the pouch into a graduated biohazard container and open the drainage port. Note the color, consistency, odor, and amount of fluid. If ordered, obtain a culture specimen and send it to the laboratory immediately. (Always follow the Centers for Disease Control and Prevention's [CDC] standard precautions when handling infectious drainage.)
• Use a tissue or clean gauze pad to wipe the bottom of the pouch and the drainage port. This prevents skin irritation or possible odor from any residual drainage. Reseal the port.
• Change the pouch only if it leaks or fails to adhere. More frequent changes are un- necessary and can irritate the patient's skin. Check and empty the pouch frequently to prevent overfilling and leakage; empty when it is one-third full. The pouch should be able to remain adhered for at least 3 days.

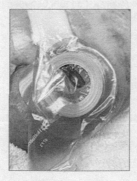

When dressing a surgical wound, use sterile technique and sterile supplies to prevent contamination. Change the dressing as often as needed to absorb drainage and keep the surrounding skin dry; however, remember that a wound heals best at body temperature. Changing the dressing lowers the temperature at the wound site, which slows healing until the site returns to normal body temperature. Assess the incision for signs of infection, drainage, pain, or surrounding redness with each dressing change. Recent trends to prevent SSIs include the application of silver dressings or negative pressure wound therapy devices to closed incisions. Silver dressings aid in the prevention of infection. A negative pressure system prevents breakdown of the closed incision and supports surrounding tissues. Negative pressure wound therapy has become the mainstay for many types of surgical and other open wounds. This can be started in acute care, and the patient can manage this method at home.

Patient education

Patient education is an important component of the care plan for patients with surgical wounds. By the time they are discharged, the patient needs to understand—and demonstrate—the ability to perform proper wound care. Start with an assessment of the patient's knowledge. Then begin your teaching with a discussion of basic asepsis and hand-washing techniques. The balance of your teaching depends on the type of surgery, the type of dressing, and the location of the wound. (See *Teaching about surgical wound care*.)

Teaching about surgical wound care

Surgical patients need to know the ways that can promote healing and prevent infection. Be sure to discuss:
• signs and symptoms of wound infection to report to the practitioner immediately, such as increased tenderness, deep or increased pain at the wound site, fever, or edema (especially if it occurs between postoperative days 3 and 5).
• how to take an accurate temperature reading.
• proper wound care, such as the importance of keeping the incision clean and dry; proper hand-washing technique; and the supplies and methods used to clean the wound.
• wound dressings, including the type, where to obtain them, and how to apply them.
• care of drains, including dressing change, measuring and recording output, and what to do if the drain becomes dislodged or stops functioning.
• types and levels of permissible activity, such as lifting restrictions (if applicable), when the patient may shower or bathe, and when they can expect to return to work.
• importance of adequate dietary and fluid intake to promote healing.
• avoidance of smoking.
• follow-up appointments.

Potential complications

Surgery results in a controlled form of acute wound. The patient's environment, the type and severity of the wound, and preoperative and postoperative care are all under the control of the health care team. Consequently, most surgical wounds heal without incident; however, some complications that might arise include infection, hemorrhage, and dehiscence and evisceration.

Infection

Wound infection or SSI is the most common wound complication as well as the second most common health care–associated infection. Infection occurs when bacterial count is greater than 10^5 per gram of tissue and impacts all phases of wound healing. SSIs occur within 30 days of surgery or within 1 year in a site where there is an implant. The CDC define SSIs as superficial, deep incisional, and organ space.

Prevention guidelines by the CDC include specific timing and choice of antibiotics, avoidance of hair removal unless absolutely necessary, tight glucose control, topical antimicrobials for bathing and preoperative skin preparation, and normothermia for colon procedures. Preventing wound infection requires meticulous attention to sterile techniques when caring for an acute wound. (See *Acute wound complications in patients following bariatric surgery*.)

 Handle with care

Acute wound complications in patients following bariatric surgery

Patients following bariatric surgery are at an increased risk for acute wound complications, including infection, dehiscence caused by increased tension on wound edges at the time of wound closure, and hematoma formation caused by pooled blood.

These complications may be the result of many factors, including the following:
- difficulty level of operation
- lengthier operation time, which increases the chances of contamination
- hypoperfusion of adipose tissue
- perioperative hyperglycemia
- increased trauma (e.g., the more forceful retraction needed during surgery may cause necrosis of the abdominal wall)
- excess fat, weight of the abdominal wall, and blood or serous fluid that may increase tension on the wound edges
    Steps to help prevent complications
- Assess the incision site and vital signs frequently.
- Use an abdominal binder over the surgical site to support the incision. Ensure that this is the correct size based on body dimensions.
- Encourage the patient to use deep breathing and spirometry to improve oxygenation.
- Assess nutritional status and promote adequate intake of protein, carbohydrates, and vitamins.

Mean to intervene

For a surgical patient, wound infection is a significant and serious event requiring prompt intervention. Interventions typically ordered in cases of postoperative infection include the following:

- obtaining a wound culture and sensitivity test
- administering antibiotics
- irrigating the wound
- dressing the wound and loosely filling any dead space, if necessary (antimicrobial dressings, such as silver dressings or medical grade honey, may also be ordered)
- monitoring wound drainage, pain, odor, condition of periwound skin, and fever

Hemorrhage

Hemorrhage may occur from damage to blood vessels. Postoperatively, it may happen in either internal or external sites. Monitor the patient receiving anticoagulation therapy carefully. The most common locations of significant internal hemorrhages are as follows:

- posterior nasal passages
- pulmonary vessels
- spleen
- liver
- stomach
- uterus

Hemorrhage may also occur at the site of a large artery injury or aneurysm. Hemorrhage in one of these areas significantly reduces the volume of circulating blood and precipitates hypovolemia. Nursing interventions include administering intravenous (IV) fluids to maintain blood pressure and urine output and determining the source of bleeding. If the hemorrhage originates externally—for example, from the wound itself or from damage to the fragile, newly developed blood vessels—place pressure or a pressure dressing on the site of the bleeding, monitor the patient's vital signs, and notify the health care provider for specific treatment orders.

Dehiscence and evisceration

As mentioned earlier, dehiscence may be a complication of infection. Dehiscence is most likely to occur when collagen fibers aren't mature enough to hold the incision closed without sutures. The first sign of dehiscence may be an abscess, a gush of serosanguineous fluid from the wound, or a report from the patient of a "popping" sensation after sneezing, coughing, or retching. Complete dehiscence leads to evisceration, in which underlying tissues protrude through the wound opening. Abdominal wounds are more likely to dehisce and eviscerate than thoracic wounds are.

An ounce of prevention

To prevent wound dehiscence and evisceration, teach the patient to support the incision with a pillow or cushion before changing position, coughing, or sneezing.

If dehiscence or evisceration occurs, take the following steps:

- Stay with the patient; keep them still and have a colleague notify the health care provider.
- If the patient has an abdominal wound, help them into a low Fowler position with the knees bent to reduce abdominal tension.
- If evisceration is evident, cover extruding tissues with gauze dressings saturated with sterile normal saline solution, and notify the surgeon.

Ostomy care

A patient with a urostomy, colostomy, or ileostomy wears an external pouch over the ostomy site, usually attached with a barrier wafer. The pouch collects urine or fecal matter, helps control odor, and protects the stoma and peristomal skin. Most disposable pouching systems can be used for 3 to 7 days unless a leak develops.

When selecting a pouching system, choose one that delivers the best adhesive seal and skin protection for that patient. Other considerations include the stoma's location and structure, consistency of the effluent, availability and cost of supplies, amount of time the patient will wear the pouch, any known adhesive allergy, and the personal preferences of the patient.

For colostomies or ileostomies, the best time to change a pouching system is first thing in the morning or 2 to 4 hours after meals, when the bowel is least active. After a few months, most patients can predict the time that it is best for them.

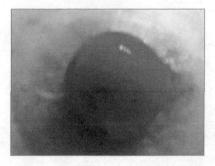

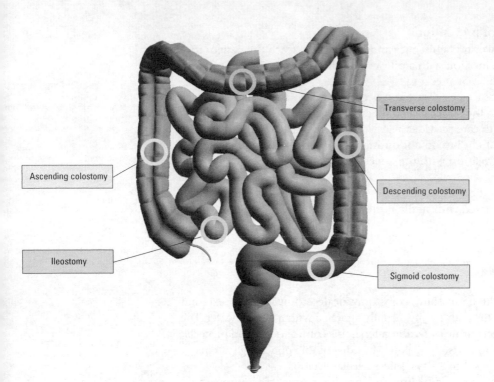

Comparing ostomy pouching systems

Manufactured in many shapes and sizes, ostomy pouches are fashioned for comfort, safety, and easy application. Characteristics of systems are as follows:

- One-piece or two-piece (two-piece systems have a barrier wafer to which the pouch attaches)

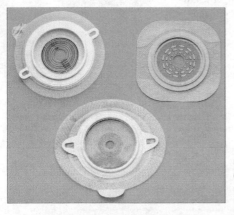

Carmel, J. E., Colwell, J. C., & Goldberg, M. T. (2021). *Wound, Ostomy, and Continence Nurses Society Core Curriculum: Ostomy management.* Lippincott Williams & Wilkins.

- Disposable reusable (occasionally people elect to use a reusable system that is washed and reused)
- Drainable (spigot or open end) or closed end

Patients who must empty the pouch often (because of diarrhea or a new colostomy or ileostomy) should use a drainable pouch with a skin barrier. One-piece, disposable, cut-to-fit pouches are the most economical for a patient with a new ostomy.

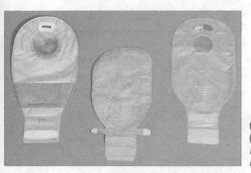

Carmel, J. E., Colwell, J. C., & Goldberg, M. T. (2021). *Wound, Ostomy, and Continence Nurses Society Core Curriculum: Ostomy management.* Lippincott Williams & Wilkins.

Disposable closed-end pouches, made of transparent or opaque odor-proof plastic, may come with a carbon filter for gas release. A patient with a regular bowel elimination pattern may choose this style for additional security and confidence.

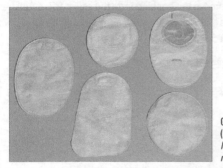

Carmel, J. E., Colwell, J. C., & Goldberg, M. T. (2021). *Wound, Ostomy, and Continence Nurses Society Core Curriculum: Ostomy management.* Lippincott Williams & Wilkins.

A two-piece, disposable, drainable pouch with a separate skin barrier permits frequent changes of the pouch while minimizing barrier removal.

Urostomy pouches have a spout on the end that can be connected to straight drainage for overnight or leg bag collection.

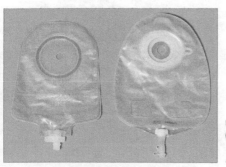

Carmel, J. E., Colwell, J. C., & Goldberg, M. T. (2021). *Wound, Ostomy, and Continence Nurses Society Core Curriculum: Ostomy management.* Lippincott Williams & Wilkins.

Applying a skin barrier and pouch

Fitting a skin barrier and ostomy pouch properly can be done in a few steps. Shown here is a two-piece pouching system, which is commonly used.

1 Measure the stoma using a measuring guide.

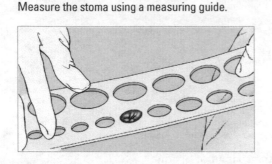

2 Trace the appropriate circle carefully on the back of the skin barrier.

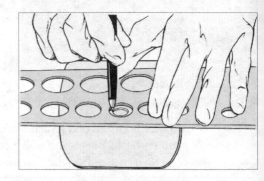

3 Cut the circular opening in the skin barrier. Bevel the edges to keep them from irritating the patient. Be sure to size the opening correctly to prevent peristomal skin breakdown (approximately one-eighth inch larger than the stoma).

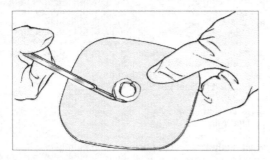

4 Remove the backing from the skin barrier. Apply a barrier ring or paste if needed along the edge of the circular opening.

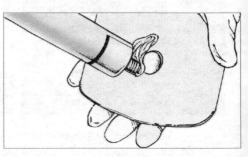

5 Center the skin barrier over the stoma, adhesive side down, and gently press it to the skin.

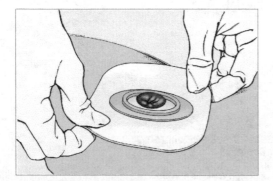

6 Gently press the pouch opening onto the ring until it snaps into place.

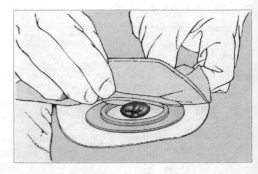

Wounds from infection

Abscess

Skin abscess is a local collection of pus and/or blood. It is usually managed with incision and drainage, often with a local anesthetic. These usually require the dead space to be filled to prevent the skin surface from healing before the deeper tissue. A drainage tube can be used to drain an internal abscess or for fluid collection. These are often placed with radiologic guidance and can stay in place for prolonged periods. The patient will need education on irrigation, site care, dressing change, monitoring output, and follow-up appointments.

Necrotizing fasciitis

Necrotizing fasciitis is a serious, rapidly spreading infection of the fascia that can destroy soft tissue. Emergency aggressive surgical debridement is needed to manage this condition as it can rapidly lead to septic shock and organ failure. Patients affected by necrotizing fasciitis may have other health conditions that decrease their ability to fight infection, such as diabetes.

Traumatic wounds

A traumatic wound is a sudden, unplanned injury to the skin that can range from minor (such as a skinned knee) to severe (such as a gunshot wound).

Types of traumatic wounds

Traumatic wounds include abrasions, lacerations, skin tears (discussed in Chapter 4), bites, and blunt or penetrating trauma wounds.

Abrasions

An abrasion occurs when a mechanical force, such as the friction of skin rubbing against a hard surface, scrapes away a partial-thickness area of the skin. Unless an unusually large amount of skin is involved or an infection develops, an abrasion is one of the least complicated traumatic wounds. Abrasions can vary in size and depth and can be impregnated with dirt or debris.

Lacerations

A laceration is a tear in the skin that's caused by a sharp object, such as metal, glass, or wood. It can also be caused by blunt trauma that produces high shearing force. A laceration has jagged, irregular edges, and its severity depends on its cause, size, depth, and location.

Bites

When assessing a bite wound, it's important to quickly discover the bite's source—cat, dog, bat, snake, spider, human? This helps the health care team determine which bacteria or toxins may be present and the likely type of tissue trauma.

Hannibal the cannibal?

A human bite can cause a puncture wound and introduce into the wound any of the innumerable organisms present in the human mouth. *Staphylococcus aureus* and streptococci are two such organisms that can be transmitted to the wound or into the patient's bloodstream. Other serious diseases that can be transmitted in this way include human immunodeficiency virus (HIV) infection, hepatitis B, hepatitis C, syphilis, and tuberculosis. Some evidence suggests that a human bite can also cause necrotizing fasciitis (rapidly progressing skin infection usually caused by two types of organisms).

Animal house

A bite from a dog, cat, or rodent can introduce deadly infectious diseases, such as rabies, into a wound. Pointed teeth can cause deep tissue damage. A dog can generate up to 200 psi of pressure when biting, and if shaking the head at the same time (which is usually the case), strong torsional force is brought to bear. Together, these forces can cause a significant amount of tissue damage from crushing and avulsion.

Penetrating trauma wounds

A penetrating trauma wound is a puncture wound. This type of wound may be caused by an accident or a personal attack, such as a stabbing or gunshot wound. It can result in soft tissue injury and possible bone, muscle, tendon, blood vessel, or nerve injury. Blunt trauma can cause a large amount of tissue destruction. The underlying injury may be worse than the wound appears.

Knife strife

A stab wound is a low-velocity wound that generally presents as a classic puncture wound or laceration. In some cases, it may involve organ damage beneath the wound site. X-rays, computed tomography scanning, and magnetic resonance imaging are used to evaluate possible organ damage. If the weapon used was contaminated, the patient is at risk for local infection, sepsis, and tetanus.

Smoking gun

A gunshot wound is a high-velocity wound. Factors that affect the severity of tissue damage include the caliber of the weapon, the velocity of the projectile, and the patient's position at the time of injury.

In most cases, a small-caliber weapon firing a relatively low-velocity projectile creates a small, clean punctuate lesion with little or no bleeding. If the projectile is no longer in the patient's body, treat this lesion as you would treat any other open wound.

A large-caliber, relatively high-velocity projectile typically causes massive tissue destruction, a large gaping wound, profuse bleeding, and wound contamination. In this case, the patient usually requires immediate surgical intervention. After surgery, treat the wound as a surgical wound.

Assessment and care

Time is critical when caring for a patient with a traumatic wound. First, assess airway, breathing, and circulation (ABCs). Although focusing first on the injury itself may seem natural, a patent airway and pumping heart take priority.

Next, turn your attention to the wound. Control bleeding by applying firm, direct pressure, and elevate the patient's extremities. If bleeding continues, you may need to compress a pressure point above the wound. Then assess the wound's condition, noting its length, width, and depth; edema; exudate; tissue perfusion; sensory and motor function; and the presence of foreign bodies or fracture. Specific wound management and cleaning depend on the type of wound and degree of contamination. (See *Caring for a patient with a traumatic wound*.)

Get wise to wounds

Caring for a patient with a traumatic wound

When treating a patient with a traumatic wound, always begin by assessing the ABCs—airway, breathing, and circulation. Move on to the wound itself only after confirming the ABCs are stable. Here are the basic steps to follow when caring for each type of traumatic wound.

(continued)

Caring for a patient with a traumatic wound *(continued)*

Abrasion

• Flush the area of the abrasion with normal saline solution, wound cleaning solution, or warm water for 5 to 10 minutes.
• Use a sterile 4″ × 4″ gauze pad moistened with normal saline solution to remove dirt or gravel, and gently cleanse around the wound.
• If the wound is extremely dirty, it may need to be scrubbed with a surgical brush. This should be ordered and supervised by a practitioner. Be as gentle as possible, and keep in mind that this is a painful process for your patient. Ensure adequate pain management if your patient needs this procedure.
• Allow a small wound to dry and form a scab. Cover larger wounds with a nonadherent pad or petroleum gauze and a light dressing. Apply antibacterial ointment if ordered. Silver absorptive dressing sheets may be used for large, involved areas. These can stay in place up to 7 days or until saturated. Follow product directions for application.

Laceration

• Cleanse the wound gently or irrigate if necessary. See Appendix 2 for wound cleansing and wound irrigation procedures.
• Assist the practitioner in suturing the wound if necessary; apply Steri-Strips if suturing isn't needed.
• Apply dressing as ordered.

Bite

• Immediately irrigate the wound with copious amounts of normal saline solution. Don't immerse and soak the wound because this may allow bacteria to float back into the tissue.
• Clean the wound with sterile 4″ × 4″ gauze pads and an antiseptic solution such as povidone-iodine.
• Assist with debridement, if ordered.
• Apply a loose dressing. If the bite is on an extremity, elevate it to reduce swelling.
• Ask the patient about the source of the bite to determine whether there is a risk of rabies. Administer rabies and tetanus shots as needed.

Penetrating wound

• If the wound is minor, allow it to bleed for a few minutes before cleaning it. A larger puncture wound may require irrigation.
• Cover the wound with a dry dressing.
• If the wound contains an embedded foreign object, such as a shard of glass or metal, stabilize the object until the practitioner can remove it. When the object is removed and bleeding is under control, clean the wound as you would a laceration.
• Administer tetanus vaccine as needed.

Special considerations

When caring for a patient with a traumatic wound, pay particular attention to the following aspects of care:

- Cleanse wounds well to remove surface bacteria and debris from the wound base. Use sterile, normal saline. Cleanse with gauze pads or irrigate well until the wound base is clean. High-pressure irrigation can seriously interfere with healing by destroying cells and forcing bacteria into the tissue.
- Use sterile, normal saline solution or commercially available wound cleansers to remove debris when cleaning the wound. Never use hydrogen peroxide or alcohol.
- Never use a cotton ball or a cotton-filled gauze pad to clean a wound because cotton fibers left in the wound may cause contamination or a foreign body reaction.
- If the health care provider plans to debride the wound to remove dead tissue and reduce the risk of infection and scarring, loosely fill the wound with fluffed gauze pads moistened with normal saline solution (see Appendix 7) until it's time for the procedure.
- Monitor the wound closely for signs of developing infection, such as warm, red skin or purulent discharge from the wound. Infection in a traumatic wound can delay healing, increase scarring, and trigger systemic infections such as septicemia.
- Inspect the dressing regularly. If edema develops, adjust the dressing to ensure adequate circulation to the affected area of the wound.

Understanding compartment syndrome

In compartment syndrome, edema or bleeding increases pressure within a muscle compartment (arm or leg) to the point at which circulation (both arterial inflow and venous outflow) to muscles and nerves within the compartment is impaired. It can occur as a result of burns, direct injury and pressure, fractures, and snake envenomation. This condition is limb-threatening and requires immediate intervention.

Symptoms

- Intense, deep, throbbing pain that doesn't improve with analgesia
- Numbness and tingling distal to the affected muscle
- Absent peripheral pulses in the affected extremity
- Pallor or mottling of the affected area
- Decreased movement, muscle strength, and sensation in the affected extremity

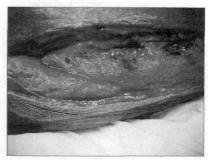

Treatments

- Positioning of the affected extremity at heart level
- Removal of constrictive clothing and dressings
- Analgesics
- Neurovascular status monitoring to detect changes in circulation and nerve function
- Intracompartmental pressure monitoring and Doppler ultrasound to assess blood flow
- Emergency fasciotomy to allow muscle to expand and decrease compartment pressure
- Wound management after fasciotomy focuses on maintaining a moist wound environment. Gauze dressings or negative pressure wound therapy are used until edema resolves and granulation occurs over visible muscle. Then, the wound is closed or a skin graft is placed.

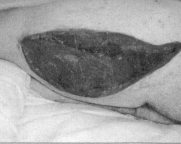

Burns

A burn is an acute wound caused by exposure to thermal extremes, electricity, caustic chemicals, or radiation. The degree of tissue damage caused by a burn depends on the strength of the source and the duration of contact or exposure. Most burns are managed in the outpatient setting depending on the severity and patient's overall condition.

Types of burns

Thermal burns

The most common type of burn, thermal burns, can result from virtually any misuse or mishandling of fire or a combustible product. Playing with matches, pouring gasoline into a hot lawnmower, and setting off fireworks are some common examples of ways in which burns occur. Thermal burns can also result from kitchen accidents, fires, automobile accidents, or physical abuse. Although it's less common, exposure to extreme cold can also cause thermal burns.

Electrical burns

Electrical burns result from contact with flowing electrical current. Household current, high-voltage transmission lines, and lightning are sources of electrical burns.

Chemical burns

Chemical burns most commonly result from contact (skin contact or inhalation) with a caustic agent, such as an acid, an alkali, or a vesicant. Alkaline chemicals generally cause more serious burns than acid substances because they penetrate the contact area more deeply.

Radiation burns

The most common radiation burn is sunburn, which follows excessive exposure to the sun. Almost all other burns due to radiation exposure occur as a result of radiation treatment or in specific industries that use or process radioactive materials.

Factors that affect healing

Factors that affect treatment and healing include:
- burn location—burns on the face, hands, feet, and genitalia are most serious due to the possible loss of function.
- burn configuration—edema due to a circumferential burn (completely encircling an extremity) can slow or stop circulation to the extremity; burns on the neck can obstruct the airway, and burns on the chest can interfere with normal respiration by inhibiting expansion.
- preexisting medical conditions—note disorders that impair peripheral circulation, especially diabetes, PVD, and chronic alcohol misuse.
- other injuries sustained at the time of the burn.
- patient age—patients younger than age 4 or older than age 60 are at higher risk for complications and consequently a higher mortality rate.
- pulmonary injury—inhaling smoke or superheated air damages lung tissue.

Assessment

Conduct your initial assessment as soon as possible after the burn occurs. First, assess the patient's ABCs. Then determine the patient's level of consciousness and mobility. Next, assess the burn, including its size, depth, severity, and causative factor.

Memory jogger

To remember the proper sequence for the initial assessment of a burn patient, remember your ABCs and add D and E.

Airway—Assess the patient's airway, remove any obstruction, and treat any obstructive condition.

Breathing—Observe the motion of the patient's chest. Auscultate the depth, rate, and characteristics of the patient's breathing.

Circulation—Palpate the patient's pulse at the carotid artery and then at the distal pulse points in the wrist,

posterior tibial area, and foot. Loss of distal pulse may indicate shock or constriction of an extremity.

Disability—Assess the patient's level of consciousness and ability to function before attempting to move or transfer them.

Expose—Remove burned clothing from burned areas of the patient's body and thoroughly examine the skin beneath.

Determining size

Determine burn size as part of your initial assessment. Typically, burn size is expressed as a percentage of total body surface area (TBSA). The Rule of Nines and the Lund-Browder Classification are two useful tools for providing reasonably standardized and quick estimates of the percentage of TBSA affected. (See *Estimating burn size*.)

Estimating burn size

Because body surface area (BSA) varies with age, two different methods are used to estimate burn size in adult and pediatric patients.

Rule of Nines
You can quickly estimate the extent of an adult patient's burn by using the Rule of Nines. This method quantifies BSA in multiples of nine, thus the name. To use this method, mentally transfer the burns on your patient to the body charts depicted. Add the corresponding percentages for each body section burned. Use the total—a rough estimate of burn extent—to calculate initial fluid replacement needs.

Lund-Browder Classification
The Rule of Nines isn't accurate for infants or children because their body shapes differ from those of adults and so their TBSAs do too. For example, an infant's head accounts for about 17% of the total BSA compared with 7% for an adult. Instead, use the Lund-Browder Classification to determine burn size for infants and children.

Estimating burn size

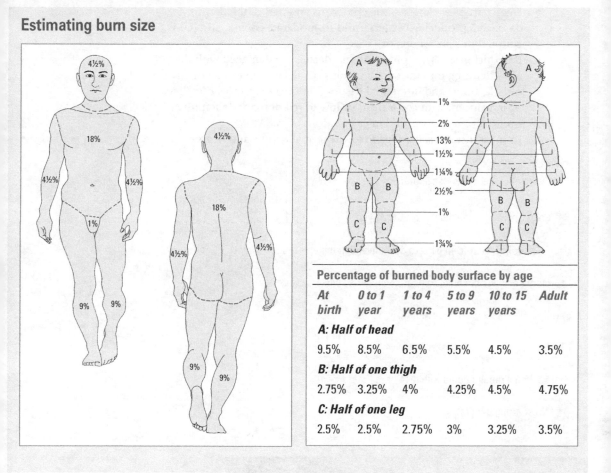

Percentage of burned body surface by age					
At birth	*0 to 1 year*	*1 to 4 years*	*5 to 9 years*	*10 to 15 years*	*Adult*
A: Half of head					
9.5%	8.5%	6.5%	5.5%	4.5%	3.5%
B: Half of one thigh					
2.75%	3.25%	4%	4.25%	4.5%	4.75%
C: Half of one leg					
2.5%	2.5%	2.75%	3%	3.25%	3.5%

Determining depth

During the initial assessment, determine the depth of tissue damage. A partial-thickness burn damages the epidermis and part of the dermis. A full-thickness burn involves the epidermis, dermis, and subcutaneous tissue.

Four degrees of separation

The traditional method of gauging burn severity classified burn depth by degree. Today, most assessment findings use the following depth of tissue damage to describe a burn (American Burn Association, 2022):

- Superficial—Usually dry and red and may be painful; sunburn is an example; not counted in calculations of TBSA
- Superficial partial thickness—Damage to the epidermis and first third of dermis, causing erythema and pain; counted in calculations of TBSA

- Deep partial thickness—The epidermis and part of the dermis are damaged, producing blisters, mild-to-moderate edema, and pain; counted in calculations of TBSA
- Full thickness—The epidermis and dermis are damaged with damage extending into the subcutaneous tissue layer; may also involve muscle, bone, and interstitial tissues. The area may appear leathery or translucent with color from yellow to red or black depending on involvement; counted in calculations of TBSA

In most instances, damage involves several depths and degrees.

In superficial partial-thickness burns:

Epidermis and some dermis are destroyed.

Thin-walled, fluid-filled blisters develop within minutes of the injury.

Nerve endings become exposed to the air as blisters break.

Pain and tactile response remain intact.

Barrier function of the skin is lost.

Epithelial repair occurs within 14 days.

No scarring occurs.

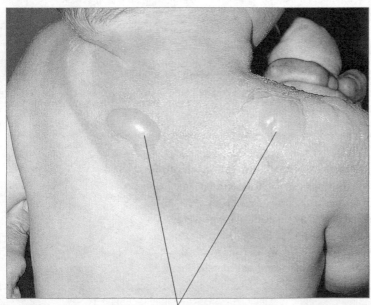

This photo shows a child with a superficial partial-thickness sunburn. Note the thin-walled, fluid-filled blisters.

Thin-walled blisters

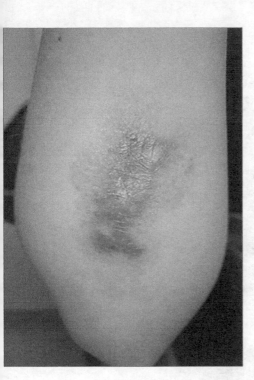

This is another example of a superficial partial-thickness burn

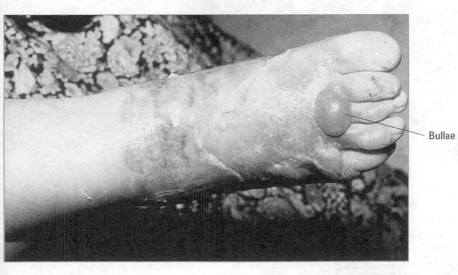

Bullae

This photo shows a deep partial-thickness burn. Note the white, waxy appearance. In this instance, the large bullae will most likely be ruptured.

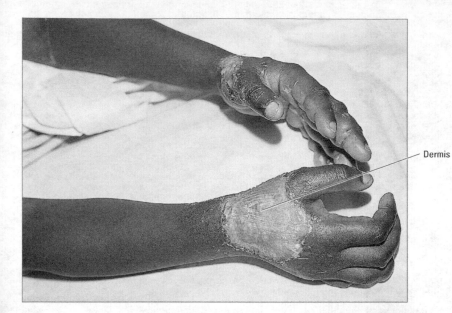

Dermis

You can see the dermis in this deep partial-thickness burn.

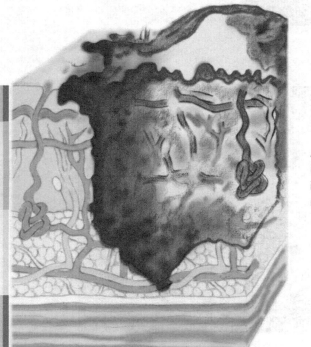

Epidermis

Dermis

Subcutaneous tissue

Muscle

A third-degree burn results in an increased calorie demand, which increases the patient's metabolic rate.

Determining severity

A combination of the burn mechanism, depth, extent, and anatomic location determines the overall severity of the burn injury, providing guidance for the preferred disposition and care of these patients.

Major

Major burns meet one or more of the following criteria:

- More than 20% of TBSA in adults; more than 10% in children and older adults
- Full-thickness burns on more than 5% of TBSA
- Clinically significant burns on the face, eyes, ears, genitalia, or major joints
- Burns complicated by major trauma, respiratory damage, and/or clinically significant associated injuries
- High-voltage burns
- Any burn in a high-risk patient

Moderate

Moderate burns meet one or more of the following criteria:

- Full-thickness burns on 2% to 5% of TBSA.
- Deep partial-thickness burns on 10% to 20% of TBSA in adults; 5% to 10% in children or older adults

Minor

Minor burns meet one or more of the following criteria:

- full-thickness burns on less than 2% of TBSA
- deep partial-thickness burns on less than 10% of TBSA in adults; less than 5% in children or older adults

Burn care

Care for a patient with a burn depends on the type and severity of the burn, the patient's general health before the injury, and whether another injury was sustained concurrent with the burn. In general, treatment seeks to reduce pain; remove dirt, debris, and dead tissue; preserve function; minimize deformity; and provide a dressing that promotes healing. In some cases, treatment includes skin grafting.

Minor to moderate burns

In minor to moderate burns, the first step is to stop the burning process and relieve pain. Remove smoldering clothing and provide pain medication as ordered. When cleaning minor burns, use cool running water and mild antibacterial soap; never use hydrogen peroxide or povidone-iodine (or products containing these agents) because they can cause further tissue damage. Cover the burns with dry, sterile towels.

Something to talk about

As soon as the patient's condition stabilizes and other injuries are ruled out, the health care provider may order an opioid analgesic, such as morphine or Dilaudid. Nonsteroidal antiinflammatory drugs (NSAIDs) may be used alone or along with narcotics for pain management. The patient may also receive medications for anxiety. Be sure to talk to the patient as you work. Emotional support and reassurance are important aspects of care and may reduce the patient's need for analgesia.

Wrapping it up

After the practitioner debrides devitalized tissue, if necessary, cover the wound with an antimicrobial and a nonadhesive bulky dressing. If ordered, administer tetanus prophylaxis. Some health care providers prescribe a slow-release silver dressing that can remain in place for up to 7 days. These help prevent infection, provide increased comfort for the patient, decrease dressing changes, and decrease time of caregiving.

Comparing topical dressings

Type	Description and uses	Nursing considerations
Silver sulfadiazine 1% (antibacterial)	Apply in a thick layer one to two times a day to maintain bactericidal activity. Cover with a light dressing. Cleanse burn with each dressing change.	Do not use with sulfa allergy or pregnancy.
Mafenide acetate, Sulfamylon (topical antibacterial)	Broad-spectrum antimicrobial that can penetrate eschar. Apply three to four times a day. Leave open to air. Use on small burns. May be very painful. Often used on nose and ears.	Softens eschar to help debride. Use with extreme caution with sulfa allergy.
Bacitracin (topical antibacterial)	Apply three to four times a day. Can be used for small wounds for up to 1 week.	Often used on the face
Silver (antibacterial), e.g., Acticoat	Decrease dressing frequency due to sustained release of silver into wound and associated pain, so now frequently chosen for burn care. Useful for partial-thickness wounds. Maintains moist environment. Follow manufacturer's instructions for dressing change frequency. Cut to the size of the wound or burn.	Conforms to body
Medicinal honey	Effective against broad spectrum of organisms, particularly pseudomonas, which are common in burns.	Avoid with allergy to the product.
Biologic dressings	Provide temporary coverage while awaiting permanent closure. Xenografts (pig skin) or allografts (preserved cadaver skin) are commonly used.	Monitor for drainage and signs of rejection.
Biosynthetic dressings	Most commonly used is Biobrane, a porcine dermal collagen bound with silicone and nylon. Used on clean partial-thickness burns or donor sites. Check after 48 hours for adherence then leave the membrane in place up to 14 days later when graft is placed.	Apply gauze, wrap, and elastic bandages to support the area.

Moderate to major burns

In moderate to major burns, immediately assess the patient's ABCs. Be especially alert for signs of smoke inhalation and pulmonary damage, for example, singed nasal hairs, mucosal burns, changes in the patient's voice, coughing, wheezing, soot in the mouth or nose, or darkened sputum. If necessary, assist with endotracheal intubation and administer 100% oxygen. When the patient's ABCs are stable, take a brief history of the burn and draw blood samples as ordered for diagnostic tests.

Next, stop residual burning and control bleeding. Remove any smoldering clothing. If material is stuck to the patient's skin, soak it with saline solution before you attempt to remove it. Remove all jewelry and any other constricting apparel. Then cover the burns with a clean, dry, sterile bed sheet. Remember, never cover large burns with saline-soaked dressings because this can drastically lower body temperature.

Solution resolution

Begin IV therapy as ordered to prevent hypovolemic shock and help maintain cardiac output. A patient with serious burns needs significant fluid replacement—especially during the first 24 hours after the injury. The health care provider may order a combination of crystalloids such as lactated Ringer solution.

What goes in must come out

Closely monitor the patient's intake and output and check vital signs often. Finally, be prepared to assist in emergency escharotomy if the patient's burns threaten circulation.

Electrical burns

Tissue damage from electrical burns is difficult to assess because internal damage along the conduction pathway is commonly greater than the surface burn indicates. If possible, determine the voltage involved. This information helps the health care team assess possible internal damage more accurately.

Keep in mind that a current passing through the body can induce ventricular fibrillation, cardiac arrest, or respiratory arrest—all life-threatening conditions requiring immediate intervention. (See *Electric shock*.)

Electric shock

When an electric current passes through the body, the damage it does depends on:
- intensity of the current (measured in amperes).
- resistance of the tissues it passes through.
- kind of current (alternating current, direct current, or a combination of both).
- frequency and duration of the current's flow.

(continued)

Electric shock *(continued)*

Electric current can cause injury in three ways:
- True electrical injury caused by a current that passes through the body
- Arc or flash burns caused by a current that doesn't pass through the body
- Thermal surface burns caused by associated heat and flames
  The patient's prognosis depends on:
- site of the injury.
- extent of damage.
- general health prior to the injury.
- speed and adequacy of treatment.

Chemical burns

When treating a patient with a chemical burn, begin by irrigating the wound with plenty of sterile water or normal saline solution for 30 minutes or more. Alkalis usually produce more severe burns than acids; however, the severity of the burn is usually determined by the length of time that the chemical was in contact with the patient's skin.

If the patient's eyes are involved, flush them with plenty of water or saline solution until the pH is neutralized. This is determined by testing the pH of the eye surface. Often, 1 to 2 L of fluid will be needed. Arrange for an ophthalmologic examination. Finally, note the type of chemical involved and the presence of any noxious fumes.

If the patient is to be transferred to a burn care unit soon after the accident, wrap them in a sterile sheet first and then a blanket for warmth and elevate the burned extremity to minimize edema.

Special considerations

When caring for a patient with a burn, the patient may require referral to a burn center if they meet specific criteria. (See *American Burn Association burn transfer criteria*.)

American Burn Association burn transfer criteria

1. Partial-thickness burns greater than 10% TBSA
2. Burns that involve the face, hands, feet, genitalia, perineum, or major joints
3. Full-thickness burns
4. High-voltage electrical injuries, including lightning injury
5. Chemical injuries
6. Suspected Inhalation injury
7. Burn injury in patients with preexisting medical disorders that could complicate management, prolong recovery, or affect mortality
8. Any patient with concomitant injuries
9. Pediatric burns
10. Burn injury in patients who will require special social, emotional, or rehabilitative intervention

Excerpted from American Burn Association. (2022). Advanced burn life support. *Guidelines for burn patient referral.* https://ameriburn.org/wp-content/uploads/2022/11/one-page-guidelines-for-burn-patient-referral-10.pdf

When caring for a patient with a burn, also remember the following:

- Assess the patient's home situation to ensure adequate assistance with mobility, wound care, and transportation to outpatient visits if the patient does not require hospitalization.
- Assess the patient's level of pain, including nonverbal indications, and administer analgesics as ordered.
- Keep the patient calm, provide periods of uninterrupted rest between procedures, and use nonpharmacologic pain relief measures as appropriate. Administer antianxiety medications if prescribed, and monitor the patient's response.
- Burn patients have very high metabolic rates and very high nutrition requirements. Assess intake, and implement the nutrition plan of care.
- Administer histamine-2 blockers or proton pump inhibitors as ordered to reduce the risk of ulcer formation.
- Prepare the patient for possible grafting as indicated.

Potential complications

Potential complications that may arise include:

- hypovolemic shock
- fluid overload
- pulmonary edema
- pruritus (can be managed with antihistamines, lubrication of the skin, or medications used for neuropathic pain)
- infection
  Be sure to monitor the patient's vital signs and hemodynamic parameters and assess for signs and symptoms of infection, such as fever, elevated WBC count, and changes in burn wound appearance or drainage.

Skin grafting

Skin grafting consists of taking healthy tissue—from either the patient (autograft) or a donor (allograft)—and applying it to an area damaged by burns, traumatic injury, or surgery. Keep in mind that a patient who has received an autograft requires care for two wounds: one at the graft site and one at the donor site.

Skin grafting may be necessary to repair defects caused by burns, trauma, or surgery. Depending on the graft's complexity, the procedure may be performed under local or general anesthesia and in some cases may be performed as an outpatient procedure.

The surgeon may choose skin grafting as the preferred treatment option if:
- primary closure isn't possible or cosmetically acceptable.
- primary closure would interfere with function.
- the wound is on a weight-bearing surface of the body.
- a skin tumor is excised, and the site needs to be monitored for recurrence.
  Three types of skin grafts exist:
- split-thickness grafts—consisting of the epidermis and a small portion of the dermis
- full-thickness grafts—consisting of the epidermis and all of the dermis
- composite grafts—consisting of the epidermis, dermis, and underlying tissues (such as muscle, cartilage, and bone)

Secret of success

The success or failure of any skin graft depends on revascularization. Initially, a skin graft survives by direct contact with the underlying tissue, receiving oxygen and nutrients through existing blood vessels. However, the graft will die unless new blood vessels develop. For split-thickness grafts, revascularization usually takes 3 to 5 days; for full-thickness grafts, it may take up to 2 weeks.

Skin substitutes

There are many temporary and permanent wound coverings available for burns and acute and chronic wounds. They protect the wound from fluid loss and infection, decrease dressing changes, and provide a moist environment to promote healing. Biologic tissues include allograft, xenograft, and human amnion membrane. Biobrane (see earlier table, *Comparing topical dressings*) is a synthetic material. Dermal constructs include AlloDerm. Integra and Permacol are examples of dermal scaffoldings. Apligraf and OrCel are examples of full skin substitutes. Read the operative note or discuss the specific substitute used with the health care provider for specific care based on the type of wound and the specific substitute.

Fall harvest

The graft is taken, or harvested, from an area of healthy tissue on the patient's body. Therefore, it is important to provide meticulous skin care to preserve potential donor sites. Also, because graft survival depends on close contact with underlying tissue, the recipient site—the wound—should be made of healthy granulation tissue that is free from eschar, debris, and infection.

Survival of the fittest

After a patient receives a skin graft, all aspects of care focus on promoting graft survival. Help the patient find comfortable positions for relaxing and sleeping that prevent them from lying on the area of the graft. If feasible, keep the graft elevated and immobilized. When needed, modify your routine to accommodate healing. For example, never use a blood pressure cuff over a graft site. Administer analgesics as necessary; however, remember to teach the patient techniques to reduce pain that don't involve medication (such as relaxation techniques).

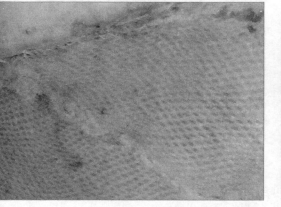 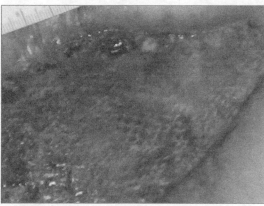

Always use sterile techniques when changing dressings, and work gently to avoid dislodging the graft. Negative pressure wound therapy may be the surgeon's choice for managing the postoperative wound. This is placed in surgery immediately after the skin graft is placed and left intact for 5 days. After removal, wound management is determined by how well the skin graft has adhered to the wound. If further dressings are needed, change the gauze and apply the prescribed topical agent; then cover the area with a gauze bandage.

In autografting, tissue is removed from the patient's body using a dermatome, an instrument that cuts uniform, split-thickness skin portions. Consequently, the donor site is a partial-thickness wound, which may bleed, drain, and cause pain. Depending on the graft's thickness, tissue may be obtained from the donor site again in as few as 10 days.

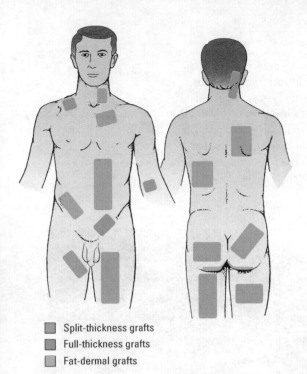

Split-thickness grafts
Full-thickness grafts
Fat-dermal grafts

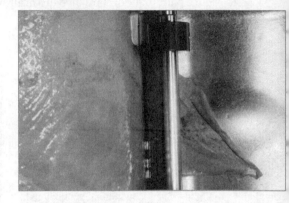

Usually, a moisture vapor–permeable dressing (transparent film dressing) or semiocclusive gauze, such as Vaseline gauze, is applied postoperatively to protect new epithelial proliferation. Some of these partial-thickness wounds can be covered with disposable negative pressure wound therapy devices, which will manage drainage and protect site during healing.

Assess the dressing over the donor site and monitor for signs of infection. Initially, some patients have moderate amounts of serosanguineous drainage from this site.

Dressing the wound

- Wash your hands and put on sterile gloves.
- Remove the outer gauze dressings within 24 hours.
- Inspect the semiocclusive gauze dressing for signs of infection; then leave it open to the air to speed drying and healing. If using a film dressing, follow the surgeon's instructions. Reinforce with gauze, if needed, for leakage.
- Apply a skin emollient daily to completely healed donor sites to keep skin tissue pliable, remove crusts, and decrease itching.

There's no place like home

As the patient prepares to go home, discuss proper care with them. Explain that the instructions for dressing care should be followed exactly as given. If they feel the dressing needs to be changed, they should call the practitioner and never attempt it themselves. Emphasize that immobilizing the area of the graft is essential for speedy and complete healing. Later, as healing progresses, the patient can apply cream to the graft site several times a day to keep the skin pliable and help the scar mature.

Sun exposure can affect graft pigmentation. Explain this to the patient and suggest that they limit the amount of time they spend in the sun. Also suggest that they use sunblock any time they plan to be outdoors.

Finally, many patients express concern about scarring and appearance. Explain that if scarring continues to be a problem when the graft completely heals, the patient can discuss plastic surgery options with the health care provider.

Quick quiz

1. After abdominal surgery, your patient says that they felt something "pop" when getting back into bed. You examine the wound and find bowel protruding. You should first place the patient:
    A.   in a high Fowler position.
    B.   in a low Fowler position.
    C.   flat in bed.
    D.   on their left side.

Answer: B. Place the patient in a low Fowler position to reduce tension on the wound.

2. What's the first step in caring for a patient with a traumatic wound?
    A.   Transport the patient to the hospital.
    B.   Take a blood pressure measurement.
    C.   Apply pressure bandages.
    D.   Assess airway, breathing, and circulation.

Answer: D. Your first priority is to assess the patient's airway, breathing, and circulation.

3. When assessing your patient's burns, you note damage to the epidermis, dermis, and subcutaneous tissue. What type of burn is this?
    A.   Superficial partial thickness
    B.   Deep partial thickness
    C.   Full thickness
    D.   Deep full thickness

Answer: C. In a full-thickness burn, the epidermis, dermis, and subcutaneous tissue are damaged. The burn may also involve muscle, bone, and interstitial tissue.

4.   Your patient has deep partial- and full-thickness burn injuries to the posterior portion of both legs as well as their entire left and right arms. Using the Rule of Nines, what percentage of total BSA is involved?
    A.   18%
    B.   27%
    C.   36%
    D.   45%

Answer: C. The posterior portion of both legs constitutes 18% of BSA and the entire left and right arms constitute another 18% for a total of 36%.

5.   Which intervention can best protect the skin around a heavily draining surgical incision from irritation due to wound drainage?
    A.   Pouching the wound
    B.   Applying packing and gauze dressings
    C.   Applying a hydrocolloid dressing
    D.   Applying an occlusive dressing

Answer: A. Pouching prevents irritation of surrounding tissue when there's copious drainage from an incision.

6.   Your patient had an open hemicolectomy 2 weeks ago. What might you see on a closed surgical incision after staple removal?
    A.   Dermabond
    B.   Butterfly closures
    C.   Steri-Strips
    D.   Gauze dressing

Answer: C. Steri-Strips are the most common method of holding a wound closed after staple or suture removal.

7.   Your patient has a surgical wound that has been closed for 8 days. During your wound assessment, you palpate a ridge along the incision line. This ridge may indicate:
    A.   normal healing.
    B.   wound dehiscence.
    C.   wound evisceration.
    D.   wound tunneling.

Answer: A. This ridge, known as the *healing ridge*, is a sign that normal healing is progressing.

Scoring

☆☆☆ If you answered all seven questions correctly, strut your stuff! You've demonstrated an acute understanding of the chapter.

☆☆ If you answered five or six questions correctly, you deserve a hand! Your surgical approach to studying has served you well.

☆ If you answered fewer than five questions correctly, that's OK! After a quick review, you'll be healed in no time.

Select references

American Burn Association. (n.d.). *Advanced burn life support.* Burn center referral criteria. Retrieved July 12, 2022, from https://ameriburn.org/wp-content/uploads/2017/05/burncenterreferralcriteria.pdf

American Burn Association. (2022). *Guidelines for burn patient referral.* https://ameriburn.org/resources/burnreferral/

Brindle, T., & Creehan, S. (2022). Management of surgical wounds. In L. L. McNichol, C. R. Ratliff, & S. S. Yates (Eds.), *Wound, Ostomy, and Continence Nurses Society core curriculum: Wound management* (2nd ed., pp. 737–774). Wolters Kluwer.

Delmore, B., Cohen, J., O'Neill, D., Chu, A., Pham, V., & Chiu, E. (2017). Reducing postsurgical wound complications: A critical review. *Advances in Skin & Wound Care, 30*(6), 272–285. https://doi.org/10.1097/01.ASW.0000516426.62418.48

Glat, P. M., & Davenport, T. (2017). Current techniques for burn reconstruction using dehydrated amnion/chorion membrane allografts as an adjunctive treatment along the reconstructive ladder. *Annals of Plastic Surgery, 78*(2 Suppl 1), S14–S18. https://doi.org/10.1097/SAP.0000000000000980

Herndon, D. N. (Ed.). (2018). *Total burn care* (5th ed.). Elsevier.

Holmes, T., & Daniels, F. *Removing stitches (Sutures).* Retrieved July 12, 2022, from https://www.emedicinehealth.com/removing_stitches/article_em.htm

ISBI Practice Guidelines Committee; Steering Subcommittee; Advisory Subcommittee. (2016). ISBI practice guidelines for burn care. *Burns, 42*(5), 953–1021. https://doi.org/10.1016/j.burns.2016.05.013

Maliyar, K., Persaud-Jaimangal, R., Sibbald, R. G. (2020). Associations among skin surface pH, temperature, and bacterial burden in wounds. *Advances in Skin & Wound Care, 33*(4), 180–185. https://doi.org/10.1097/01.ASW.0000655488.33274.d0

Marré, D. (Ed.). (2018). *Fundamental topics in plastic surgery.* Thieme. https://doi.org/10.1055/b-006-160145

Mlambo, S. S., Parkar, H., Naude, L., & Cromarty, A. D. (2022). Treatment of acute wounds and injuries: Cuts, bites, bruises and sprains. *South African Pharmaceutical Journal, 89*(1), 12–18. https://hdl.handle.net/10520/ejc-mp_sapj_v89_n1_a5

Middelkoop, E., & Sheridan, R. L. (2018). Skin substitutes and 'the next level'. In D. Herndon (Ed.), *Total burn care* (5th ed., pp. 167–173). Elsevier.

Mier, Y. (2021). Thermal wounds: Burns and frostbite injuries. In L. L. McNichol, C. R. Ratliff, & S. S. Yates (Eds.), *Wound, Ostomy, and Continence Nurses Society core curriculum: Wound management* (2nd ed., pp. 695–721). Wolters Kluwer.

Niederstatter, I. M., Schiefer, J. L., & Fuchs, P. C. (2021). Surgical strategies to promote cutaneous healing. *Medical Sciences, 9*(2), 45. https://doi.org/10.3390/medsc9020045

Owen, T., Ramsay, A., Yiasemidou, M., Hardie, C., Ashmore, D., Macklin, C., Bandyopaddhyay, D., Patel, B., Burke, J., & Jayne, D. (2020). The surgical management of cutaneous abscesses: A UK cross-sectional survey. *Annals of Medicine and Surgery, 60,* 654–659. https://doi.org/10.1016/j.amsu.2020.11.068

Singer, A., & Boyce, S. (2017). Burn wound healing and tissue engineering. *Journal of Burn Care and Research, 38*(3), e605–e613. https://doi.org/10.1097/BCR.0000000000000538

Smith & Nephew. (n.d.). *More wound care products.* Retrieved July 11, 2022, from https://www.smith-nephew.com/key-products/advanced-wound-management/other-wound-care-products/

Texas EMS Trauma & Acute Care Foundation Trauma Division. (2016). *Burn clinical practice guideline.* http://tetaf.org/wp-content/uploads/2016/01/Burn-Practice-Guideline.pdf

Turner, R. (2019). Acute lacerations assessment and non-surgical management. *Australian Journal of General Practitioners, 48*(9), 585–588. https://doi.org/10.31128/AJGP-06-19-4962

Wax, M. (2021, December 23). *Split-thickness skin grafts. Overview, graft selection, donor site selection.* Retrieved July 13, 2022, from https://emedicine.medscape.com/article/876290-overview#a1; https://emedicine.medscape.com/article/876290-overview#a2; https://emedicine.medscape.com/article/876290-overview#a3

Chapter 6

Pressure injuries

Just the facts

In this chapter, you'll learn about:

◆ pressure injury definition, etiology, and staging criteria
◆ pressure injury assessment and risk factors
◆ nursing interventions to prevent and treat pressure injuries

A look at pressure injuries

Pressure injuries are a serious health problem across all health care settings. Although incidence data vary widely as a result of study design and differing health care settings, the Agency for Healthcare Research and Quality (AHRQ, 2014) estimates that almost 2.5 million people in the United States develop pressure injuries each year. In certain groups, such as patients in intensive care units, those with spinal cord injuries, and those in nursing homes, the risk for pressure injury may be even greater.

Pressure injuries are considered a largely preventable condition. As a result, in 2008, Medicare reduced reimbursement to hospitals for care associated with hospital-acquired pressure injuries. In order to reduce pressure injuries in health care facilities, multifaceted evidence-based pressure injury prevention plans need to be instituted. To determine compliance with these plans, regular monitoring of pressure injury rates is conducted within individual health care settings and reported to governmental and regulatory agencies.

Because a pressure injury can become a chronic wound that may be hard to heal, prevention and early intervention are critical for more effective management. Patients who have had prior pressure injuries may also be at higher risk for future pressure injuries.

It has been estimated that the annual cost for hospital-acquired pressure injuries is a staggering $26.8 billion (Padula & Delarmente, 2019). Pressure injuries account for approximately 60,000 deaths annually (National Pressure Injury Advisory Panel [NPIAP], n.d.-a).

The closer you get

Collaboration among government agencies, insurers, and health care professionals is imperative to ensure quality care in the prevention and treatment of pressure injuries. Therefore, many national health care initiatives include measures that address pressure injuries. For example, *Healthy People 2030* (a report of the nation's near-term health care goals) includes a goal of reducing the rate of pressure injury–related hospitalizations among older adults. The National Database of Nursing Quality Indicators (NDNQI) also considers pressure injuries as a nurse-sensitive indicator and tracks pressure injury prevalence and prevention strategies as measures of the quality of nursing care.

Definition

The National Pressure Injury Advisory Panel (NPIAP), European Pressure Ulcer Advisory Panel (EPUAP), and Pan Pacific Pressure Injury Alliance (PPPIA) define a pressure injury as: "localized damage to the skin and underlying soft tissue usually over a bony prominence or related to a medical or other device. The injury can present as intact skin or an open ulcer and may be painful. The injury occurs as a result of intense and/or prolonged pressure or pressure in combination with shear. The tolerance of soft tissue for pressure and shear may also be affected by microclimate, nutrition, perfusion, comorbidities, and condition of the soft tissue" (Haesler, 2019, p. 16).

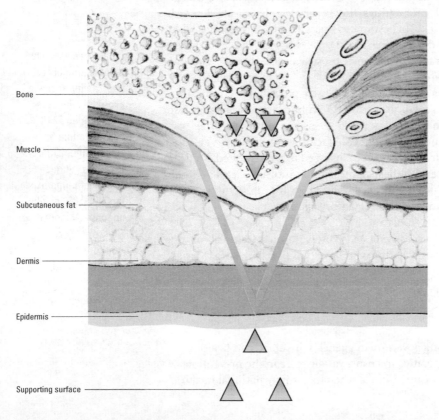

Bone

Muscle

Subcutaneous fat

Dermis

Epidermis

Supporting surface

Now appearing on stage

Staging reflects the depth and extent of tissue involvement and can range from nonblanchable erythema to the deep destruction of tissue and underlying structures such as occurs in deeper wounds like stage 4 pressure injuries. Keep in mind that although staging is useful for classifying pressure injuries, it is only one part of a comprehensive assessment. This staging system should not be used to describe other types of wounds or tissue injuries such as arterial wounds, venous wounds, diabetic wounds, skin tears, or incontinence-related skin changes. Staging pressure injuries falls within the scope of practice for a registered nurse.

Healthy Skin – Lightly Pigmented   **Healthy Skin – Darkly Pigmented**

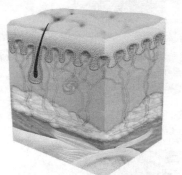   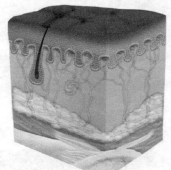

Used with permission of the National Pressure Injury Advisory Panel, 2020. Copyright © NPIAP.

Note that when describing healing pressure injuries, reverse staging of pressure injuries is not done. For example, as a stage 4 pressure injury heals, it would not be reversed to a stage 3 and so on, because the tissue lost would not be replaced with normal anatomic tissue. The wound should be identified as a "healing stage 4 pressure injury."

Why is accurate staging of pressure injuries important?

Documenting the stage of the pressure injury is critical. The stage and appearance of the pressure injury determine treatment, and often, third-party payment is based on the stage. If you are uncertain of the stage of the pressure injury, document what type of tissue you see in the wound and request a wound care consult from a wound care professional. Many health care agencies have standing orders or protocols that are used to guide patient care and treatment based on the stage of the pressure injury. Remember, since pressure injury development is a quality indicator, it is important to assess and stage all pressure injuries found upon admission to a health care facility or service. Any pressure injury discovered at admission would be considered a pressure injury present upon admission and therefore would not be considered a nosocomial pressure injury.

NPIAP Pressure Injury Classification System

Stage 1: Nonblanchable erythema of intact skin

"Intact skin with a localized area of nonblanchable erythema, which may appear differently in darkly pigmented skin. Presence of blanchable erythema or changes in sensation, temperature, or firmness may precede visual changes. Color changes do not include purple or maroon discoloration; these may indicate deep tissue injury."

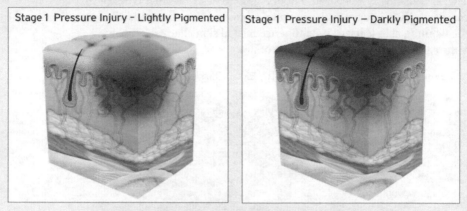

Stage 1 Pressure Injury – Lightly Pigmented

Stage 1 Pressure Injury – Darkly Pigmented

Used with permission of the National Pressure Injury Advisory Panel, 2020. Copyright © NPIAP.

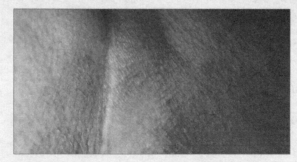

"Darkly pigmented skin may not have visible blanching; therefore, in patients with darker skin tones, stage 1 pressure injuries may be more difficult to detect."

Blanchable erythema

Erythema (redness) results from capillary dilation near the skin's surface. Blanchable erythema is redness that blanches (turns white) when pressed with a fingertip and then immediately turns red again when pressure is removed. Tissue exhibiting blanchable erythema usually resumes its normal color and suffers no long-term damage; however, it can signal risk for future tissue damage. The term "reactive hyperemia" is a type of blanching erythema. Reactive hyperemia is a compensatory mechanism by the body to overcome the tissue deformation and ischemia caused by pressure.

Remember: If blanchable erythema exists, this is *not* a stage 1 pressure injury.

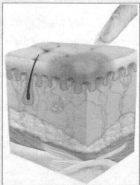

Used with permission of the National Pressure Injury Advisory Panel, 2020. Copyright © NPIAP.

Stage 1: Nonblanchable erythema of intact skin

In patients with darker skin tones, any type of erythema may be harder to discern. Use bright light and look for taut, shiny patches of skin that may have a purple or deep red hue. Also, assess the area carefully for localized heat, induration, or edema, which can be better indicators of impending or current tissue damage than erythema.

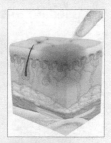

Nonblanchable erythema

In patients at high risk for pressure injuries, nonblanchable tissue can develop quickly and it signifies a stage 1 pressure injury. The redness associated with nonblanchable erythema is more intense and doesn't change when compressed with a finger. Nonblanchable erythema can be the first sign of tissue destruction. If recognized and treated early, nonblanchable erythema may be reversible.

Used with permission of the National Pressure Injury Advisory Panel, 2020. Copyright © NPIAP.

Remember to look for other signs of impending or existing tissue damage in patients with darker skin tones in whom erythema may not be as easily visible.

Source: Definitions were taken from https://npiap.com/page/PressureInjury/Stages

Stage 2 pressure injury: Partial-thickness skin loss with exposed dermis

"Partial-thickness loss of skin with exposed dermis. The wound bed is viable, pink or red, moist, and may also present as an intact or ruptured serum-filled blister. Adipose (fat) is not visible, and deeper tissues are not visible. Granulation tissue, slough, and eschar are not present. These injuries commonly result from adverse microclimate and shear in the skin over the pelvis and shear in the heel. This stage should not be used to describe moisture-associated skin damage (MASD) including incontinence-associated dermatitis (IAD), intertriginous dermatitis (ITD), medical adhesive-related skin injury (MARSI), or traumatic wounds (skin tears, burns, and abrasions)."

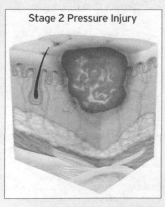

Stage 2 Pressure Injury

Used with permission of the National Pressure Injury Advisory Panel, 2020. Copyright © NPIAP.

(continued)

Stage 2 pressure injury: Partial-thickness skin loss with exposed dermis *(continued)*

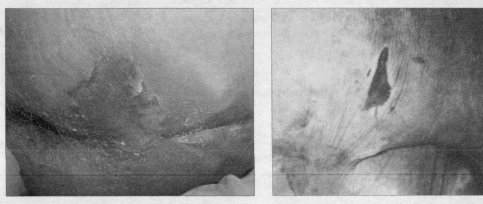

Used with permission of the National Pressure Injury Advisory Panel, 2020. Copyright © NPIAP.

Source: Definitions were taken from https://npiap.com/page/PressureInjury/Stages

Stage 3 pressure injury: Full-thickness skin loss

"Full-thickness loss of skin, in which adipose tissue is visible in the injury and granulation tissue and epibole (rolled wound edges) are often present. Slough and/or eschar may be visible. The depth of tissue damage varies by anatomic location; areas of significant adiposity can develop deep wounds. Undermining and tunneling may occur. Fascia, muscle, tendon, ligament, cartilage and/or bone are not exposed. If slough or eschar obscures the extent of tissue loss, this is an unstageable pressure injury."

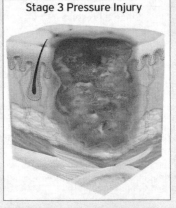

Stage 3 Pressure Injury

Used with permission of the National Pressure Injury Advisory Panel, 2020. Copyright © NPIAP.

Stage 3 pressure injury: Full-thickness skin loss

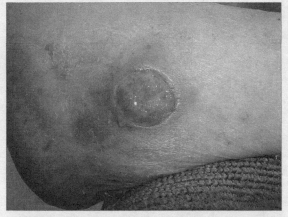

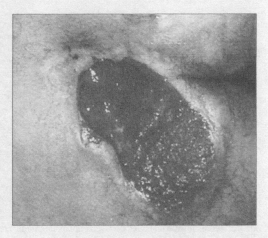

Used with permission of the National Pressure Injury Advisory
Panel, 2020. Copyright © NPIAP.

Source: Definitions were taken from https://npiap.com/page/PressureInjury/Stages

Stage 4 pressure injury: Full-thickness skin and tissue loss

"Full-thickness skin and tissue loss with exposed or directly palpable fascia, muscle, tendon, ligament, cartilage, or bone in the injury. Slough and/or eschar may be visible. Epibole is present. Undermining and/or tunneling often occur. Depth varies by anatomic location. If slough or eschar obscures the extent of tissue loss, this is an unstageable pressure injury."

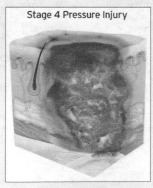

Stage 4 Pressure Injury

Used with permission of the
National Pressure Injury Advisory
Panel, 2020. Copyright © NPIAP.

(continued)

Stage 4 pressure injury: Full-thickness skin and tissue loss *(continued)*

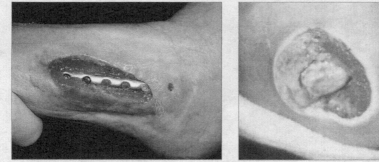

Used with permission of the National Pressure
Injury Advisory Panel, 2020. Copyright © NPIAP.

Source: Definitions were taken from https://npiap.com/page/PressureInjury/Stages

Unstageable pressure injury: Obscured full-thickness skin and tissue loss

"Full-thickness skin and tissue loss in which the extent of tissue damage within the ulcer cannot be confirmed because it is obscured by slough or eschar. If slough or eschar is removed, a stage 3 or stage 4 pressure injury will be revealed. Stable eschar (i.e., dry, adherent, intact without erythema or fluctuance) on the heel or ischemic limb *should not* be softened or removed."

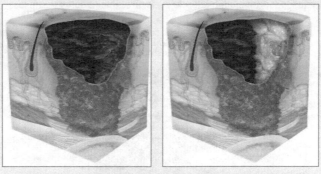

Used with permission of the National Pressure Injury Advisory Panel, 2020.
Copyright © NPIAP.

Unstageable pressure injury: Obscured full-thickness skin and tissue loss

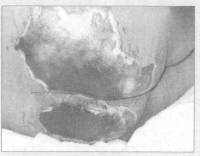

Source: Definitions were taken from https://npiap.com/page/PressureInjury/Stages

Deep tissue pressure injury: Persistent nonblanchable, deep red, maroon, or purple discoloration

"Intact or nonintact skin with localized area of persistent nonblanchable, deep red, maroon, purple discoloration or epidermal separation revealing a dark wound bed or blood-filled blister. Pain and temperature change often precede skin color changes. Discoloration may appear differently in darkly pigmented skin. This injury results from intense and/or prolonged pressure and shear forces at the bone–muscle interface. The wound may evolve rapidly to reveal the actual extent of tissue injury or may resolve without tissue loss. If necrotic tissue, subcutaneous tissue, granulation tissue, fascia, muscle, or other underlying structures are visible, this indicates a full-thickness pressure injury (unstageable, stage 3, or stage 4). Do not use 'deep tissue pressure injury' to describe vascular, traumatic, neuropathic, or dermatologic conditions."

In patients with darkly pigmented skin, remember to look carefully for localized heat, induration, or edema, which can be better indicators of impending or current tissue damage than erythema.

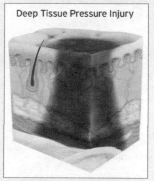

Deep Tissue Pressure Injury

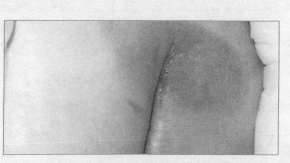

Used with permission of the
National Pressure Injury Advisory
Panel, 2020. Copyright © NPIAP.

Source: Definitions were taken from https://npiap.com/page/PressureInjury/Stages

Additional pressure injury definitions

Device-related pressure injury

"Device-related pressure injuries result from medical devices, equipment, furniture or everyday objects that have applied pressure to the skin. Medical device-related pressure injuries result from the use of devices designed and applied for diagnostic or therapeutic purposes. The resultant pressure injury generally conforms to the pattern or shape of the device. The term 'device related' describes the etiology of the pressure injury and not the extent of skin or tissue loss. The injury should be staged using the staging system."

Mucosal membrane pressure injury

"Mucosal membrane pressure injuries are pressure injuries of the moist membranes, usually in respiratory, gastrointestinal and genitourinary tracts. Mucosal membrane pressure injuries are usually caused by medical devices exerting sustained pressure and/or shear forces on the mucosa. Due to the anatomy of the tissue, these wounds cannot be staged using the pressure injury staging system."

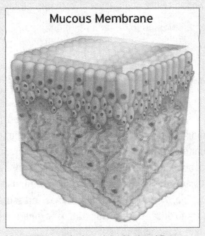

Mucous Membrane

Used with permission of the National Pressure Injury Advisory Panel, 2020. Copyright © NPIAP.

Source: Definitions were taken from https://npiap.com/page/PressureInjury/Stages

Location, location, location

The most common sites for pressure injuries to develop are the sacrum, coccyx, trochanters, ischial tuberosities, and heels.

However, any bony prominence where deformation of soft tissue can occur may result in a pressure injury. Pressure injuries can also develop on any soft tissue subjected to prolonged pressure or under medical devices. (See *Pressure points*.)

Pressure points

These illustrations show the areas at highest risk for **pressure injuries** when the patient is in different positions.

Occipital bone   Scapula   Vertebra   Sacrum   Coccyx   Calcaneus

Frontal bone   Mandible   Humerus   Sternum   Tuberosity of pelvis   Patella   Tibia

Scapula   Ribs   Iliac crest   Greater trochanter of femur   Lateral knee   Lateral malleolus   Medial malleolus

Used with permission from Taylor, C. R., Lillis, C., LeMone, P., & Lynn, P. (2008). *Fundamentals of nursing: The art and science of nursing care* (6th ed.). Lippincott Williams & Wilkins. Copyright © 2008 Lippincott Williams & Wilkins.

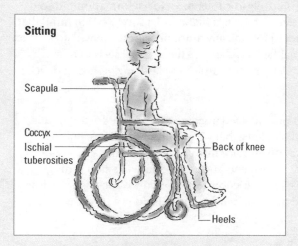

Sitting

Scapula

Coccyx
Ischial tuberosities

Back of knee

Heels

How do pressure injuries occur?

Pressure: Mechanical loads and deformation

The primary cause of pressure injuries is sustained mechanical loads applied to soft tissue, usually over a bony prominence. These mechanical loads result in damage to the tissue as a result of deformation of the skin and/or deeper tissues. The sustained deformation of the cells, blood vessels, and tissues is the driving force behind the development of a pressure injury. This deformation sets in motion many intersecting pathophysiologic pathways that result in tissue ischemia, tissue edema (as a result of inflammatory mediators), capillary distortion, reduced nutrient delivery to tissues, and obstruction of the lymphatics.

The magnitude and duration of these mechanical loads as well as the type of load (e.g., pressure, shear) are also important players. In pressure injury formation, an inverse relationship exists between time and pressure, meaning that pressure injuries can occur after a short period of intense pressure or due to a long period of lower sustained pressure. Furthermore, after the time–pressure threshold for damage passes, damage can still occur, even after the pressure is relieved.

Tissue tolerance

The ability of the individual patient's skin and underlying tissue to tolerate mechanical loads is also an important contributor to the development of pressure injuries.

Different tissues have different abilities to tolerate pressure. Muscle and fat have comparatively low tolerances for deformation-induced damage, whereas skin may have a higher tolerance. Keep in mind that the ability of tissues to tolerate any amount of pressure will depend on internal and external factors related to the patient, such as microclimate, nutrition, underlying comorbidities, and any perfusion deficits.

Friction

Friction is another potentially damaging mechanical force, but it is not considered a direct force that contributes to pressure injuries. Friction develops as one surface moves across another surface—for example, repetitive movements such as the patient's skin sliding across the bed sheet. Pure friction-related wounds such as abrasions are not considered pressure injuries and should not be staged using the staging system.

What about shear?

Shear is a mechanical force that occurs parallel—rather than perpendicular—to an area of tissue. In this illustration, gravity pulls the body down the incline of the bed and can contribute to pressure injury development. Shearing force is most likely to occur during repositioning or when a patient slides down after being placed in a high Fowler position. However, simply elevating the head of the bed increases shear and pressure in the sacral and coccygeal areas because gravity pulls the body down, but the skin on the back resists the motion due to friction between the skin and the sheets. The result is that the skeleton (and attached tissues) actually slides somewhat beneath the skin (evidenced by the puckering or wrinkling of skin in the gluteal area), generating shearing force between outer layers of tissue and deeper layers. The force generated is enough to obstruct, tear, or stretch blood vessels. Shearing forces can result in extensive and deep tissue damage. At the sacrum, shearing forces may contribute to tunneling or deep undermining at the wound edges that can be found in deeper pressure injuries such as stage 3 or 4 pressure injuries.

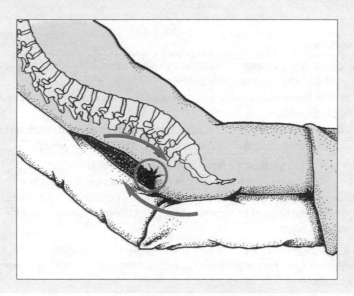

Moisture

The microclimate of the skin affects its structure and function as well as its response to mechanical load, so it is important to consider regarding the potential for pressure injury development. Prolonged exposure to moisture can waterlog, or macerate, skin. Maceration contributes to pressure injury formation by softening the epidermal and dermal layers. Macerated epidermis erodes more easily, degenerates, and can eventually slough off. In addition, damp skin adheres to bed linen more readily, making the effects of friction more profound. Consequently, moist skin is more likely to ulcerate than dry skin. Excessive moisture can result from perspiration, wound drainage, bathing, and/ or fecal or urinary incontinence. Remember that not all wounds that occur as a result of moisture are pressure injuries. (See Chapter 4 for more information on moisture-associated skin damage.)

Risk factors

There is no single risk factor that leads to pressure injury but instead a complicated interplay of factors. Some important factors that increase the risk of pressure injury development include advancing age; immobility; incontinence; poor nutrition; deficits in perfusion, circulation, and oxygenation; obesity; and diabetes mellitus. Patients at high risk, whether in acute care, long-term care, or at home, should be assessed regularly for pressure injuries.

Risk factor	Considerations
Advanced age	• Skin becomes more fragile as epidermal turnover slows, vascularization decreases, and skin layers adhere less tightly to one another. • Less lean body mass and less subcutaneous tissue cushioning bony areas may lead to tissue damage from shear and pressure. • Common problems in older adults such as poor nutrition, poor hydration, and impaired respiratory or immune systems may also contribute to pressure injury development.
Immobility	• Considered the greatest risk factor for pressure injury development • The person's ability to move in response to the sensation of pressure as well as the frequency with which the position is changed should always be considered in risk assessment. • Identifying the patient's underlying conditions that impact mobility is important when determining pressure injury risk.
Incontinence	• Increases a patient's exposure to moisture and over time, increases the risk of skin breakdown • Both urinary and fecal incontinence create problems as a result of excessive moisture and chemical irritation. • Due to pathogens in the stool, fecal incontinence can cause more skin damage than urinary incontinence.
Perfusion, circulation, and oxygenation impairment	• Studies have demonstrated that patients with perfusion and circulation deficits are at a higher risk for pressure injuries. Because there are a large number of clinical conditions that can affect perfusion and circulation, clinical judgment is needed to determine the potential impact on the risk for pressure injury development. • Smoking, peripheral vascular disease, cardiac disease, low blood pressure, and anemia are some clinical conditions to consider when assessing risk.
Nutrition	• Proper nutrition is vitally important to tissue integrity. • Nutrition is important to both pressure injury prevention and treatment. • Both inadequate nutritional intake and undernutrition have been found to be associated with pressure injury development. • A strong correlation exists between poor nutrition and poor pressure injury healing.

Diabetes mellitus	• Considered a strong risk factor for pressure injuries as it is both a microvascular and macrovascular disease.
	• Sensory (peripheral neuropathy) impairment and vascular deficits are strong risk factors.
Obesity	• Regardless of excess weight, patients may not have optimal nutrition and may be prone to developing protein calorie malnutrition during metabolic stress (even if they have excess body fat storage).
	• Adipose tissue has decreased vascularity.
	• May be unable to change position or move independently easily due to obesity
	• May be more susceptible to skin moisture in skin folds, promoting growth of organisms that can lead to infections

Risk factor assessment

Several validated pressure injury risk assessment tools are available to help determine a patient's risk of pressure injuries. The AHRQ recommends use of either the Norton Scale or Braden Scale.

The Norton Scale, developed over 50 years ago, measures pressure injury risk based on the following risk categories:

- physical condition
- mental state
- activity level
- mobility
- incontinence

The Braden Scale for Predicting Pressure Sore Risk is the most widely used and researched pressure injury risk assessment tool globally and the most common tool used across all health care settings.

The Braden Scale measures seven pressure injury risk factors on six subscales. Each subscale aligns with a risk factor and includes:

- sensory perception
- moisture
- activity
- mobility
- nutrition
- friction/shear

The lowest possible total score is 6 and the highest possible score is 23. Lower scores indicate higher pressure injury risk. A score of 18 or lower is what is commonly considered "at risk for pressure injury development." Remember, when developing a plan of care, your interventions should be targeted on the patient's subscale scores.

Risky business

Braden score	
15–18	At risk
13–14	Moderate risk
10–12	High risk
9 or less	Very high risk

Reproduced with permission from the Centre for Policy of Ageing (formerly NCCOP), London, UK.

Let's look at a patient example using the Braden Scale to determine pressure injury risk.

C.H. is a 75-year-old male admitted to your unit with a diagnosis of urinary tract infection. The patient is alert and oriented × 3 and is able to provide his past medical history. On assessment, you note that the patient has difficulty walking even short distances, and he tells you that he has limited sensation in both of his feet due to his diabetes. As a result, he tells you that he spends the majority of his day sitting in a recliner. He also tells you that he has not been eating well for the past month due to a lack of appetite, and he has lost 5 lb.

Using the Braden Scale, score each subscale:

Subscale	Score	Meaning
Sensory perception	3	Patient has decreased sensation (neuropathy) of the feet.
Moisture	4	No problem identified
Activity	3	Patient reports difficulty walking short distances.
Mobility	3	Mobility is slightly limited.
Nutrition	1	Patient has not been eating well for the past month and exhibits weight loss.
Friction/shear	3	No problem identified
Total score	17	At risk

This patient is at risk for a pressure injury based on the scoring criteria.

Practice point: subscales

Let's look more closely at the patient's Braden Scale score. When we look closely, the total score doesn't tell the whole story. It doesn't tell us which risk factors were the most significant for this patient.

Nutritional intake was rated as "very poor;" for this patient, this is a significant pressure injury risk factor that must be addressed with a nutritionist/dietitian consult. In addition, the patient has limited walking and is spending prolonged time periods in a chair, compromising activity and mobility. A chair cushion is a prevention strategy to consider for this patient as well as a physical therapy consult.

When calculating a patient's pressure injury risk score, each category receives a value based on the patient's condition. The sum of these values determines the patient's score and level of risk. However, the scores of each subscale are equally important when determining pressure injury risk for the patient. The subscale score provides a clue as to the most vulnerable area for the patient. This will help in planning pressure injury prevention strategies that will best match the individual needs of the patient.

How often?

Most health care agencies require an assessment score for every patient upon admission and have set guidelines for how frequently thereafter. For example, many acute care hospital policies require reassessment of patients every day or every shift. Patients should also be reassessed when there is a change in overall condition.

Prevention

Pressure injury prevention focuses on mitigating development by accurately assessing the patient's prevailing risk factors and then addressing these risk factors through the implementation of appropriate evidence-based pressure injury prevention strategies. See Appendix 3 for a pressure injury prevention algorithm.

Managing pressure

Managing the intensity and duration of mechanical load is key to preventing pressure injuries, especially for patients with limited mobility. Other prevention strategies include reducing friction and shear, minimizing moisture, maximizing nutritional status, and controlling chronic illnesses that contribute to pressure injury development, such as diabetes. Recently, prophylactic dressings made of soft silicone multilayered foam have been recommended over bony prominences in patients at high risk to prevent pressure injuries. Regular skin assessment and pressure injury risk assessment are vital parts of the prevention plan. Remember that early changes in darkly pigmented skin may not be easily visible, so these patients need especially careful assessment with attention to such factors as changes in temperature, pain, or skin texture (e.g., bogginess, edema).

Positioning

Repositioning schedules should be individualized to meet the patient's condition. No set time interval is recommended, but many facilities choose to reposition most patients every 2 hours. Any time you reposition the patient, look for telltale areas of reddened skin and make sure the new position offloads these areas.

Avoid the use of doughnut-shaped supports or ring cushions as these can reduce blood flow to an even wider expanse of tissue. If the affected area is on an extremity, use pillows to support the limb and reduce pressure. Avoid raising the head of the bed more than 30 degrees whenever clinically possible to prevent tissue damage due to friction and shearing force.

Baby steps

Inactivity increases a patient's risk of pressure injury development. To the degree that the patient is physically able, activity should be encouraged and incorporated into the daily plan of care. A physical therapist can assist with developing an activity plan appropriate for the patient.

Positioning a patient in bed

When the patient is positioned on the side, it is better to allow the weight to be evenly distributed between the sacrum and trochanter. When possible, the patient should not be positioned directly on the greater trochanter of the femur. Instead, position the patient at a 20- to 30-degree angle. Use a pillow or foam wedge to maintain the position. This position ensures pressure is evenly distributed between the trochanter and sacrum.

Five pillows or a combination of pillows and wedges is needed for adequate repositioning. A pillow under the head, on the abdomen for the arms, and between the knees to minimize the pressure exerted when one limb lies atop the other are three of the five. A pillow or wedge behind the upper back and behind the thighs assists in keeping the patient turned.

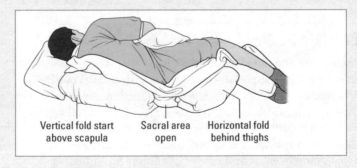

| Vertical fold start above scapula | Sacral area open | Horizontal fold behind thighs |

Suspending the heel is ideal

Heels should be elevated off the bed mattress in order to decrease pressure on them. Suspend the patient's foot so that the bony prominence on the heel is suspended and off of the pillow. A pillow or pressure redistribution cushion placed under the patient's calves (not under the knees) facilitates a comfortable position while suspending the foot. Remember to take care to avoid knee contraction. Patients with a high risk for developing heel pressure injuries may need special products designed to suspend the heel fully and redistribute pressure such as foam, gel, or air-filled boots. Any boots or devices should be removed daily to assess the skin for any impending damage to the lower legs or heels. Be sure that the straps that secure the boots are not positioned in such a way to cause pressure.

Positioning a seated patient

Sitting in a chair or wheelchair tends to focus the patient's weight on relatively small surface areas. Much of this weight is focused on the small area of tissue covering the ischial tuberosities. Pressure injuries occurring over the ischial tuberosities are usually associated with prolonged sitting. Proper posture and alignment help ensure that the weight of the patient's body is distributed as evenly as possible.

Proper posture preferred

Proper posture alone can significantly reduce the patient's pressure injury risk on the ankles, elbows, forearms, wrists, ischial tuberosities, and knees. Be sure to include these points when explaining proper posture to the patient:

- Sit with the back erect and against the back of the chair, thighs parallel to the floor, knees comfortably parted, and arms horizontal and supported by the arms of the chair. (This posture distributes weight evenly over the available body surface area.)
- Keep feet flat on the floor or on the wheelchair footrests to protect the heels from focused pressure.
- Avoid slouching, which causes shearing force and friction and places increased pressure on the sacrum and coccyx as well as the back.
- Keep thighs and arms parallel to ensure that weight is evenly distributed all along the thighs and forearms instead of being focused on the ischial tuberosities and elbows, respectively.
- Keep knees and ankles apart to protect from rubbing together.

Put your feet up

If the patient is sitting in a chair and likes to use an ottoman or footstool, check to see if the knees are positioned above the level of the hips. If so, it means that weight has shifted from the back of the thighs to the ischial tuberosities. The same problem—knees above hips—can occur if the chair itself is too short for the patient. In this case, use of a different footstool or chair is recommended.

Repositioning in the chair

Patients at risk should reposition themselves while sitting if they are able. Repositioning intervals should be geared and timed with regard to the individual needs of the patient. Patients can perform wheelchair pushups and weight shifts to intermittently relieve pressure on the buttocks and sacrum; however, this requires a fair amount of upper body strength. A reclined position in the chair is recommended to reduce pressure on the ischial tuberosities. In patients at high risk for pressure injuries, it is recommended that the amount of time seated in a chair be limited.

For patients who spend longer periods of time in a wheelchair and are at risk for pressure injuries (e.g., patients with spinal cord injuries), it is recommended that the patient be referred to a seating specialist for specialized pressure mapping and cushion selection.

Support aids and cushions

A vast array of support surfaces and cushioning devices are available for use in all settings to aid in repositioning and to redistribute pressure such as specialty beds, mattresses, and seating options that employ foams, gels, and air. These devices make it possible to tailor a comprehensive and individualized system of supports for the patient. Remember, effective care depends on knowledge of the classes and types of products available. (See *Pressure redistribution devices*.)

Pressure redistribution devices

Special beds, mattresses, and seating pads help redistribute pressure when a patient is confined to one position for long periods.

Comparing support surface characteristics

Reactive surfaces may be powered or nonpowered and change their load properties in response to the applied load (the individual's movement, size, and weight). Meanwhile, active surfaces are powered surfaces that have the ability to change their load distribution with or without applied load, such as the body surface.

Specialty support surfaces (beds and mattresses) distribute load over the contact areas of the body. They work by managing tissue load and microclimate. Check specific product information to determine what is the best for the individualized patient's needs.

A word about standards testing for support surfaces: The Rehabilitation Engineering and Assistive Technology Society of North America (RESNA), in collaboration with the American National Standards Institute (ANSI) and the NPIAP, has published standards to test the characteristics of mattresses and support surfaces. These standards are used to guide manufacturers in new product development and to ensure quality standards are met by manufacturers. More information on this initiative can be found on the NPIAP website.

Important points

The EPUAP, NPIAP, and PPPIA in *Prevention and Treatment of Pressure Ulcers/Injuries: Clinical Practice Guideline* (Haesler, 2019, p. 156) suggested that a support surface should be selected based on the following factors:

- Level of mobility and inactivity of the individual
- The need to influence microclimate and shear reduction
- The individual's size and weight
- The number, severity, and location of existing pressure injuries
- The individual's risk for developing new pressure injuries

Pressure redistribution devices

Other considerations

- Many surfaces are contraindicated with unstable cervical, thoracic, or lumbar spine injuries.
- Consider fall risk and bed height when selecting the appropriate bed.

Need help deciding?

An algorithm, developed by the Wound, Ostomy, and Continence Nurses Society™, is available as a resource to help guide the clinician to the appropriate support surface at https://algorithm.wocn.org/#home.

Specialty beds and mattresses

Air-fluidized therapy bed

In an air-fluidized therapy bed, an air-fluidized chamber contains silicone-coated beads that create air and fluid support. When air is pumped through the beads, they act like liquid, and a third of the patient's body floats above the surface while the rest is immersed in the bed so that more surface area is in contact with the beads to decrease pressure on body points.

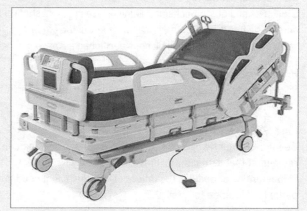

The fluid-like surface of an air-fluidized therapy bed redistributes pressure on the skin by forcing air through the beads. It conforms to the body as the patient sinks into the surface.

It helps prevent pressure injuries and promotes wound healing. Because this is a high-air loss surface,

it promotes evaporation and is especially useful when skin maceration is a problem. However, a risk of dehydration with the use of high-air loss beds exists.

Low-air loss beds and mattresses

Low-air loss therapy beds and mattresses contain segmented air cushions that inflate to help redistribute pressure on skin surfaces and to minimize shearing force during repositioning. The beds also help manage heat and humidity, maintaining a healthy microclimate for the skin. Mattresses with low-air loss technology can also be placed on a standard hospital bed frame.

For patients with multiple stage 2 pressure injuries or multiple stage 3 or 4 pressure injuries on the trunk and pelvis involving more than one turning surface, a low-air loss mattress or bed or air-fluidized therapy should be considered.

Other considerations

Beds or mattresses that have the "turn-assist" feature are helpful in preventing back injuries among staff and facilitating the turning of patients, but manual turning is still imperative to redistribute pressure. Continuous lateral rotation therapy (CLRT) beds that rotate are used to improve pulmonary function in patients who are critically ill and will alter the patient's position during the rotation; however, this *does not* constitute repositioning the patient for pressure injury prevention. Patients on CLRT still need to be manually repositioned.

Mattress overlays

The most common mattress overlays used in pressure injury prevention are made of foam, air, and gel. If the patient's weight completely compresses a mattress overlay, the overlay won't help. Follow the manufacturer's instructions for

(continued)

Pressure redistribution devices *(continued)*

weight limit. Palm or hand checks are not advised by the NPIAP as there is no research to support this potentially unsafe practice.

Alternating-pressure mattresses

An alternating-pressure mattress is also a mattress overlay that can redistribute pressure using cyclic changes that create alternating low- and high-pressure areas.

Mechanical lifting devices

Lift sheets and other mechanical lifting devices prevent shearing by lifting the patient rather than dragging the patient across the bed. Check with the manufacturer of the product to determine if the lift sheet used with the lifting device is safe to be left under the patient once positioned as these can become a source of pressure.

Positioning devices

Pillows, wedges, and conformational positioning devices can also be used to assist with proper repositioning of the patient while in bed.

False security

Be informed but be cautious as well. Using these devices can instill a false sense of security. It is important to remember that as helpful as these devices may be, they aren't substitutes for attentive care. Patients require individual turning schedules regardless of the equipment used, and this schedule depends on your assessment of the patient's tolerance for pressure.

Seating considerations

Both patients who are ambulatory and at risk for pressure injury and who use wheelchairs should use seat cushions to distribute weight over the largest possible surface area. Patients who use wheelchairs require especially durable seat cushions that can stand up to the rigors of daily use. Cushions are made of foam, gel, or air bladders.

Many wheelchair-seating clinics now use computers to create custom seating systems tailored to fit the physiology and needs of each patient. For patients with spinal cord injuries, the selection of wheelchair seating is based on pressure evaluation, lifestyle, postural stability, continence, and cost. Custom seats and cushions are more expensive, but these may be a good choice for the patient. Encourage patients who use wheelchairs to replace seat cushions as soon as their current one begins to deteriorate.

Managing nutrition

Proper nutrition, including a balanced dietary intake and maintaining proper weight, is essential to both pressure injury prevention and healing. For all patients at risk for pressure injuries or with existing pressure injuries, nutritional screening should be conducted and a nutritional consult with a registered dietitian or nutritionist should be initiated (Munoz et al., 2020).

Dietary intake

Protein is particularly important to skin maintenance and wound healing. The patient needs a balanced diet that includes about 1 to

1.5 g/kg/day of protein. This is especially important for older adults. Sources of protein can include meats, milk, cheese, and eggs. When needed, protein supplements can be added to the diet to boost protein intake. Keep in mind that the patient's kidney function should be assessed to determine if high levels of protein are appropriate.

Body weight

Low body weight can be a problem for many patients with existing pressure injuries or at risk for them. An underlying illness or anorexia can make eating undesirable or impossible. Weighing the patient weekly is one way to monitor the results of nutritional interventions; however, don't base your nutritional assessment solely on weight. If the patient's history includes an unintentional weight loss of 10 lb (4.5 kg) or more during the previous 6 months, a nutrition consult should be obtained with a registered dietitian or nutritionist. Keep in mind that body weight may be skewed in certain patients, such as a patient with heart failure or anasarca, so it may not be a reliable indicator of nutritional status. Therefore, when assessing nutritional risk, a holistic approach should be taken. See Appendix 4.

Complications

Complications, such as bleeding or infection, may develop during the care of a patient with a pressure injury. If a pressure injury begins to bleed, apply direct pressure to the site. If the bleeding continues despite pressure, notify the practitioner. Be alert for foul-smelling drainage, a temperature over 101°F (38.3°C), increased pain from the injury site, or erythema that increases on the skin surrounding the pressure injury. If you notice any of these symptoms, notify the health care provider.

Treatment

Treatment of pressure injuries follows basic steps common to all wound care.

A key element in all pressure injury treatment plans is identifying and treating the underlying pathophysiology whenever possible. In the case of pressure injuries, since pressure is usually the primary causative agent, alleviating pressure is imperative for healing to occur. However, you will recall that many intrinsic factors such as poor nutrition, impaired tissue tolerance, and impaired perfusion can also negatively influence pressure injury healing.

Remember to include the patient and caregiver in the treatment plan to improve the potential for wound healing. See Chapter 3, "Wound Bed Preparation," and Chapter 9, "Wound Management."

Patient education

Remember that the goal of patient education is to improve the outcome. For any care plan to succeed after the patient leaves the health care facility, they and their caregiver must understand the care plan, be physically and financially capable of carrying it out at home, and value both the information and the outcomes. Therefore, education and goal establishment should take into consideration the preferences and lifestyles of the patient and their family whenever possible.

Teach the patient and family how to prevent pressure injuries and what to do when they occur. (See *Pressure injury dos and don'ts.*) For example, explain the importance of repositioning and demonstrate what a 20- to 30-degree laterally inclined position looks like. If assistive devices for repositioning are required, make sure the appropriate types of devices are identified and where they can be obtained.

Get wise to wounds

Pressure injury dos and don'ts

With proper skin care and frequent position changes, patients and their caregivers can keep the patient's skin healthy—a crucial element in pressure injury prevention. Here are some important dos and don'ts to pass along:

Do...

• reposition the patient at a frequency based on the patient's individual needs and condition. In general, an every-2-hour repositioning schedule should be followed; however, this should be altered as needed to meet the goals for the patient. Position the patient on their right side, then left side, then back. Lying on the stomach is also fine if it is tolerated by the patient.
• use pillows and positioning devices for support. Small weight shifts can also be used to offload vulnerable areas of skin.
• check the skin for early signs of pressure injury at least daily.
• use a mirror to view bony prominences that can't be inspected directly, such as the shoulders, coccyx, hips, elbows, heels, and back of the head.
• report any skin changes to the health care provider.
• follow the prescribed mobility program based on the patient's abilities, including range-of-motion exercises.
• maintain a balanced nutritional plan including adequate fluid intake. Consult a registered dietitian or nutritionist as needed for development of an individualized nutritional plan.
• cleanse the skin after incontinence episodes to reduce the harmful effects of stool and/or urine on the skin.
• moisturize skin regularly to maintain skin integrity.

Don't...

• use commercial soaps or skin products that dry or irritate skin.
• massage reddened areas.
• position the patient over wrinkled bed sheets as wrinkles can be a source of pressure.

Dressings at home

If the patient needs to apply dressings at home, make sure the proper application and removal techniques are taught. Refer all discharged patients with a high risk for pressure injury formation or existing pressure injuries to home health care agencies for further assessment and evaluation.

Nag about nutrition

Ensuring proper nutrition can be difficult, but the patient and family need to know how important proper nutrition is to both preventing pressure injuries and the healing process. Provide materials on nutrition and maintaining an ideal weight as appropriate. A consult with a registered dietitian or nutritionist should be arranged for all patients at risk for or with an existing pressure injury.

In the name of progress

Pressure injuries require regular reassessments in order to determine wound improvement or deterioration. Progress can be measured by the reduction in necrotic tissue and drainage and the increase in granulation tissue and epithelial growth. Clean, vascularized pressure injuries should show some evidence of improvement within 2 weeks. If they don't and the patient has followed the guidelines for nutrition, repositioning, use of support surfaces, and wound care, it's time to reevaluate the care plan and a consult or reconsult with a wound care practitioner may be indicated.

The NPIAP has developed the Pressure Ulcer Scale for Healing (PUSH) tool that can be utilized to measure a wound's healing and response to interventions. Recent studies have shown that this tool is easy to use and reliable. It's a validated tool for assessing pressure injury healing rates. (See Appendix 5 for more information on the *PUSH tool*.)

Pressure injury controversies

Are all pressure injuries the result of poor or inadequate nursing care? This debate is ongoing; however, research seems to support that some pressure injuries are unavoidable, especially among high-risk patients. Sometimes pressure injuries develop despite the consistent use of all pressure injury prevention strategies. If documentation clearly notes that everything possible is being implemented to prevent pressure injuries and the patient is in serious or critical condition, a newly acquired pressure injury may have been unavoidable. However, it should be noted that to date, the term "unavoidable pressure injury" is not recognized by regulatory agencies in acute care settings. This term, however, is recognized and has regulatory support in the long-term care setting.

Skin failure is another condition recognized by wound care experts, and research into this phenomenon is ongoing. Skin failure may be an acute phenomenon associated with critical illness or associated with the end of life. Examples of wounds associated with the end of life are the Trombley–Brennan Terminal Tissue Injury and the Kennedy Terminal Ulcer. The Kennedy Terminal Ulcer is described as a wound that develops rapidly and is typically found on the sacral area. It is usually butterfly shaped and may be red, purple, or yellow in color. It is usually seen in the hours or days before death. More research is still needed in this area in order to better distinguish a wound caused by skin failure or a pressure injury.

Quick quiz

1. Match the illustrations of pressure injuries with their correct stage.

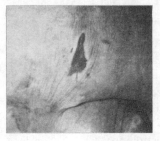

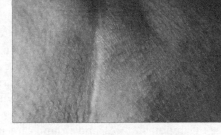

A.   Stage 1

B.   Stage 2

C.   Stage 3

D.   Stage 4

1.

2.

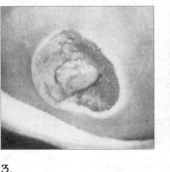

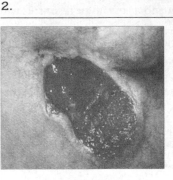

3.

4.

Answer: 1. B; 2. A; 3. D; 4. C

2. What is the first step when treating a patient's pressure injury?
    A.   Providing a moist wound environment
    B.   Thoroughly assessing the systemic and local risk factors
    C.   Lightly filling areas of undermining
    D.   Preventing infection

Answer: B. A full assessment of the patient's underlying risk factors is the first step.

3. An older adult patient is admitted to your nursing unit. What is the best way to assess the patient for pressure injury risk?
    A. The PUSH tool
    B. The patient's ability to reposition themselves in bed
    C. Your experience with other similar patients
    D. The Braden Pressure Sore Risk Assessment Scale

Answer: D. The Braden Pressure Sore Risk Assessment Scale is commonly used to assess pressure injury risk.

4. Which intervention is most appropriate for offloading the heels?
    A. Flexing the knees
    B. Placing a doughnut-shaped cushion under the feet
    C. Suspending the heels by placing a pillow under the calves
    D. Putting a pressure-reducing foam mattress under the heels

Answer: C. Suspending the heels using a pillow under the calves is the best way to protect heels from pressure injury.

5. Which body position simultaneously relieves pressure on the sacrum and trochanter?
    A. Prone
    B. Supine
    C. 30-degree lateral position
    D. High Fowler

Answer: C. The 30-degree lateral position is the best way to relieve pressure on both the sacrum and the trochanter.

6. A nurse assesses a newly admitted patient and identifies Braden subscores of 2 in each of the six categories. What are the priority nursing interventions? Select all that apply.
    A. Reassess the patient in 2 weeks.
    B. Consult with a dietitian.
    C. Manage skin moisture and incontinence.
    D. Institute an appropriate repositioning schedule.

Answer: B, C, and D. If the patient has scores of 2 in each of the six categories, the patient's total Braden Score is 12. A score of 12 indicates high risk for pressure injury development. Consulting with a dietitian, managing skin moisture and incontinence, and instituting an appropriate repositioning schedule are appropriate interventions for the nurse to take. This patient should be reassessed daily.

7. Registered dietitians, physical therapists, and occupational therapists can help prevent pressure injuries in patients at high risk. True or false?

Answer: True. Pressure injury prediction, prevention, and treatment require a multidisciplinary plan of care. Adequate dietary intake and maintaining patient mobility are important aspects of care.

8. All pressure injuries are avoidable and the result of poor nursing care. True or false?

Answer: False. New evidence has determined that some pressure injuries may be unavoidable due to the clinical status of the patient. It is important to implement all possible nursing interventions to prevent pressure injuries even in the most critically ill patients or patients at the end of life.

Scoring

☆☆☆ If you answered all eight questions correctly, congratulations! You've certainly demonstrated that you can handle the pressure.

☆☆ If you answered five or six questions correctly, nicely done! You're near the top of the pressure gradient.

☆ If you answered fewer than five questions correctly, don't despair! You'll reposition yourself soon.

Select references

Agency for Healthcare Research and Quality. (2014). *Preventing pressure ulcers in hospitals.* https://www.ahrq.gov/sites/default/files/publications/files/putoolkit.pdf

Ayello, E. A., Levine, J. M., Langemo, D., Kennedy-Evans, K. L., Brennan, M. R., & Sibbald, R. G. (2019). Reexamining the literature on terminal ulcers, SCALE, skin failure, and unavoidable pressure injuries. *Advances in Skin & Wound Care, 32*(3), 109–121. https://doi.org/10.1097/01.ASW.0000553112.55505.5f

Baranoski, S., & Ayello, E. A. (Eds.). (2020). *Wound care essentials: Practice principles* (5th ed.). Wolters Kluwer.

Borchert, K. (2021). Pressure injury prevention: Implementing and maintaining a successful plan and program. In L. L. McNichol, C. R. Ratliff, & S. S. Yates (Eds.), *Wound, Ostomy and Continence Nurses Society core curriculum: Wound management* (2nd ed., pp. 395–423). Wolters Kluwer.

Bryant, R. A., & Nix, D. P. (Eds.). (2016). *Acute & chronic wounds: Current management concepts* (5th ed.). Mosby-Elsevier.

Edsberg, L. (2021). Pressure and shear injuries. In L. L. McNichol, C. R. Ratliff, & S. S. Yates (Eds.), *Wound, Ostomy and Continence Nurses Society core curriculum: Wound management* (2nd ed., pp. 372–394). Wolters Kluwer. https://bookshelf.vitalsource.com/#/books/9781975164614/

Haesler, E. (Ed.). (2019). *European Pressure Ulcer Advisory Panel, National Pressure Injury Advisory Panel and Pan Pacific Pressure Injury Alliance. Prevention and treatment of pressure ulcers/injuries: Clinical practice guideline.* Cambridge Media.

Langemo, D., & Parish, L. C. (2022). The past, present, and future of skin failure. *Advances in Skin & Wound Care, 35*(2), 81–83. https://doi.org/10.1097/01.ASW.0000803596.89726.6e

Mackey, D., & Watts, C. (2021). Therapeutic surfaces for bed and chair. In L. L. McNichol, C. R. Ratliff, & S. S. Yates (Eds.), *Wound, Ostomy and Continence Nurses Society core curriculum: Wound management* (2nd ed., pp. 372–394). Wolters Kluwer. https://bookshelf.vitalsource.com/#/books/9781975164614/

Munoz, N., Posthauer, M. E., Cereda, E., Schols, J., & Haesler, E. (2020). The role of nutrition for pressure injury prevention and healing: The 2019 international clinical practice guideline recommendations. *Advances in Skin & Wound Care, 33*(3), 123–136. https://doi.org/10.1097/01.ASW.0000653144.90739.ad

National Pressure Injury Advisory Panel. (n.d.-a). *Pressure injury fact sheet.* https://npiap.com/store/viewproduct.aspx?id=14427618&hhSearchTerms=%22pressure+and+injury+and+fact%22

National Pressure Injury Advisory Panel. (n.d.-b). *Support surface standards initiative (S3I).* https://npiap.com/page/S3I

Padula, W. V., & Delarmente, B. A. (2019). The national cost of hospital-acquired pressure injuries in the United States. *International Wound Journal, 16*(3), 634–640. https://doi.org/10.1111/iwj.13071

Pickham, D., Berte, N., Pihulic, M., Valdez, A., Mayer, B., & Desai, M. (2018). Effect of a wearable patient sensor on care delivery for preventing pressure injuries in acutely ill adults: A pragmatic randomized clinical trial (LS-HAPI study). *International Journal of Nursing Studies, 80*, 12–19. https://doi.org/10.1016/j.ijnurstu.2017.12.012

Pittman, J., Beeson, T., Dillon, J., Yang, Z., Mravec, M., Malloy, C., & Cuddigan, J. (2021). Hospital-acquired pressure injuries and acute skin failure in critical care: A case-control study. *Journal of Wound, Ostomy, and Continence Nursing, 48*(1), 20–30. https://doi.org/10.1097/WON.0000000000000734

Wound, Ostomy, and Continence Nurses Society. (n.d.). *An evidence- and consensus-based support surface algorithm.* https://algorithm.wocn.org/#home

Chapter 7

Lower extremity ulcers: vascular and neuropathic

Just the facts

In this chapter, you'll learn about:

- ◆ causes, assessment, prevention, and interventions for lower extremity venous disease (LEVD)
- ◆ causes, assessment, prevention, and interventions for lower extremity arterial disease (LEAD)
- ◆ causes, assessment, prevention, and interventions for lower extremity lymphatic issues
- ◆ causes, assessment, prevention, and interventions for lower extremity neuropathic disease (LEND)

The vascular system

The vascular system is composed of arteries, veins, capillaries, and lymphatics. Pressure from the beating heart carries blood away from the heart through the arteries into progressively smaller vessels until they connect to the capillaries. On the other side of the capillaries, small veins receive blood and pass it into progressively larger veins on its return trip to the heart. The lymphatic system is a separate system of vessels that collects waste products and delivers them to the venous system.

Disorders that affect the lymphatic vessels (blood vessels outside the heart) are known collectively as peripheral vascular disease (PVD). Vascular ulcers are chronic wounds that stem from PVD in the venous, arterial, and lymphatic systems. Venous and arterial ulcers are most common in the distal lower extremities, whereas lymphatic ulcers occur in the arms or the legs.

A look at lower extremity vascular ulcers

Lower extremity (vascular) ulcers are common in the United States, affecting as many as 2% of adults each year; they are more prevalent in older adults (Singer et al., 2017). Current evidence indicates that as many as 15% of older adults in the United States will develop a lower extremity ulcer (Singer et al., 2017). Lower extremity vascular ulcers are typically broken into two groups, leg and foot ulcers, and can include venous, arterial, and lymphatic ulcers as well as neuropathic ulcers and pressure injuries. Chronic ulcers are defined as those that fail to heal or show any signs of healing after 4 weeks.

Types of vascular ulcers

Type of ulcer	Typical location	Clinical findings	Image of the wound
Venous	• Anywhere from ankle to midcalf • Most common on the medial aspect of the ankle above the malleolus	• Irregular shape that can be large • Can drain heavily but can also become dry, crusted, or moist with slightly macerated borders • Shallow wound base covered with beefy red granulation tissue, yellow film, or gray necrotic tissue (black necrotic tissue is rarely present except in acute injury.)	
Arterial	Tips of toes, corners of nail beds on toes, over bony prominences, and between the toes	• Pale or mottled wound, generally small in size and can look "punched out" • Well-demarcated wound edges • Dry wound base with no granulation tissue due to impaired blood flow to tissue • Presence of necrotic tissue (common) or hard, dark, dry, and leathery eschar • Surrounding skin that feels cooler than normal on palpation	
Lymphatic	Arms and legs, most commonly ankle area; these ulcers are rare.	• Shallow ulcer bed that may be oozing, moist, or blistered • Firm, fibrotic surrounding skin thickened by edema • Possible cellulitis	

As many as 90% of all leg ulcers are venous ulcers and most commonly occur on the lower extremities between the malleoli and calves, also known as the gaiter area (Schneider et al., 2021).

Venous ulcers

Venous ulcers arise when valves in the leg veins become damaged. Damage to the valves results in dilation of the veins and retrograde blood flow as the body cannot efficiently circulate blood back to the heart. As blood remains in the veins of the leg, this can result in a buildup of pressure as well as the leakage of fluid, resulting in edema. Trauma to the leg, ankle, or foot can result in the development of an open wound or venous ulcer.

Venous disorders are the most common type of vascular conditions and encompass venous insufficiency, venous disease, and other conditions such as venous thromboembolism. The primary cause of venous insufficiency is hypertension in the venous system or obstructions from blood clots, whereas venous disease is a progressive disorder that leads to damaged veins and at worst, ulceration.

Vein anatomy and function

In the circulatory system, arteries carry blood away from the heart and veins carry blood back to the heart. Capillaries connect these two systems. On the venous side, venules are the small veins that receive blood from the capillaries and deliver it to the larger veins for its return trip to the heart.

Types of veins

In the lower portion of the body where venous ulcers develop, there are three major types of veins: superficial veins, perforator veins, and deep veins.

Skin deep

Superficial veins lie just beneath the skin and drain into deep veins through perforator veins. Varicose veins are superficial veins that have become stretched and tortuous.

Central connectors

Perforator veins connect the superficial veins to the deep veins. Their name is derived from the fact that they perforate the deep fasciae as they connect superficial veins to the deep venous system.

U-turns

Deep veins receive venous blood from the perforator veins and return it to the heart. The major deep veins in the leg include the posterior tibial veins, anterior tibial veins, peroneal veins, and the popliteal veins. Each of these veins parallels a corresponding artery. (See *Major lower limb veins*.)

Major lower limb veins

Venous ulcers most commonly occur in the lower extremities. This illustration shows the major veins in this part of the body.

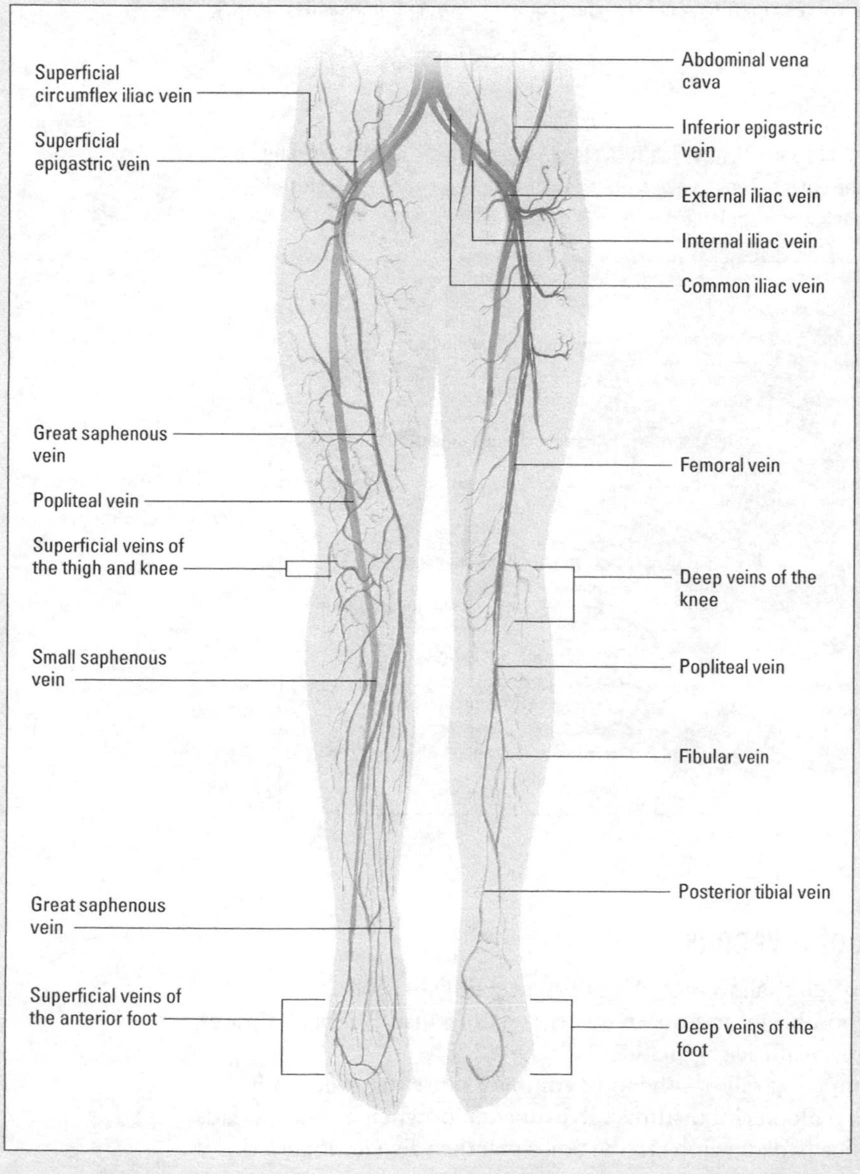

Superficial circumflex iliac vein

Superficial epigastric vein

Abdominal vena cava

Inferior epigastric vein

External iliac vein

Internal iliac vein

Common iliac vein

Great saphenous vein

Popliteal vein

Superficial veins of the thigh and knee

Femoral vein

Deep veins of the knee

Small saphenous vein

Popliteal vein

Fibular vein

Great saphenous vein

Posterior tibial vein

Superficial veins of the anterior foot

Deep veins of the foot

Vein walls and valves

Compared to arteries of the same size, veins have thinner walls and wider diameters. Vein walls have three distinct layers: an inner, endothelial layer (tunica intima); a middle layer of smooth muscle (tunica media); and an outer, supportive layer (tunica adventitia).

Veins also have a unique system of cup-shaped valves. The valves function to keep blood flowing in one direction—toward the heart. Deep veins have more of these valves than superficial veins, and veins in the lower leg have more of these valves than veins in the thigh. In perforator veins, the valves open toward the deep veins. (See *A close look at a vein.*)

A close look at a vein

This cross-section of a vein clearly illustrates the three layers of the vein wall and its unique cup-shaped valves. These valves open toward the heart and when closed, prevent blood from flowing backward.

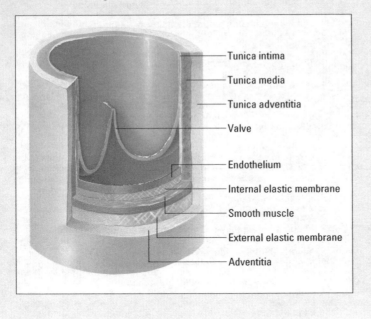

- Tunica intima
- Tunica media
- Tunica adventitia
- Valve
- Endothelium
- Internal elastic membrane
- Smooth muscle
- External elastic membrane
- Adventitia

Development of a venous ulcer

When leg veins fail to propel a sufficient supply of blood back to the heart, blood begins to pool in the legs (venous insufficiency). Causes of venous insufficiency include:

- incompetent valves—the most common cause that can result when a blood clot disrupts valve function or when a vein distends (venous hypertension) to the point that the valve no longer closes completely.

- inadequate calf muscle function.
- poor range of motion of the ankle.
- damaged perforator veins.

Risk factors for venous insufficiency

Major risk factors for venous insufficiency include:
- older age.
- female sex.
- obesity.
- prolonged sitting or standing.
- family history.
- lower leg trauma.
- venous thromboembolism (deep vein thrombosis).
- pregnancy.

Signs of venous insufficiency

Signs of venous insufficiency are progressive and classified.
- Edema is one of the first signs and can be pitting or nonpitting.

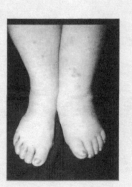
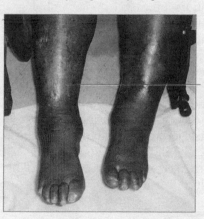

Swelling of the lower legs with brown discoloration and small ulcers characterize venous insufficiency.

- Telangiectasia—the superficial veins just below the skin's surface become dilated, producing a weblike appearance of the skin, sometimes referred to as spider veins.
- Hyperpigmentation in the calves and around the gaiter area (between the malleoli and calves) due to buildup of hemosiderin is the result of breakdown of red blood cells that have leaked into tissue, sometimes referred to as brown staining.

(continued)

Signs of venous insufficiency *(continued)*

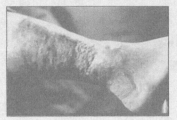

- Atrophie blanche appears as round spots of ivory-white plaque in the skin, usually surrounded by hyperpigmentation.
- Lipodermatosclerosis is a hardening condition of the skin caused by inflammation of the fat that can cause a constriction around the lower leg, giving the appearance of an upside-down champagne bottle.
- Venous eczema is characterized by red, flaky, and sometimes raised areas referred to as stasis dermatitis.
- Venous ulceration is the most severe consequence of venous disease, resulting in tissue loss.

Symptoms of venous insufficiency

Many patients with venous insufficiency report dull, aching pain or heaviness that is relieved by elevation of the leg. Itching, throbbing, burning, and muscle cramps during walking or exercising (venous claudication) are other commonly reported symptoms. Feelings of irritability and fatigue may be prevalent.

Physical activity is crucial to adequate venous return. Leg muscle paralysis or prolonged inactivity such as bed rest during hospitalization can drastically hinder the amount of blood returning to the heart. The blood then pools in the legs, causing swelling and putting patients at risk for blood clots. During hospitalization, patients should have some type of venous embolism prevention in place, such as stockings or pumps. When discharged, higher compression will be necessary to manage the venous insufficiency.

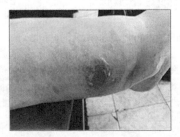

Care considerations

The goal of nursing care is to protect the affected skin by covering the wound with nonadherent dressings. Compression therapy should also be emphasized as this is considered the standard of care for both preventing and treating venous leg ulcers. Patients should be encouraged to walk and exercise and stop any smoking. Many walking and smoking cessation programs are readily available. Exercise can improve calf muscle function to help improve blood flow in the leg. Often, patients with venous insufficiency will need revascularization procedures to enhance blood flow.

A closer look at venous ulcers

Venous ulcers most commonly occur above the medial malleolus. These ulcers have irregular borders and typically appear moist.

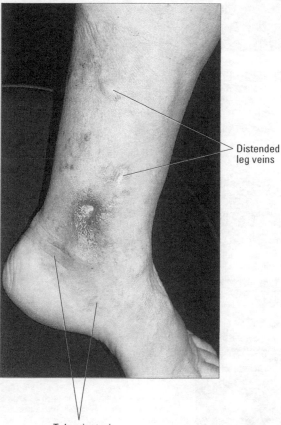

Distended leg veins

Telangiectasis

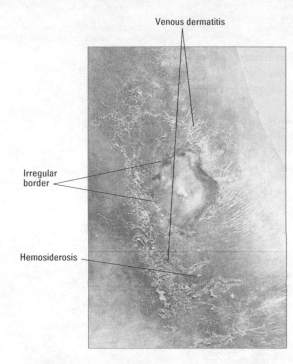

Venous dermatitis

Irregular border

Hemosiderosis

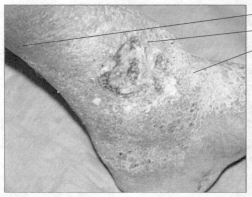

Hemosiderosis

Lipodermatosclerosis

Venous dermatitis

Moist, beefy red wound base

Diagnostic tests

Diagnostic tests for venous ulcers include plethysmography, venous duplex scanning, and venography.

Plethysmography

Plethysmography records changes in the volumes and sizes of extremities by measuring changes in blood volume. Types of plethysmography include:

- air plethysmography—uses an inflatable pneumatic cuff placed around the limb to obtain volume measurements and standing and walking pressures. It gives an overall assessment of the venous functioning but is not specific to the exact location of reflux.
- photoplethysmography—uses infrared light transmitted through the skin to measure venous reflux and filling times; delayed healing can be predicted by abnormal filling times. Duplex ultrasonography is necessary to accurately find the location of reflux.

Duplex ultrasonography

Venous duplex scanning is used to assess venous patency and reflux by measuring and recording venous pressures along an extremity as its veins are compressed and released. An experienced technician can use venous duplex scanning to identify thrombosis within a vein and determine whether it is acute or chronic as well as to assess venous reflux and the status of valve function. The test is more accurate than venography, reproducible, noninvasive, and less expensive than venography.

Venography

Venography is the radiographic examination of a vein that has been injected with a contrast medium. In the past, this was the only test available to evaluate venous thrombosis; however, with the advent of newer noninvasive tests, venography is rarely used today since it is expensive, uncomfortable for the patient, and can be associated with deep vein thrombosis and complications related to the administration of contrast.

Treatment

Effective treatment of a venous ulcer involves caring for the wound and managing the underlying venous disease. Controlling edema is the most important goal in managing chronic venous insufficiency. Methods to control edema include elevation of the affected limb, compression therapy, and sometimes medication or surgery. Wound care involves selecting the best dressing for the venous ulcer.

Elevation of the limb

An effective method of reducing edema is to elevate the leg and allow gravity to drain fluid from it. This is best accomplished with the patient in bed with the legs elevated above the level of the heart. However, a patient with a cardiac or pulmonary condition may find this position intolerable. In this case, any elevation that the patient can tolerate is beneficial.

Compression therapy

Compression therapy is the most effective way of managing edema. A general rule is that higher compression is better than lower compression and some compression is better than none. Compression bandages and stockings are used when a patient can't elevate the affected limb and is ambulatory. Various rigid and more flexible types of compression bandages are available. However, before adding compression therapy to the patient's treatment regimen, rule out congestive heart failure and assess their ankle-brachial index (ABI) to ensure the adequacy of arterial blood supply.

Paste bandages (Unna boot)

A commercially prepared, inelastic, sometimes medicated gauze compression bandage, the paste bandage is one of the oldest treatments for venous ulcers.

The paste bandage consists of a gauze roll impregnated with zinc oxide, glycerin, and sometimes calamine. It is placed over the skin from the metatarsal heads to just below the knee. Any concavity over the ulcer is filled with an additional dressing. This dressing is covered with cotton dressings to pad the wound and to absorb drainage. An elastic bandage is wrapped around the outside to provide compression. As the dressing dries, it becomes semirigid. (See *How to wrap a paste bandage*.)

How to wrap a paste bandage

To wrap a paste bandage, follow these steps:

1. Clean the patient's skin thoroughly and then flex their knee.
2. With the patient's foot positioned at a right angle to their leg (have the patient point their toes toward their nose), wrap the impregnated gauze bandage firmly—not tightly—around the foot. Make sure the dressing covers the heel.
3. Continue wrapping upward, overlapping the layers by 50% with each turn. Make sure the dressing circles the patient's leg at an angle to avoid compromising their circulation. Smooth the boot with your free hand as you go, as shown here.

How to wrap a paste bandage

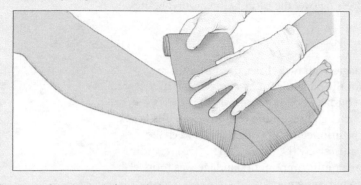

4. Stop wrapping about 1 in (2.5 cm) below the patient's knee. If constriction develops as the dressing becomes stiff, make a 2-in (5.1-cm) slit in the boot just below the knee.
5. If drainage is excessive, wrap a roll gauze dressing over the boot.
6. Finally, wrap the boot with an elastic bandage in a spiral as the paste layer was applied. Consider a cohesive outer wrap but do not use ACE-type bandages as these provide inadequate levels of sustainable compression.

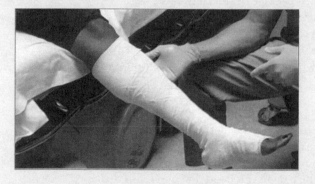

Although a paste bandage provides compression, protection, and a moist environment for healing, its most significant feature is its rigidity. Calf muscle contractions are key to the effectiveness of any lower extremity compression system. As the patient walks, the rigid dressing restricts outward movement of the calf muscle, directing more of the contraction force inward and improving the function of the calf muscle pump and in turn venous circulation. Therefore, the paste bandage is much less effective for a sedentary patient or one who is bed-bound. Regardless of which compression system is used, one suggestion for patients who are sedentary is to teach a rocking-chair motion to simulate walking and facilitate the calf pump muscle response.

If the patient finds the firmness against the ulcer uncomfortable, or there is breakthrough drainage, place a hydrocolloid, alginate, hydrofiber, honey, or foam dressing over the ulcer before applying the paste bandage.

Layered compression bandages

Layered compression bandages with two, three, or four layers are some of the best options for the patient with a venous ulcer. In these bandages, the first layer is cotton, wool, or foam, which protects the skin and absorbs moisture. Depending on the composition, this layer can be pulled apart and repositioned to fill concavities and create a more uniform fit. A Cochrane review (O'Meara et al., 2012) regarding compression indicated that a multicomponent bandage was more effective than a single-component system.

Compression stockings

Compression stockings are essential for long-term management of lower extremity venous disease. They're available in four classes of pressure, ranging from 15 mm Hg to greater than 40 mm Hg for patients with lymphedema. Each package of stockings has a list of indications on the label; however, most health care professionals rely on their own experience when choosing a class for a patient based on that patient's specific concerns. Be aware that a patient with arthritis, back problems, or obesity may have difficulty putting on compression stockings.

CircAid Thera–Boot

If the Unna boot or compression stockings aren't viable options, a CircAid Thera-Boot may be the answer. This dressing provides about 30 to 40 mm Hg of compression and is easier to put on than compression stockings as long as the patient can bend down to reach their legs. It can also continue compression even if there is a change in the size of the affected limb. The CircAid Thera-Boot is made of a non-elastic, semirigid material and has easy-to-use straps that secure the dressing in place. It is washable and reusable and can be removed at night and then put back on in the morning.

Elastic bandages

Elastic bandages are inexpensive wraps that may be used for compression. They may be long stretch or short stretch.

The long...

A long-stretch bandage stretches to more than 140% of its length. Long-stretch bandages provide low working pressure and high resting pressure. A long-stretch bandage exerts a specific amount of pressure all the time, whether the patient is active or resting, and may provide more pressure than is desirable during periods of rest.

...and short of it

A short-stretch bandage has limited elastic stretch, typically less than 90% of its length. When stretched to its limit, a short-stretch bandage becomes semirigid, providing compression while the patient is active. When the patient rests, the dressing provides less compression, protecting the skin from unnecessary pressure. This type of bandage provides high working pressure and low resting pressure.

Graduated compression support stockings

As their name suggests, graduated compression support stockings provide a pressure gradient that is greatest at the ankle and lowest at the top of the stocking. This compression is consistent with the hydrostatic pressure in leg veins, which is greatest at the ankle and diminishes up the leg. These stockings exert 100% of their pressure at the ankle, 70% at the calf, and 40% at the thigh level, producing a pressure gradient that helps reduce venous reflux. Knee-high-length stockings are all that's necessary to treat edema caused by venous hypertension.

Compression pumps may be used in conjunction with support stockings. These devices are available with sleeves that intermittently inflate. They may have a single chamber or separate bladders that inflate sequentially.

Medications are rarely prescribed to treat venous ulcers. Antibiotics may be ordered to treat an infection. In most instances, they are given systemically because topical antibiotics aren't effective in treating wound infections; in fact, they may interfere with healing. If the patient is a candidate for skin grafting, topical antimicrobials may be used to kill surface bacteria before the procedure.

Diuretics shouldn't be prescribed to treat edema in cases of venous insufficiency because edema is typically treated in these cases with compression and limb elevation. If the patient has concomitant heart failure, diuretics may be prescribed to treat this. Because diuretics can cause volume depletion and serious metabolic disorders, monitor the patient closely.

Surgery

Venous ulcers are chronic, and they heal slowly and recur frequently. Consequently, surgery is rarely a viable treatment. Large surface defects may require repair by skin grafting; however, this is a temporary solution. The underlying problem of venous hypertension remains, and in time, edema beneath the scar tissue breaks down the scar and creates another ulcer.

Replacement parts

Valve transplant, which involves replacing a section of a vein containing a defective valve with a section of vein containing a healthy valve, is performed selectively and almost never for a patient with venous ulcers. This is because, by the time an ulcer forms, venous disease is so pervasive that replacing a single valve won't help.

Endovenous thermal ablation

Saphenous vein ablation and perforator ablation is the injection of a sclerosant foam to ablate the faulty perforator or treat the associated interconnected superficial veins to redirect blood flow to healthy veins, thereby improving ulcer healing. Obliteration in the form of radiofrequency or laser therapies is becoming the treatment of choice in the treatment of reflux within the superficial venous system.

Wound care

Choosing the proper dressing is an important part of wound care because it affects wound healing. Occlusive dressings are typically selected for venous ulcers because they promote growth of granulation tissue and reepithelialization. If an ulcer contains necrotic debris, a moist gauze dressing or hydrocolloid dressing can be used to provide autolytic debridement. It is appropriate to select a dressing that promotes moist wound healing even though venous ulcers typically produce copious amounts of drainage. Hydrocolloid dressings and some foam dressings retain moisture in the wound while absorbing light to moderate drainage. More absorbent dressings can be used for venous ulcers with moderate to heavy drainage.

And introducing...

Newer therapies can also aid in healing chronic venous ulcers. Studies show that cellular tissue products are effective for healing venous ulcerations.

Treatment of venous ulcers

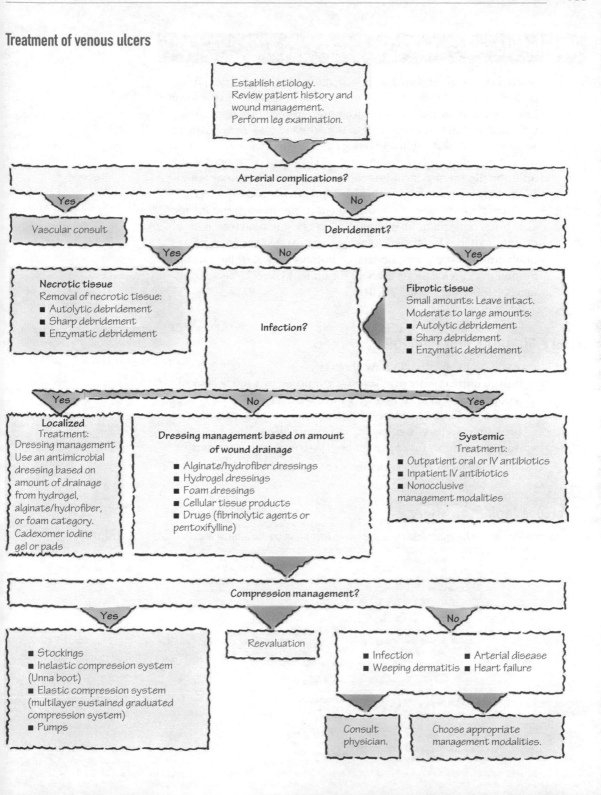

Establish etiology.
Review patient history and
wound management.
Perform leg examination.

Arterial complications?

Yes → Vascular consult

No → **Debridement?**

Yes →
Necrotic tissue
Removal of necrotic tissue:
- Autolytic debridement
- Sharp debridement
- Enzymatic debridement

No → **Infection?**

Yes →
Fibrotic tissue
Small amounts: Leave intact.
Moderate to large amounts:
- Autolytic debridement
- Sharp debridement
- Enzymatic debridement

Yes →
Localized
Treatment:
Dressing management
Use an antimicrobial
dressing based on
amount of drainage
from hydrogel,
alginate/hydrofiber,
or foam category.
Cadexomer iodine
gel or pads

No →
**Dressing management based on amount
of wound drainage**
- Alginate/hydrofiber dressings
- Hydrogel dressings
- Foam dressings
- Cellular tissue products
- Drugs (fibrinolytic agents or
pentoxifylline)

Yes →
Systemic
Treatment:
- Outpatient oral or IV antibiotics
- Inpatient IV antibiotics
- Nonocclusive
management modalities

Compression management?

Yes →
- Stockings
- Inelastic compression system
(Unna boot)
- Elastic compression system
(multilayer sustained graduated
compression system)
- Pumps

Reevaluation

No →
- Infection   - Arterial disease
- Weeping dermatitis - Heart failure

Consult
physician.

Choose appropriate
management modalities.

Arterial ulcers

Arterial ulcers, also referred to as ischemic ulcers, result from poor perfusion to the lower extremities. Disruptions in blood to the lower limbs result in the inability to deliver nutrient-rich blood to tissues, resulting in a cascade of changes to the skin and underlying tissue. More specifically, the skin and tissues of the lower leg are deprived of oxygen, resulting in necrosis and the development of an open wound. Additionally, trauma, including minor scrapes and cuts, may fail to adequately heal, resulting in the development of an arterial ulcer.

Arterial ulcers most commonly occur in the area around the toes. The most common cause of arterial ulcers is atherosclerosis. Other causes of arterial insufficiency include arterial stenosis (narrowing) or obstruction (from thrombosis, emboli, vasculitis, or Raynaud phenomenon). Arterial ulcers account for up to 15% to 20% of all leg ulcers (Isoherranen et al., 2020).

Artery anatomy and function

Like vein walls, artery walls have three layers:
- tunica intima (innermost layer)—composed of a single layer of endothelial cells on a layer of connective tissue
- tunica media (middle layer)—composed of a thick layer of smooth muscle cells, collagen, and elastic fibers
- tunica adventitia (strong outer layer)—composed of connective tissue, collagen, and elastic fibers (See *A close look at an artery.*)

A close look at an artery

This cross-section of an artery illustrates the layers that make up the arterial wall.

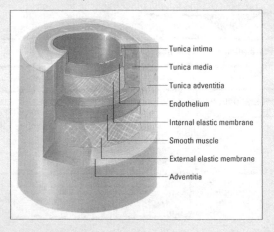

- Tunica intima
- Tunica media
- Tunica adventitia
- Endothelium
- Internal elastic membrane
- Smooth muscle
- External elastic membrane
- Adventitia

Arteries carry blood leaving the heart to every functioning cell in the body. Their strong, muscular walls allow expansion and relaxation with each heart beat, smoothing the powerful pulse to an almost constant pressure by the time blood reaches the capillaries. The lower portion of the body receives its arterial flow through the abdominal aorta and the major arteries that branch from it. (See *Major lower limb arteries.*)

Major lower limb arteries

This illustration identifies the major arteries in the lower portion of the body.

Development of an arterial ulcer

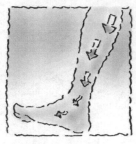 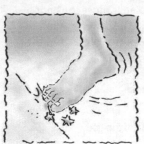 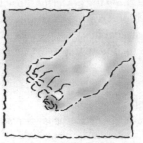

1 Arterial flow is diminished.

2 Trauma occurs to an area with arterial insufficiency.

3 Reduced blood flow impairs healing, resulting in a chronic wound, meaning, healing will not take place or takes place over many weeks to months.

Causes

Arterial insufficiency occurs when arterial blood flow is interrupted by an obstruction or arterial stenosis (narrowing of an artery). Occlusion can occur in any artery—from the aorta to a capillary—and can result from acute trauma or a chronic ailment.

The origins of occlusion

The most common cause of occlusion is atherosclerosis. Patients at the highest risk for atherosclerosis include males, people who smoke, and individuals with diabetes mellitus, hyperlipidemia, or hypertension. Advanced age places patients at even greater risk. (See *Aging and arterial insufficiency.*)

 Handle with care

Aging and arterial insufficiency

When assessing older patients, be alert for signs of arterial insufficiency. As aging occurs, the tunica intima thickens and loses elasticity. Thickening of the intima is one cause of arterial stenosis, which puts older adults at greater risk for arterial insufficiency.

Warning signs

In many cases, no signs of arterial insufficiency are apparent until the affected individual experiences an injury. As the demand for additional blood flow to the site of the injury outpaces an occluded artery's ability to deliver blood, ischemia occurs. Ischemia is a reduction in the flow of blood to any organ or body part. The primary symptom of ischemia is pain, which can be severe and may progress from claudication to rest pain.

Claudication

Claudication of the legs is similar to angina of the heart in that the cause of both is an insufficient supply of oxygen. In the heart muscle, this oxygen deficiency causes the pain of angina. In leg muscles, the same deficiency causes the pain of claudication.

Claudication, which can occur in any muscle distal to a narrowed artery, is brought on by exercise and is relieved by rest. Typically, patients report claudication pain in the calf, thigh, or buttocks. It is measured by how many city blocks (or an equivalent distance) the patient can walk before needing to stop to relieve the pain. Factors that tend to shorten the distance include obesity, smoking, and progressive atherosclerotic disease.

Claudication occurs at a specific distance and is reproducible. Patients experiencing claudication don't have to sit or adopt a particular position to relieve the discomfort; merely stopping reduces the oxygen demand and relieves the pain. As arterial insufficiency progresses, the distance shortens until ultimately, the patient feels pain even when resting.

Rest pain

Rest pain commonly occurs in the foot and can occur when the patient is asleep. Getting up and walking may provide some relief; however, walking isn't the key—lowering the extremity is. Gravity helps blood flow into the foot and calf, reducing the oxygen deficit and relieving discomfort. By the time rest pain occurs, tissues in the foot are severely ischemic regardless of whether an ulcer is present. Unless arterial flow is restored, the patient may need amputation.

Assessment

Assessment of arterial ulcers requires collecting a thorough patient history and performing a physical examination.

History

A patient history reveals whether the patient's wound is an arterial ulcer caused by arterial insufficiency. Obtain answers to such questions as the following:

- Has the patient experienced any pain?
- If they describe intermittent claudication, how far can they walk before pain occurs?
- If the patient says they have pain while resting, when did they first notice it and what measures do they take to relieve the pain?
- If the pain is in the foot, does getting up or hanging that foot over the edge of the bed help relieve the pain?

- What position is most comfortable for the patient? (Many patients spend their nights sleeping in a chair because the arterial pressure in the leg is too low to perfuse tissues while the leg is extended.)
- Ask the patient about smoking as well. If they smoke, determine how long they've been smoking and how much they smoke.

Physical examination

Start your examination by inspecting the common sites of arterial ulcers: the tips of the toes, the corners of the nail beds on the toes, over bony prominences, and between the toes. The edges of arterial ulcers are well demarcated. Because there is little blood flow to the tissue, the base of the ulcer is pale and dry with no granulation tissue present. You may see an area of wet necrosis or a dry scab. The skin surrounding the ulcer will feel cooler than normal on palpation. (See *Other signs of arterial insufficiency.*)

Other signs of arterial insufficiency

Arterial ulcers most commonly occur in the area around the toes. In a patient with arterial insufficiency, the foot usually turns deep red when dependent and the nails may be thick and ridged. In addition, pulses may be faint or absent; the skin is cool, pale, and shiny; and the patient may report pain in their legs and feet.

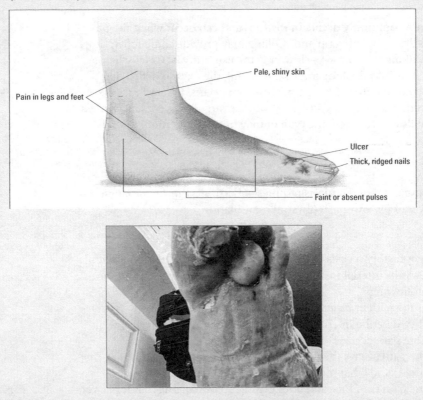

Identifying dependent rubor

- Dependent rubor is a change in color of the skin to a deep bluish red when the patient places the foot in a dependent position due to ischemia. This may be more difficult to observe in patients with darker skin tones.
- The lower extremity appears slender from lack of blood flow to muscle.
- Thin, pale, brittle, or crumbly yellow nails are present. Nails may be thickened as a result of arterial insufficiency or from fungal infection.

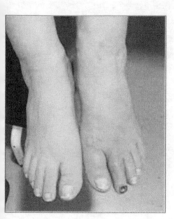

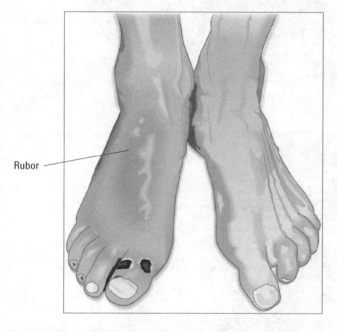

Rubor

To elicit this sign during a physical examination:

- Elevate the foot with the ulcer to a 30-degree angle. If the foot is ischemic, the skin will be pale.
- Ask the patient to lower the foot into a dependent position. Ischemic skin becomes deep red as the tissue fills with blood. This may be more difficult to observe in patients with darker skin tones. If it's observable, this dramatic color change signifies severe tissue ischemia.

A closer look at arterial ulcers

Arterial ulcers usually have well-demarcated edges. Because of decreased blood flow, the base of the ulcer is typically pale and dry and granulation tissue may be absent. On examination, you may notice an area of wet necrosis or a dry scab. The skin surrounding the ulcer will feel cooler than normal.

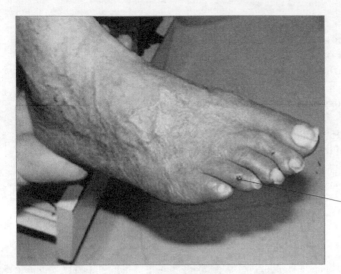

Arterial toe ulcer

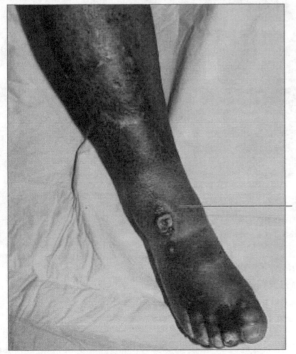

Ulcers on lower leg and
second toe resulting from
critical limb ischemia

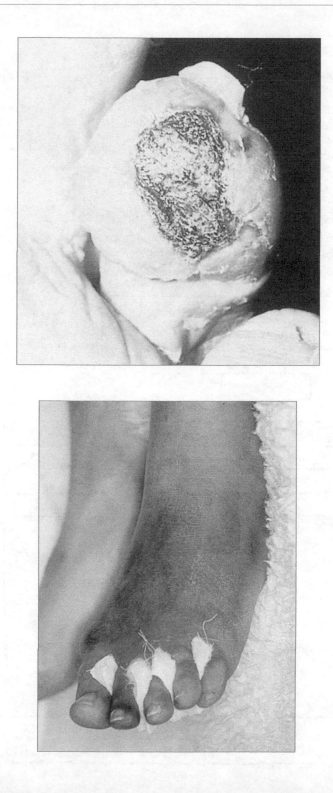

Care considerations

The goal of nursing care for patients with arterial ulcers is to improve circulation while also controlling pain. Nurses should use occlusive dressings to reduce infection while also controlling exudate and fostering debridement of the wound. These dressings will provide a moist environment for wound healing. Patients with arterial ulcers may require surgical intervention to manage the wound, including stenting and bypass grafting. Pain management is also imperative as these ulcers because of significant ischemic pain.

Treatment of arterial ulcers

Do not debride arterial ulcers. The hard covering (eschar) should not be disturbed; it should be protected. Be careful not to disturb the already compromised arteries.

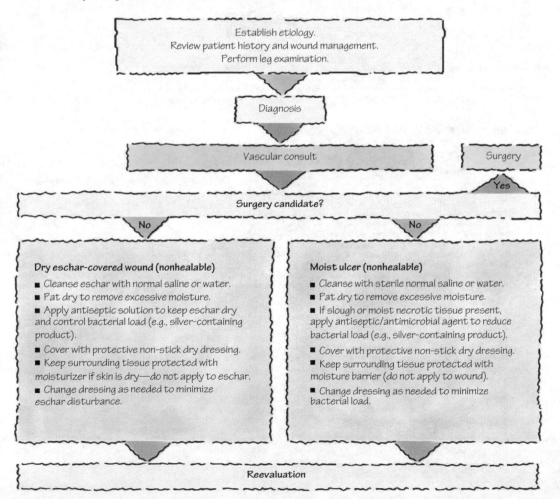

Establish etiology.
Review patient history and wound management.
Perform leg examination.

Diagnosis

Vascular consult — Surgery

Surgery candidate?

Yes

No — No

Dry eschar-covered wound (nonhealable)

- Cleanse eschar with normal saline or water.
- Pat dry to remove excessive moisture.
- Apply antiseptic solution to keep eschar dry and control bacterial load (e.g., silver-containing product).
- Cover with protective non-stick dry dressing.
- Keep surrounding tissue protected with moisturizer if skin is dry—do not apply to eschar.
- Change dressing as needed to minimize eschar disturbance.

Moist ulcer (nonhealable)

- Cleanse with sterile normal saline or water.
- Pat dry to remove excessive moisture.
- If slough or moist necrotic tissue present, apply antiseptic/antimicrobial agent to reduce bacterial load (e.g., silver-containing product).
- Cover with protective non-stick dry dressing.
- Keep surrounding tissue protected with moisture barrier (do not apply to wound).
- Change dressing as needed to minimize bacterial load.

Reevaluation

Focused examination of the arterial system

Perform a focused examination of the arterial system. Palpate the femoral, popliteal, posterior tibial, and dorsalis pedis pulses in each leg and compare your findings. (See *Assessing lower extremity pulses*.) Keep in mind that an absent dorsalis pedis pulse may not be an abnormal finding. Under normal conditions, some patients don't have a palpable dorsalis pedis pulse. Pulses can be palpated when the pressure is about 70 mm Hg. If there's no palpable pulse, the pressure is probably less than 70 mm Hg. Pulses aren't palpable in a foot with an arterial ulcer.

Assessing lower extremity pulses

Assessing pulses is an effective way to evaluate arterial blood flow to the lower extremities. These illustrations show where to position your fingers when palpating for pulses of the lower extremities. Use your index and middle fingers to apply pressure.

Femoral pulse

Press firmly at a point inferior to the inguinal ligament. For patients with excess weight, palpate in the groin crease halfway between the pubic bone and hip bone.

Popliteal pulse

Press firmly in the popliteal fossa at the back of the knee.

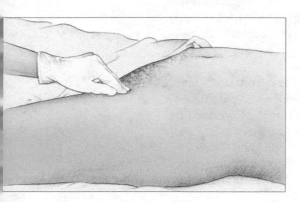

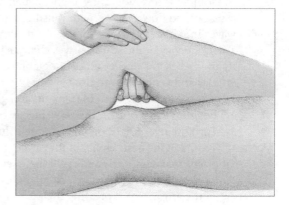

Posterior tibial pulse

Apply pressure behind and slightly below the medial malleolus.

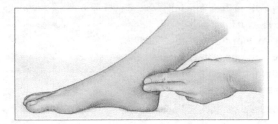

Dorsalis pedis pulse

Place your fingers on the medial dorsum of the foot while the patient points the toes downward. The pulse is difficult to palpate here and may seem absent in healthy patients. Sometimes, it helps to dorsiflex the foot to "pop up" the artery that lies between the first and second metatarsal bones.

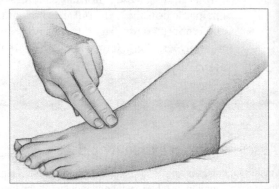

Using Doppler to assess blood flow

In Doppler ultrasonography, high-frequency sound waves are used to assess blood flow. A handheld transducer, or probe, directs the sound waves into a vessel, where they strike moving red blood cells (RBCs). The frequency of the sound waves changes in proportion to the velocity of the RBCs. Doppler ultrasonography can be used to assess both arterial and venous blood flow.

1. Apply a small amount of transmission gel to the ultrasound probe.
2. Position the probe on the skin directly over the selected artery.
3. Turn the instrument on, and set the volume to the lowest setting.
4. To obtain the best signal, tilt the probe at a 45-degree angle from the artery, making sure that the gel is between the skin and the probe.
5. Slowly move the probe in a circular motion to locate the center of the artery. Avoid pressing the probe too heavily on the artery to avoid compressing it.
6. Listen for a triphasic, biphasic, or monophasic sound, which occurs when the Doppler signal isolates an artery.
7. Count the signal for 60 seconds to determine the pulse rate.

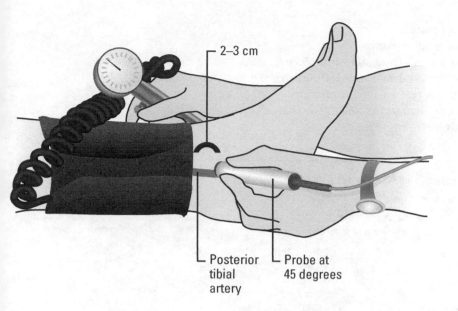

2–3 cm

Posterior tibial artery

Probe at 45 degrees

Measuring ankle–brachial index

The ABI is a value derived from blood pressure measurements. It shows the progress or improvement of arterial disease. Each value in the index is a ratio of the blood pressure measurement in the affected limb to the highest systolic pressure in the brachial arteries.

Steps

1. Place the patient in a supine position with the legs at heart level.
2. Measure and record both brachial blood pressures.
3. Wrap the blood pressure cuff around one ankle just above the malleolus with the cuff bladder centered over the posterior tibial artery.
4. Apply ultrasound transmission gel to a Doppler transducer.
5. Hold the Doppler transducer over the dorsalis pedis artery at a 45-degree angle.
6. Inflate the blood pressure cuff until the Doppler signal disappears.
7. Slowly deflate the cuff until the Doppler signal returns. Record this pressure as the dorsalis pedis pressure.
8. Repeat this same procedure over the posterior tibial artery. Record this pressure as the posterior tibial pressure.
9. Calculate the ABI by dividing the highest ankle pressure by the highest brachial systolic pressure.
10. Repeat the process on the contralateral limb.

Interpretation of results

- ABI greater than 0.9 = normal
- ABI 0.71 to 0.9 = mild arterial insufficiency
- ABI 0.41 to 0.7 = moderate arterial insufficiency
- ABI 0 to 0.40 = severe arterial insufficiency

The ABI may not be accurate in patients who have diabetes or arterial medial calcinosis.

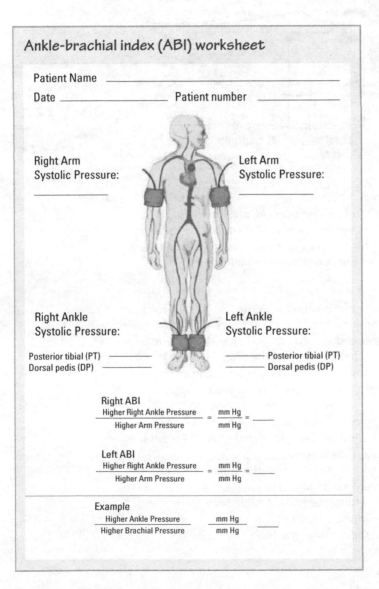

Ankle-brachial index (ABI) worksheet

Patient Name _____

Date _____ Patient number _____

Right Arm
Systolic Pressure:
_____

Left Arm
Systolic Pressure:
_____

Right Ankle
Systolic Pressure:

Left Ankle
Systolic Pressure:

Posterior tibial (PT) _____
Dorsal pedis (DP) _____

_____ Posterior tibial (PT)
_____ Dorsal pedis (DP)

Right ABI

$$\frac{\text{Higher Right Ankle Pressure}}{\text{Higher Arm Pressure}} = \frac{\text{mm Hg}}{\text{mm Hg}} = \underline{\quad}$$

Left ABI

$$\frac{\text{Higher Right Ankle Pressure}}{\text{Higher Arm Pressure}} = \frac{\text{mm Hg}}{\text{mm Hg}} = \underline{\quad}$$

Example

$$\frac{\text{Higher Ankle Pressure}}{\text{Higher Brachial Pressure}} = \frac{\text{mm Hg}}{\text{mm Hg}} \quad \underline{\quad}$$

Lymphatic ulcers

Lymphatic ulcers result when a part of the body afflicted with lymphedema sustains an injury. Lymphedema occurs when an obstruction in the lymphatic system causes lymphatic fluid to build up in the interstitial spaces of body tissues. In the legs, the steady seepage of fluid into interstitial tissues can result in massive edema, as shown here.

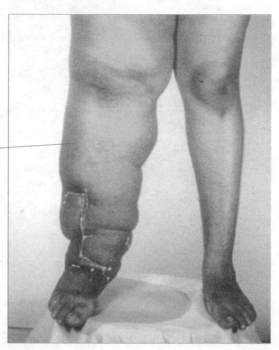

Lymphedema

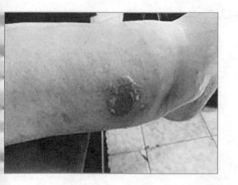

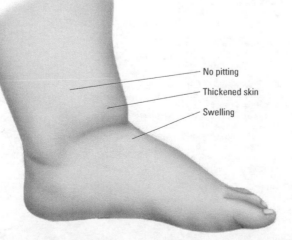

No pitting

Thickened skin

Swelling

Lymphatic system anatomy and function

The lymphatic system is a vascular network that drains lymph (a protein-rich fluid similar to plasma) from body tissues and intravascular compartments and returns it to the venous system.

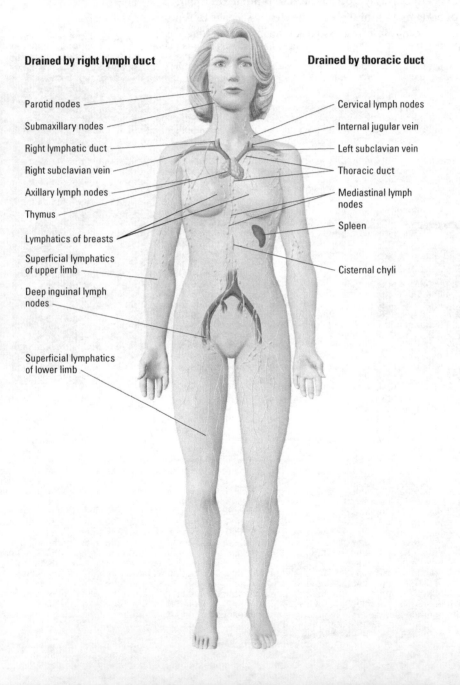

Drained by right lymph duct

Parotid nodes

Submaxillary nodes

Right lymphatic duct

Right subclavian vein

Axillary lymph nodes

Thymus

Lymphatics of breasts

Superficial lymphatics of upper limb

Deep inguinal lymph nodes

Superficial lymphatics of lower limb

Drained by thoracic duct

Cervical lymph nodes

Internal jugular vein

Left subclavian vein

Thoracic duct

Mediastinal lymph nodes

Spleen

Cisternal chyli

Lymphatic system and drainage route

The lymphatic system begins peripherally, with lymph capillaries that absorb fluid. The capillaries proceed centrally to thin vascular vessels. These vessels empty into collecting ducts, which empty into major veins at the base of the neck.

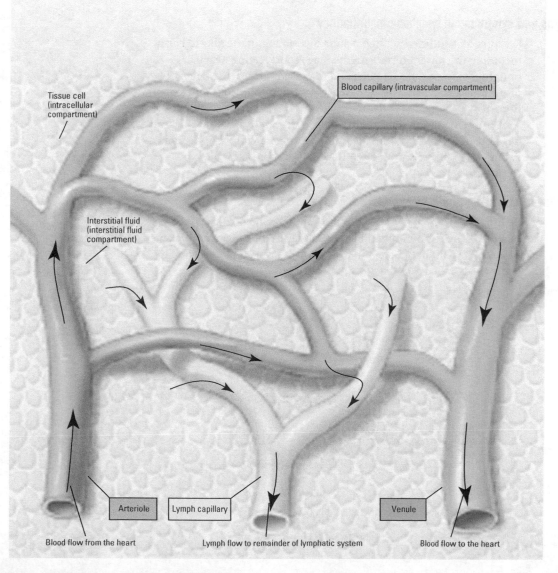

Tissue cell (intracellular compartment)

Blood capillary (intravascular compartment)

Interstitial fluid (interstitial fluid compartment)

Arteriole

Lymph capillary

Venule

Blood flow from the heart

Lymph flow to remainder of lymphatic system

Blood flow to the heart

Development of a lymphatic ulcer

- Pressure on capillaries—The skin and underlying tissue in areas with lymphedema become firm and fibrotic over time. This thickened tissue presses on capillaries, occluding blood flow and leaving the area vulnerable to ulcer formation. Because of the poor circulation, these ulcers are extremely difficult to treat.
- Skin folds from massive swelling—Skin folds can trap moisture, leading to tissue maceration and ulcer formation.
- Traumatic injury or pressure—Pressure or injury in an area with lymphedema commonly leads to an ulcer.

Signs and symptoms of lymphatic insufficiency

Lymphatic insufficiency often results in swelling of the affected area, including the lower limbs. Patients may report feeling heaviness or tightness in the affected area and may have a restricted range of motion. Patients may also experience recurrent infections and skin fibrosis.

Lymphatic ulcers commonly occur in the ankle area, but they can develop at any site of traumatic injury in an area with lymphedema. Patients with this disorder often have skin that is pale, cold, and translucent.

A closer look at lymphatic ulcers

Lymphatic ulcers are typically shallow and may be oozing, moist, or blistered. The surrounding skin is usually firm, fibrotic, and thickened by edema. Cellulitis (tissue inflammation) may also be present. Dry, warty spots called *papillomatoses* may develop.

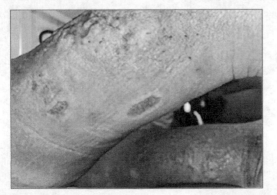

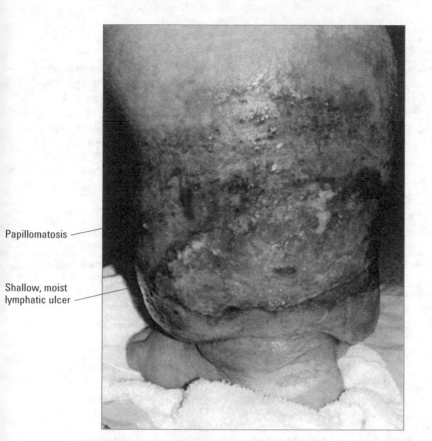

Papillomatosis

Shallow, moist
lymphatic ulcer

Care considerations

Use of an absorbent dressing is often required because these ulcers
generally have high drainage until the edema is controlled. It is important to keep the skin around the ulcers clean, dry, and moisturized.
If there is excessive drainage from the ulcer, a moisture barrier will be
needed.

Treatment of vascular ulcers

Effective treatment of a vascular ulcer involves caring for the wound as
well as managing the underlying vascular disease. The goals and treatment recommendations vary depending on the type of ulcer.

Type of ulcer	Treatment goals	Therapies and procedures	Wound care
Venous	• Control edema. • Manage underlying venous disease. • Provide appropriate wound care.	• Limb elevation to allow gravity to drain fluid from the limb • Compression bandages, layered compression bandages, elastic bandages, compression pumps, compression stockings, or graduated compression support hosiery to reduce edema • Bandaging and wrapping (paste wrap such as an Unna boot) may be used to provide compression, protection, and a moist environment for healing.	• Apply dressings to promote moist wound healing, growth of granulation tissue, and reepithelialization. • Apply growth factors to the wound bed as ordered to improve healing rate. • Consider advanced wound healing technologies such as cellular tissue products (CTPs) for a venous ulcer that fails to heal within 4 weeks of treatment.
Arterial	• Reestablish arterial flow. • Provide appropriate wound care and wound protection.	• Arterial bypass to restore arterial flow • Angioplasty (with possible stent insertion) to treat arterial stenosis	• Keep the wound dry and protected from pressure or trauma. • As ordered, apply an antiseptic or antimicrobial agent and then place small gauze pads between the toes. Change the pads daily to keep toe ulcers dry. • Never soak arterial ulcers. • If revascularization succeeds, change the type of dressing to keep moist tissue moist and dry tissue dry.
Lymphatic	• Reduce lymphedema. • Prevent infection. • Provide appropriate wound care.	• Compression pump therapy to reduce lymphedema • Referral to lymphedema specialist or physical therapy for comprehensive decongestive therapy (a form of massage) to reduce lymphedema and improve circulation • Refer for high-dose effective sustained graduated compression garments to manage chronic lymphedema	• Follow guidelines for venous ulcer care. • Choose dressings that can manage large fluid loads while protecting the surrounding skin, such as foams and other absorbent dressings. • Negative pressure wound therapy may be a good alternative to dressings for copious fluid leakage.

Neuropathic and diabetic foot ulcers

Neuropathic and diabetic foot ulcers have similar causes. Damage to the nerves in the lower extremity and foot can result in ulceration of the skin. While neuropathic injury can result from trauma, neurologic conditions, and viral infections, the most common cause of neuropathy is diabetes. As many as 25% of patients with diabetes will develop a neuropathic ulcer at some point in their lives and may require amputation (Bonham et al., 2021). Because diabetes is such a significant contributor to neuropathic ulcers, it is helpful to consider how diabetes impacts the development of these wounds.

Diabetes mellitus is a metabolic disorder characterized by hyperglycemia resulting from lack of insulin, lack of insulin effect, or both. Insulin transports glucose into cells, where it is used as fuel or stored as glycogen. Insulin stimulates protein synthesis and storage of free fatty acids in fat deposits. An insulin deficiency compromises these important functions. Diabetes can begin suddenly or develop insidiously. (See *Diabetes: The not-so-sweet facts.*)

Diabetes: The not-so-sweet facts

Diabetes has been characterized as a modern-day epidemic, and it isn't hard to understand why when you look at the statistics for the United States (Bonham et al., 2021; Lane et al., 2020; O'Connor & Varnado, 2022):
• Diabetes is the seventh leading cause of death.
• Diabetes most frequently occurs in African Americans, Hispanic Americans, Asian Americans, and Native Americans.
• Middle-aged and older adults are at the highest risk.
• Diabetes is the leading cause of kidney failure, amputations, and new cases of blindness.
• Individuals with diabetes incur 60% of all nontraumatic amputations.

High plasma glucose levels caused by diabetes can damage blood vessels and nerves. Therefore, patients with diabetes are prone to developing foot ulcers due to nerve damage and poor circulation to the lower extremities. Effective glucose control is essential for prevention and management of a potential or current chronic lower extremity wound.

Poor glucose control commonly results in a trineuropathy (three concurrent neuropathies) that dramatically increases a patient's risk of developing foot ulcers.

Causes

Diabetic neuropathy, pressure and other mechanical forces, and PVD can cause foot ulcers in patients with diabetes.

Diabetic neuropathy

Peripheral neuropathy is the primary cause of foot ulcer development among people with diabetes. Neuropathy is a nerve disorder that results in impaired or lost function in the tissues served by the affected nerve fibers. In diabetes, neuropathy may be caused by ischemia due to thickening in the tiny blood vessels that supply the nerve or by nerve demyelination (destruction of the protective myelin sheath surrounding a nerve), which slows the conduction of impulses.

Polyneuropathy, or damage to multiple types of nerves, is the most common form of neuropathy in patients with diabetes. In the foot, a trineuropathy develops that includes:

- loss of protective sensation (LOPS).
- alteration of motor structure and function.
- loss of autonomic functions (the autonomic nervous system controls smooth muscles, glands, and visceral organs). (See *Understanding diabetic trineuropathy.*)

Understanding diabetic trineuropathy

Sensory neuropathy

In sensory neuropathy, ischemia or demyelination (see illustration) causes nerve death or deterioration. When this occurs, the patient no longer feels painful stimuli and does not respond appropriately.

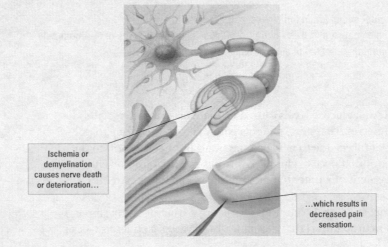

Ischemia or demyelination causes nerve death or deterioration...

...which results in decreased pain sensation.

Motor neuropathy

In motor neuropathy, intrinsic muscles deep in the plantar surface of the foot atrophy, resulting in increased arch height and clawed toes. In addition, the fat pad that normally covers the metatarsal heads migrates toward the toes, exposing the metatarsal heads to increase pressure. The risk of ulcer development is high for the upper surfaces of clawed toes, especially if the patient has poorly fitted shoes.

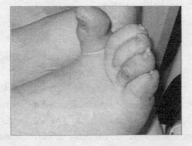

Understanding diabetic trineuropathy

The illustration shows the degenerative changes in the foot resulting from motor neuropathy. Shading indicates the areas where ulcers are most likely to develop.

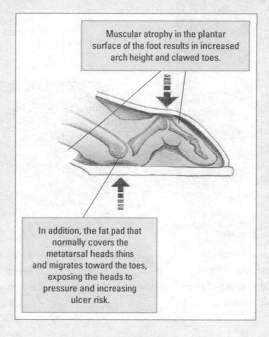

Muscular atrophy in the plantar surface of the foot results in increased arch height and clawed toes.

In addition, the fat pad that normally covers the metatarsal heads thins and migrates toward the toes, exposing the heads to pressure and increasing ulcer risk.

Autonomic neuropathy

In uncontrolled diabetes, autonomic neuropathy inhibits or destroys the sympathetic component of the autonomic nervous system, which controls vasoconstriction in peripheral blood vessels. The resulting unfettered flow of blood to the lower limbs and feet may cause osteopenia (reduction of bone volume) in the foot and ankle bones.

In Charcot disease (neuropathic osteoarthropathy), bones weakened by osteopenia sustain fractures that the patient doesn't feel because of the loss of protective sensation due to sensory neuropathy. Over time, this process causes bony dissolution that culminates with the collapse of the midfoot into a rocker bottom deformity. Charcot deformity is often misdiagnosed as an acute infection. Patients with Charcot disease are placed on non–weight-bearing status until inflammation subsides.

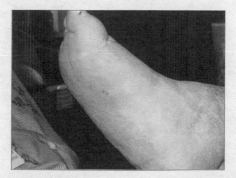

(continued)

Understanding diabetic trineuropathy *(continued)*

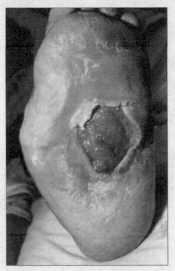

Full-thickness plantar surface neuropathic ulcer with osteomyelitis and Charcot deformity related to loss of protective sensation (LOPS).

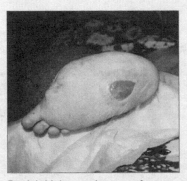

Partial-thickness plantar surface neuropathic ulcer with Charcot deformity, rocker bottom, and hallux (great toe) amputation.

In Charcot disease, bones weakened by osteopenia suffer fractures that the patient doesn't feel because of sensory neuropathy. Over time, this process causes bony destruction that culminates with the collapse of the midfoot into a rocker bottom deformity.

In uncontrolled diabetes, autonomic neuropathy inhibits or destroys the sympathetic component of the autonomic nervous system, which controls vasoconstriction in peripheral blood vessels. The resulting unrestricted flow of blood to the lower limbs and feet may cause osteopenia in foot and ankle bones.

Midfoot ulcers that result from increased plantar pressure over the rocker bottom deformity heal more slowly than ulcers on the forefoot.

Typically, impairment affects the feet and hands first and then progresses toward the knees and elbows, respectively. This presentation is called a *stocking and glove distribution*.

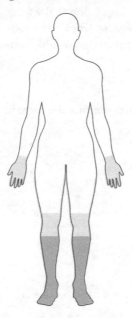

As sensory nerves degenerate and die, the patient may experience a burning or "pins-and-needles" sensation that might worsen at night.

As sensation declines, the patient is at higher risk for foot injury. Impaired sensation prevents the patient from feeling stimuli, such as pain and pressure, which normally warn of impending damage. Anything from stepping on something sharp to wearing ill-fitting shoes can result in foot injury because the patient can't feel the damage happening.

As motor nerves degenerate and die (motor neuropathy), muscles in the limbs atrophy, especially the intrinsic muscles of the feet, which causes foot drop and structural deformities. These degenerative changes increase the patient's risk of stumbling or falling and further damaging the foot.

As autonomic nerves degenerate and die (autonomic neuropathy), sweat and sebaceous glands malfunction and skin on the patient's feet dries and cracks. If fissures develop, the risk of infection rises.

Mechanical forces

Mechanical forces that can cause neuropathic foot ulcers include pressure, friction, and shear. These forces contribute to the development of callus on the plantar and medical/lateral aspects of the foot.

Pressure

Sensory neuropathy places a patient at increased risk for foot ulcers caused by pressure—especially a patient who is confined to a bed or wheelchair. Such a patient can sustain damage simply due to the feet resting for too long on a bed or a wheelchair footrest. Impaired sensation prevents the patient from feeling the discomfort that results from staying in one position too long.

Prominent plantar pressure places

As with pressure injuries, areas over bony prominences are the most common place for foot ulcers, including:

- metatarsal heads.

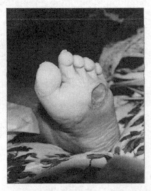

- great toe (hallux).

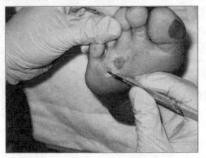

- the heel (calcaneus).

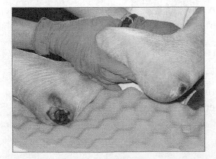

Friction and shear

Although pressure is the major mechanical force at work in the development of foot ulcers, it isn't the only one. Friction and shear can cause damage as well. A loose shoe rubbing against the foot or a foot sliding across a bed sheet can cause friction damage.

Shearly it's true

Shearing forces build up when damp skin sticks to a surface while the underlying bone and tissue move. For example, the skin of a sweating foot can cling to a shoe while the underlying tissues slide beneath the skin.

Peripheral vascular disease

A common problem in people with diabetes, PVD impairs the healing process of existing ulcers and may contribute to neuropathy. In PVD, atherosclerosis narrows the peripheral arteries, slowly reducing the flow of blood to the limbs. Poor blood flow or lack of it to the lower extremity is a major reason for an amputation. (See *How atherosclerosis impairs circulation*.) As perfusion drops, the risks of ischemia and tissue necrosis increase.

How atherosclerosis impairs circulation

In atherosclerosis, fatty deposits (cholesterol) and fibrous plaques accumulate along the walls of the arteries, narrowing the lumen and reducing the artery's elasticity. Thrombi (blood clots) form on the roughened surface of plaques and may grow large enough to block the artery's lumen.

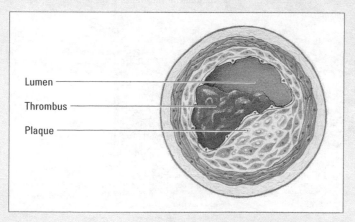

Lumen

Thrombus

Plaque

In diabetes, the arterial damage caused by atherosclerosis reduces blood flow to the lower limbs and to the nerves that innervate them. In addition to promoting ulcer development, poor perfusion slows the healing process for existing ulcers and impedes circulation of systemic antibiotics to infected areas.

Risk factors

Identifying the patient's risk factors is an important part of prevention. Loss of protective sensation is the top reason for a foot ulcer and greatest risk factor, but it isn't the only one. Other general risk factors for neuropathic ulcers include:

- structural foot deformity (such as clawed toes, rocker bottom, or hallux vagus).
- trauma and improperly fitted shoes.

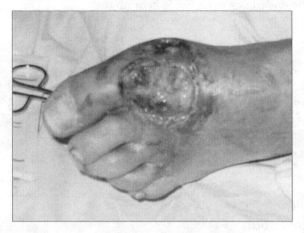

- calluses.

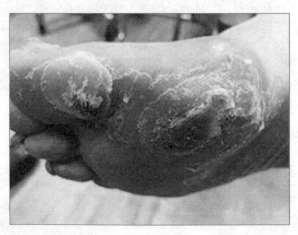

- prolonged, elevated pressure on areas of tissue.
- limited joint mobility.
- prolonged history of diabetes with poor glucose control.
- blindness or partial sight.
- chronic kidney disease.

  Risk factors for neuropathic foot ulcers may be either local or systemic. Local risk factors include:
- previous foot ulcer or amputation.
- neuropathy.
- PVD.

  Systemic risk factors include:
- age older than 65.
- hypertension.
- hyperglycemia with a hemoglobin A1c (HbA1c) level higher than 7.
- lymphedema.
- hyperlipidemia.
- obesity.
- smoking.

Prevention

Patient teaching

Neuropathic foot ulcer prevention starts with identifying the patient's risk factors and then teaching the patient how to eliminate or minimize these risks. Teach the patient about ulcer care and the importance of controlling diabetes, including the consequences of not controlling it. For example, patients should be aware that poorly controlled blood glucose levels can lead to peripheral neuropathy and vascular damage. Research indicates that tight glycemic control reduces the frequency and severity of neuropathy in patients with type 1 diabetes (Lane et al., 2020). Similar findings have been shown for patients with type 2 diabetes (Singer et al., 2017).

Proper foot care and steps to prevent ulcers, including daily examinations, skin washing and maintenance techniques, toenail care, and exercise are important pieces of information. Choosing proper socks and shoes is knowledge the individual with diabetes needs. (See *Proper foot care.*)

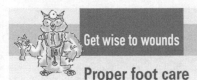

Get wise to wounds

Proper foot care

Here are some tips to teach to help ensure proper foot care.

Performing foot hygiene
- Check your feet (top and bottom) daily for injury or pressure areas (a long-handled mirror can help).
- Wash your feet with a mild soap and dry thoroughly, especially between the toes.
- Check your bath water to make sure it isn't too hot (test the water with your elbow, if able; otherwise, use a thermometer or ask a family member to help).
- Apply a moisturizing cream to prevent dry, cracking skin on your feet and to balance skin pH. Avoid moisturizing between the toes.
- Cut your toenails according to the shape of the end of the toe; see a podiatrist if they're dystrophic (deformed and thickened).
- Don't go barefooted—the risk of injury is too great.

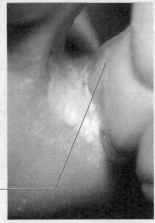

Maceration leads to skin breakdown as well as fungal infections.

Choosing socks
- Use silver-impregnated socks for tinea pedis and or onychomycosis control.
- Wear white- or light-colored socks in order to quickly detect bleeding from trauma.
- Wear socks that wick perspiration away from your feet (such as cotton-blend socks) to prevent maceration and allow ventilation; avoid 100% cotton socks.
- Use padded socks for shear and friction control, but make sure that shoes are big enough to accommodate thicker socks.

Choosing shoes
- Wear well-fitting shoes, not shoes that are too tight or loose.
- Wear shoes that breathe to reduce the risk for maceration and fungal infections.
- Wear new shoes for short periods (under 1 hour) each day initially; gradually increase the time as your feet adjust.
- Wear professionally fitted shoes if you have any foot deformities or a history of ulceration.

Proper foot care

• Wash your shoes, if possible, to destroy microorganisms.
• Check your shoes before putting them on to make sure nothing fell in that could cause harm to your foot or a change to the structure of the shoe.
• Ensure any inserts are properly fitted.
• Change your footwear two to three times throughout the day and evening to reduce time on the same pressure points.

Team effort

Current guidelines stress the importance of an evidence-based "team approach" to prevent, treat, and avoid recurrence of foot ulcers and infections. The "toe and flow" concept emphasizes a team approach with specialists to address adequate "flow" for perfusion and antibiotics as needed to be delivered to the "toe." Limb salvage teams include vascular surgeons, podiatrists, and infectious disease specialists.

Successful prevention programs for neuropathic foot ulcers begin with health promotion. The patient should play an active role in setting personal health care goals, working in partnership with the health care team to achieve those goals.

Many patients with diabetes have multiple disorders, requiring a series of interventions involving many health professionals, which may include nurses, doctors, physical therapists, occupational therapists, nutritionists, podiatrists, endocrinologists, psychologists, diabetes educators, prosthetists or orthotists, and social workers. A case manager or care coordinator is critical to coordinate the many facets of effective glucose control, prevention, treatment, and avoiding recurrence of neuropathic foot ulcers and amputation.

Assessment

An assessment of neuropathic foot ulcers includes gathering a thorough patient history and performing a physical examination with special testing of the lower extremities.

History

A thorough patient history and complete lower extremity assessment are key to assessing neuropathic foot injuries and ulcers. In addition to the basic information elicited during a traditional patient history, ask the patient about:
• date of onset of diabetes.
• management measures.
• glycemic control (using the HbA1c level as an indicator).
• medications.
• other diagnosed problems (especially hypertriglyceridemia).

- status and history of any diagnosed neuropathy.
- allergies, especially skin reactions.
- tobacco and alcohol use.
- recent changes in activity level.
- date and location of previous ulcerations.
- date the current ulcer was first noticed.
- the way in which the ulcer occurred.
- type and quality of any associated pain.

Physical examination

Use a holistic approach when performing the physical examination, which consists of a general examination and a complete lower extremity assessment. Remember that a person's overall physical health and state of mind affect wound healing.

General examination

During the general physical examination, you'll evaluate the musculoskeletal, neurologic, vascular, and integumentary systems to provide perspective for assessing the condition of the lower limbs.

Bone up

Assess these aspects of the person's musculoskeletal system:
- Posture
- Gait
- Strength, flexibility, and endurance
- Range of motion

Make connections

Assess these aspects of the person's neurologic system:
- gait
- balance
- reflexes
- sensory function

Check the flow

Assess these aspects of the person's vascular system:
- Posterior tibial and dorsalis pedis pulses
- ABI
- Toe-brachial index (TBI)

    Keep in mind that ABI isn't as reliable due to calcification in the microvasculature in people with diabetes.

Get the skin-y

Assess these aspects of the person's integumentary system:
- Texture
- Temperature
- Color
- Appendages (hair, sweat glands, sebaceous glands, nails)

Absence of hair on the legs and hypertrophic nails are suggestive of poor arterial perfusion.

Foot examination

Carefully examine the person's feet to detect and assess foot ulcers. Check the following high-risk areas of the feet for existing or impending ulcers (calluses are considered a heralding sign of a neuropathic foot ulcer):

- Plantar surfaces (soles) of the toes
- Tips of the toes
- Area between the toes
- Lateral aspect of the foot's plantar surface

Wound characteristics depend on where the injury occurs on the foot. (See *Features of neuropathic foot ulcers*.) Characteristics of surrounding skin may include:

- calluses (considered "prewounds").
- blood blisters (hemorrhage beneath a callus).
- erythema (a sign of inflammation or infection).
- induration (hardened edges).
- skin fissures (portals for bacterial entry).
- dry, scaly skin.

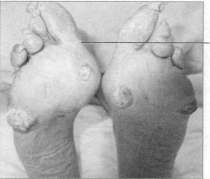

Sensory neuropathy can lead to excessive callus formation. This patient was unaware of the callus.

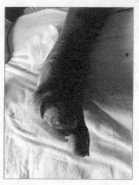

Great toe (hallux) classic injury related to peripheral neuropathy. This is often due to short-fitting shoes or traumatic injury.

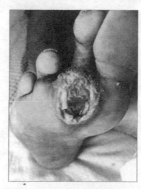

Third metatarsal neuropathic pressure/shear/friction injury with increasing callus leading to a neuropathic wound.

Features of neuropathic foot ulcers

In neuropathic foot ulcers, characteristic clinical features depend on the ulcer's location and underlying etiology.

Ulcer location	Clinical features
Plantar surface	Even wound margins
Great toe	Deep wound bed
Metatarsal head	Dry or low to moderate exudate

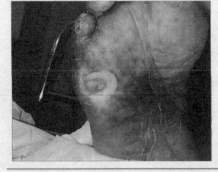

Heel	Low to moderate exudate

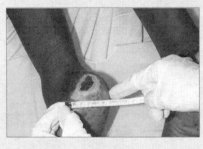

Tip or top of toe	Pale granulation with ischemia or bright-red, friable granulation tissue with infection or necrotic tissue

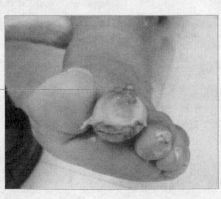

Ulcers can hide under whitish tissue such as this one. The circulation in this toe was poor, leading to eventual toe amputation.

Features of neuropathic foot ulcers

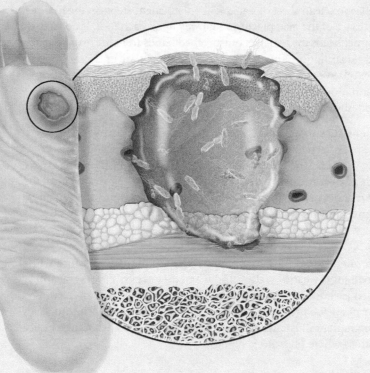

Special testing
Special tests provide a clearer picture of lower leg and foot health. These tests evaluate pressure, neurologic function, and perfusion. The results provide insight into the mechanism of injury, condition of the wound bed and surrounding tissue, prognosis for healing, and required treatment interventions.

Musculoskeletal tests
Harris mat prints and computerized pressure mapping are conducted to provide information about the plantar pressures of the foot.

Harris mat prints
Pressure over bony prominences is one cause of foot ulcers. A simple method for determining areas of increased pressure on the plantar surface of the foot is to use an ink mat.

Making an impression

In Harris mat prints, the examiner inks the bottom of the mat, which has a grid to aid the assessment of results, and places it on an evaluation template or clean sheet of paper. Then the patient steps on the ink-free top surface of the mat, placing equal weight on each foot. If needed, the examiner holds the patient's outstretched hands to help ensure equal weight distribution. The impression on the template or sheet of paper shows relative areas of pressure under the patient's foot. Darker areas on the grid indicate high-pressure areas. When a dynamic impression is required, the patient slowly walks across the mat to create the impression.

Under pressure

High-pressure areas usually correlate with calluses (prewounds) or existing wounds. The results help guide the choice of offloading devices (such as custom-fitted orthotics, shoes, padding, removable boot, or total contact cast), which provide redistribution of pressure when the patient stands or walks.

Computerized pressure mapping

Computerized pressure mapping devices test plantar pressures while the patient is wearing a shoe and when they are barefoot. The approach is similar to Harris mat prints; however, in this test, a computer maps the pressures and displays the results on a printout. A color gradient illustrates relative pressure with red and orange indicating areas where pressure is highest.

Neurologic tests

Neurologic tests for the lower extremities include deep tendon reflexes testing with a plexar, vibration perception testing with a tuning fork or biothesiometer, and Semmes–Weinstein monofilament testing for protective sensation.

Deep tendon reflexes testing

Peripheral neuropathy causes a decrease in deep tendon reflexes. Decreased deep tendon reflexes correlate with muscular atrophy, usually the intrinsic muscles of the foot in a patient with diabetes. The examiner uses the pointed end of a reflex hammer to strike the biceps, triceps, brachioradialis, patellar, and Achilles reflexes.

Tuning fork test

In this test, the examiner uses a tuning fork to assess peripheral nerve function and help identify and quantify existing neuropathy.

Name that tune

1. The examiner activates the tuning fork and holds it against a bony prominence in the affected limb (e.g., a metatarsal head or malleoli) and then records the patient's ability to sense the vibration.

2. Next, the examiner tests other bony prominences in the body (e.g., the patella or elbow) or the same prominence in the opposite limb if it's unaffected.
3. Afterward, the results are compared to assess neurologic function.

Biothesiometer

A biothesiometer is another tool used to assess the patient's vibratory perception threshold. It provides a better quantitative measurement of vibratory sense than the tuning fork. Patients with sensory neuropathy have impaired vibratory perception thresholds (less than 25 volts as measured on the biothesiometer).

Semmes–Weinstein test

The Semmes–Weinstein test helps determine the level of protective sensation in the feet. While the patient's eyes are closed, the examiner holds the Semmes–Weinstein monofilament perpendicular to the patient's foot and then presses the monofilament against the skin until it bows. The patient is then asked to identify when and where the skin has been touched. As protective sensation decreases, plantar pressures tend to rise, as does the patient's risk of ulcers at these points. (See *Performing the Semmes–Weinstein test.*)

Performing the Semmes–Weinstein test

In the Semmes–Weinstein test, the examiner uses a special monofilament to assess protective sensation in the patient's feet. This illustration shows the points to test.

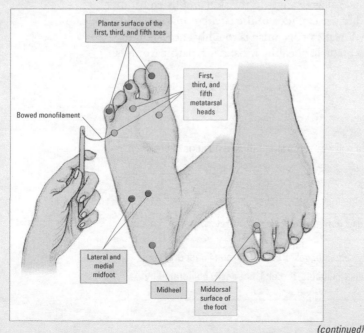

Plantar surface of the first, third, and fifth toes

First, third, and fifth metatarsal heads

Bowed monofilament

Lateral and medial midfoot

Midheel

Middorsal surface of the foot

(continued)

Performing the Semmes–Weinstein test *(continued)*

How it's done
1. Ask the patient to close their eyes.
2. Ask the patient to identify where and when they feel the monofilament touch.
3. Place the 5.07 monofilament which delivers 10 g of pressure on one of the testing points shown at right, and exert enough pressure to bow the monofilament.
4. Count "one one thousand" for touch, "two one thousand" for wait, "three one thousand" for removal.

Vascular tests

Vascular tests help assess circulation in the lower extremities. These tests include pulse palpation (Doppler preferred as palpation is not as valid), ABI, measuring toe pressures, and obtaining transcutaneous oxygen (TcPO$_2$) levels.

Pulse palpation

The initial assessment of limb perfusion includes palpating the dorsalis pedis, posterior tibial, popliteal, and femoral pulses. If it is hard to palpate a pulse due to edema, weakness, or a thready pulse, use Doppler ultrasound, which produces an audible signal coinciding with the pulse.

Hear the beat

Hold the transducer at a 45-degree angle to the skin and listen for the beats. The results provide a general idea of the circulation to each level of the limb. A palpable dorsalis pedis pulse is roughly equivalent to 80 mm Hg, which is adequate for healing most neuropathic wounds. (See *Pulse rating.*)

Pulse rating

When assessing the amplitude of a pulse, rate the strength on a numeric scale, such as this one.

Rating	Pulse characteristic
0	No palpable pulse
+1	Weak or thready pulse: hard to feel, easily obliterated by slight finger pressure
+2	Normal pulse: easily palpable, obliterated by strong finger pressure
+3	Bounding pulse: readily palpable, forceful, not easily obliterated by finger pressure

Ankle-brachial index
PVD and resulting poor perfusion are common problems for patients with diabetes. Poor perfusion increases the patient's likelihood of developing ulcers and reduces the speed with which existing ulcers heal. Although this test is less reliable in a patient with diabetes, ABI is used in conjunction with other vascular tests to determine and monitor the patient's risk of ischemia in the area of the ankle. ABI is a ratio of systolic blood pressure in the brachial artery in the arm to systolic blood pressure measured in the dorsalis pedis artery in the ankle. However, the ABI may not be accurate in patients with diabetes if the vessels being measured are calcified and therefore not compressible. A falsely high reading may be seen due to incompressible artery walls caused by medial sclerosis of the arteries.

Toe-brachial index
TBI may be a more sensitive indicator of changes in vascular integrity in the distal areas of the foot. Toe pressures are performed in the same manner as limb blood pressures, except that a much smaller, specialized cuff is used for the toe. Due to the tiny arteries in digits, the corresponding arterial pressures are lower than those measured in an arm or leg. Typical pressure in the toe is about 70% of systolic values obtained in the arm.

What the toes know
A toe pressure of 45 mm Hg or higher is needed for healing to occur. Toe pressures allow you to gauge the patient's ischemic risk profile. Generally, a toe pressure:
- higher than 55 mm Hg reflects a low risk of tissue ischemia.
- lower than 40 mm Hg reflects a high risk of ischemia.
- lower than 20 mm Hg reflects a severe risk of ischemia and impending amputation without intervention.

Transcutaneous oxygen levels
A $TcPO_2$ of 30% or higher is required for healing. $TcPO_2$ levels reflect the oxygen saturation of tissues. Typically, $TcPO_2$ levels are measured close to the ulcer. In general, a $TcPO_2$ level:
- higher than 40% reflects a low risk of tissue ischemia.
- between 20% and 30% reflects a high risk of ischemia.
- lower than 20% reflects a severe risk of ischemia.

Classification
Diabetic foot ulcers are classified according to depth, presence of ischemia, and presence of infection depending on the classification system. The Wagner Ulcer Grade Classification and the University of Texas Diabetic Foot Classification system are two commonly used classification systems.

Wagner Ulcer Grade Classification

The original Wagner Ulcer Grade Classification considers depth of penetration; however, it doesn't allow for the assessment of infection at all tissue levels. A modified version of this classification system adds levels to take into account infection and ischemia. (See *Wagner Ulcer Grade Classification.*)

Wagner Ulcer Grade Classification

In the Wagner Ulcer Grade Classification, less complex ulcers receive lower scores and more complex ulcers receive higher scores. Ulcers with higher scores may require surgical intervention or amputation. This system has been widely used since the 1970s but less so in recent years as wound depth and tissue viability are the focus.

Grade	Characteristics
0	• No open wounds • Intact skin • No presence of bony deformity, cellulitis, callus, or healed ulcers
1	• Superficial ulcer (partial thickness) without penetration to deeper layers • Bony prominence under ulcer may be present. • Deformities may be present.
2	• Deeper ulcer and may expose or probe to the bone, tendon, or joint capsule.
3	• Deep ulcer • Osteitis, abscess, joint sepsis, tendonitis, or osteomyelitis
4	• Gangrene localized to toes and/or forefoot
5	• Gangrene involving at least two thirds of the foot and requiring foot amputation

Bonham, P. A., Brunette, G., Crestodina, L., Droste, L. R., Gonzalez, A., Kelechi, T. J., Ratliff, C. R., & Varnado, M. F. (2021). *Guideline for management of patients with lower-extremity wounds due to diabetes mellitus and/or neuropathic disease* (WOCN Clinical Practice Guideline Series 3). Wound, Ostomy, Continence Nurses Society; Monteiro-Soares, M., Boyko, E. J., Jeffcoate, W., Mills, J. L., Russell, D., Morback, S., & Game, F. (2020). Diabetic foot ulcer classifications: A critical review. *Diabetes Metabolism Research and Reviews, 36*(Suppl. 1). https://doi.org/10.1002/dmrr.3272

University of Texas Diabetic Foot Classification System

The University of Texas system takes tissue infection and ischemia into consideration and provides a more detailed breakdown of classifications than the Wagner system. (See *University of Texas Diabetic Foot Classification System.*)

University of Texas Diabetic Foot Classification System

The University of Texas Diabetic Foot Classification System, developed in 1996, provides a detailed categorization of diabetic foot ulcers. Staging the ulcer from A to D reflects burdens and characteristics in the wound and grading it from 0 to 3 refers to the depth of the wound.

Staging
- Stage A: Nonischemic, clean
- Stage B: Nonischemic but infection present
- Stage C: Ischemic but not infected
- Stage D: Ischemic and infected

Grading
- Grade 0: Preulcerative or postulcerative wound with complete epithelialization
- Grade 1: Superficial wound not involving tendon, capsule, or bone
- Grade 2: Wound penetrates to tendon or capsule
- Grade 3: Wound penetrates to bone or joint

Bonham, P. A., Brunette, G., Crestodina, L., Droste, L. R., Gonzalez, A., Kelechi, T. J., Ratliff, C. R., & Varnado, M. F. (2021). *Guideline for management of patients with lower-extremity wounds due to diabetes mellitus and/or neuropathic disease* (WOCN Clinical Practice Guideline Series 3). Wound, Ostomy, Continence Nurses Society; Monteiro-Soares, M., Boyko, E. J., Jeffcoate, W., Mills, J. L., Russell, D., Morback, S., & Game, F. (2020). Diabetic foot ulcer classifications: A critical review. *Diabetes Metabolism Research and Reviews, 36*(Suppl. 1). https://doi.org/10.1002/dmrr.3272

SINBAD

Initially designed for auditing large populations of ulcers, the SINBAD (site, ischemia, neuropathy, bacterial infection, area, and depth) framework is now recommended for classification, especially for the purpose of communication between clinicians and for comparing presentation and outcomes of diabetic and neuropathic foot ulcers in different centers.

SINBAD uses six parameters and is scored from 0 to 6. A higher score indicates greater severity.

Parameter	Findings	Score
Location	Forefoot	0
	Midfoot or hindfoot	1
Area	<1 cm^2	0
	>1 cm^2	1
Depth	Skin or subcutaneous tissue	0
	Muscle, tendon, bone	1
Bacterial infection (using International Working Group on the Diabetic Foot [IWGDF] criteria)	None	0
	Present	1
Ischemia	Pedal blood flow with at least one palpable pulse	0
	Clinical evidence of reduced pedal flow	1
Neuropathy	Protective sensation intact	0
	Loss of protective sensation (LOPS)	1

Monteiro-Soares, M., Boyko, E. J., Jeffcoate, W., Mills, J. L., Russell, D., Morback, S., & Game, F. (2020). Diabetic foot ulcer classifications: A critical review. *Diabetes Metabolism Research and Reviews, 36*(Suppl. 1). https://doi.org/10.1002/dmrr.3272

The Infectious Diseases Society of America/International Working Group on Diabetic Foot (IDSA/IWGDF) suggests the following for identifying infection in a neuropathic foot wound:

Index of severity	Clinical manifestations
Uninfected	No purulence or inflammation
Mild infection	Cellulitis/erythema in periwound of ≤2 cm or presence of two or more manifestations of inflammation (purulence, erythema, tenderness, warmth, induration)
Moderate	Systemically well and metabolically stable patient, but has one or more characteristics of infection (cellulitis extending >2 cm periwound; lymphangitic streaking; inflammation beneath the superficial fascia; abscess of deep tissues; involvement of muscle, tendon, joint, or bone; or gangrene)
Severe	Patient exhibiting signs of metabolic instability or systemic toxicity (fever, chills, tachycardia, hypotension, confusion, vomiting, acidosis, and other signs)

Monteiro-Soares, M., Boyko, E. J., Jeffcoate, W., Mills, J. L., Russell, D., Morback, S., & Game, F. (2020). Diabetic foot ulcer classifications: A critical review. *Diabetes Metabolism Research and Reviews, 36*(Suppl. 1). https://doi.org/10.1002/dmrr.3272

Complications

Infection is the most common complication that impedes the healing of neuropathic foot ulcers and can cause a wound to become chronic. Other complications include:
- multiple comorbidities, including PVD, which cause a number of problems that increase the risk of ulceration and reduce the likelihood of speedy healing.
- uncontrolled hyperglycemia, which commonly signals infection and inhibits the immune system, particularly the scavenging function of neutrophils.
- psychosocial problems, such as depression and limited economic resources, which can profoundly affect the patient's nutritional status, in turn affecting the body's ability to prevent ulcers and heal existing wounds.

Infection

An infection in the wound or elsewhere consumes protein needed for healing and interferes directly by damaging the wound bed. Infections fall into two categories: non–limb-threatening or limb-threatening. Non–limb-threatening infections tend to be superficial infections involving tissues within 2 cm of the wound margin. In this type of infection, no significant tissue ischemia is present, and bone isn't palpable in the wound bed. Non–limb-threatening infection can be treated with topical antimicrobials, sharp debridement, and wound cleaning once or twice daily.

In contrast, limb-threatening infection involves tissue more than 2 cm from the wound margin, palpable bone in the wound bed, and tissue ischemia. When this occurs, hospitalization and surgical debridement of infected bone and soft tissues are necessary. Unless the infected bone is fully resected, the patient requires 4 to 8 weeks of intravenous antibiotic therapy. Baseline x-rays and laboratory inflammatory markers such as erythrocyte sedimentation rate (ESR) and C-reactive protein (CRP) can be useful in monitoring the patient's response to therapy. Most diabetic limb-threatening infections are polymicrobial with five to seven different organisms growing in the wound bed. There has been a dramatic increase in methicillin-resistant *Staphylococcus aureus* (MRSA) prevalence in hospital and community settings. MRSA is a common pathogen in diabetic foot infections and can place the patient at greater risk of amputation.

Show me a sign

Uncontrollable blood glucose or hyperglycemia may be the first sign of infection because patients with diabetes commonly fail to demonstrate the typical systemic responses. A 4-degree to 5-degree difference in temperature between similar areas on each foot is a local sign of infection. An infrared thermometer is the most reliable way to check for this difference. An infection in the wound bed commonly causes friable (easy to bleed), bright-red granulation tissue.

Oste-oh-my-elitis

Osteomyelitis, or bone infection, is common in deep wounds. A quick and reliable method for determining whether osteomyelitis is present in a diabetic ulcer bed is to palpate for bone. A palpable bone usually indicates osteomyelitis; however, osteomyelitis may be difficult to distinguish from acute Charcot neuropathic osteoarthropathy. The best way to differentiate between the two is to culture a bone fragment from the wound bed. The initial assessment of a deformed, inflamed, or unusual anatomic presentation is an ankle and foot x-ray.

Treatment for neuropathic ulcers

Successful healing depends on proper wound cleansing and correct application and removal of dressing and offloading. Topical antimicrobials, debridement biotherapies, and surgery may also be included in the care plan.

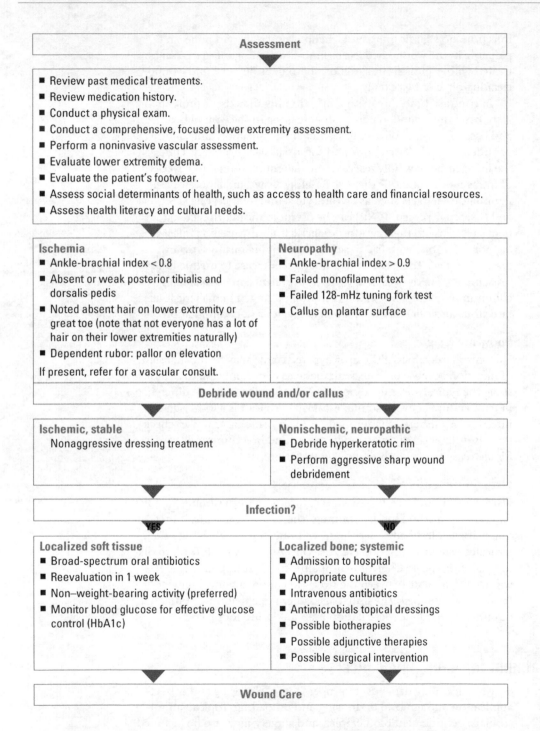

Assessment

- Review past medical treatments.
- Review medication history.
- Conduct a physical exam.
- Conduct a comprehensive, focused lower extremity assessment.
- Perform a noninvasive vascular assessment.
- Evaluate lower extremity edema.
- Evaluate the patient's footwear.
- Assess social determinants of health, such as access to health care and financial resources.
- Assess health literacy and cultural needs.

Ischemia
- Ankle-brachial index < 0.8
- Absent or weak posterior tibialis and dorsalis pedis
- Noted absent hair on lower extremity or great toe (note that not everyone has a lot of hair on their lower extremities naturally)
- Dependent rubor: pallor on elevation

If present, refer for a vascular consult.

Neuropathy
- Ankle-brachial index > 0.9
- Failed monofilament text
- Failed 128-mHz tuning fork test
- Callus on plantar surface

Debride wound and/or callus

Ischemic, stable
Nonaggressive dressing treatment

Nonischemic, neuropathic
- Debride hyperkeratotic rim
- Perform aggressive sharp wound debridement

Infection?

YES   NO

Localized soft tissue
- Broad-spectrum oral antibiotics
- Reevaluation in 1 week
- Non–weight-bearing activity (preferred)
- Monitor blood glucose for effective glucose control (HbA1c)

Localized bone; systemic
- Admission to hospital
- Appropriate cultures
- Intravenous antibiotics
- Antimicrobials topical dressings
- Possible biotherapies
- Possible adjunctive therapies
- Possible surgical intervention

Wound Care

Wound cleaning

Wound cleansing is a fundamental step in the healing process to reduce the superficial bioburden which inhibits wound healing (see Chapter 3).

For neuropathic ulcers related to diabetes, wound care is as follows.

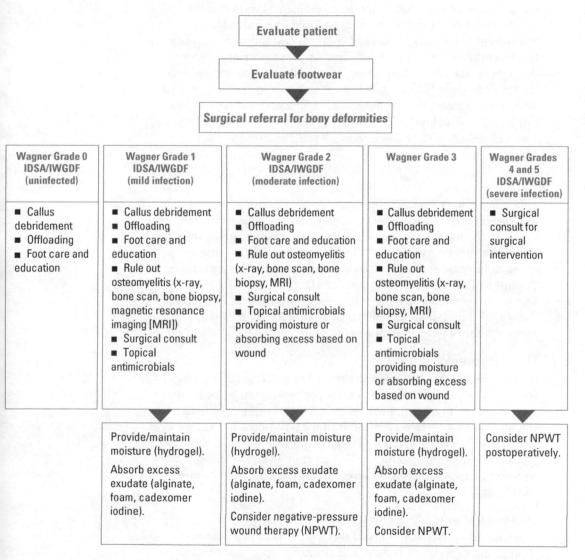

Dressings

Moist wound therapy speeds healing in diabetic and neuropathic foot ulcers. Dressings are selected based on the wound characteristics (see Chapter 9).

The dressing you choose depends on the condition of the patient's ulcer and periwound area. Diabetic and neuropathic foot ulcers tend to produce low to moderate drainage; however, if the wound bed is dry, it needs a dressing that adds moisture. Either amorphous hydrogels or sheet hydrogels may be appropriate options. Hydrogel sheets are more cost-effective but don't work as well in deeper wounds. For deep or tunneling wounds that require obliterating the dead space (loosely filled), hydrogel-impregnated gauze is an alternative to amorphous hydrogels. All hydrogel dressings add moisture to the wound bed because they're made up of as much as 95% water. Hydrogels keep the wound moist while encouraging autolytic debridement.

Offloading

Offloading plantar tissues is the cornerstone of neuropathic treatment as well as prevention for those patients at risk for recurrent breakdown. Redistributing the pressure from a focal point of injury over the larger foot surface is the goal. Offloading seeks to control, limit, or remove all intrinsic and extrinsic factors that increase plantar pressures. Examples of intrinsic risk factors include faulty biomechanics in the foot or the presence of a bony deformity. Extrinsic risk factors include trauma, ill-fitting shoes, or maintaining a position for too long, which allows for the buildup of damaging pressure.

Damage control

Because patients with neuropathy related to diabetes can no longer feel the growing discomfort that precedes tissue damage, offloading is particularly important. Both nonsurgical and surgical offloading interventions may prevent or limit the type of tissue damage that results in ulcer formation. Effective offloading is evident if the wound is improving specifically by reduction in size and depth and wound bed appearance, and there is minimal periwound callous formation.

Nonsurgical offloading interventions

Nonsurgical interventions include therapeutic footwear, custom orthotics, and casts. When considering a device, keep in mind that using a device may increase the patient's risk of falling. Be sure to provide instructions on fall prevention.

Therapeutic footwear

A patient with recurring ulcers and severe foot deformities can greatly benefit from a custom-molded shoe. Common design features of therapeutic footwear include:

- soft, breathable fabric or leather that conforms to foot deformities.
- high tops for ankle stability.
- rocker soles and bottoms for pressure and pain relief across the plantar metatarsal heads.
- a toe box with extra depth and width to accommodate deformities, such as clawed toes and hallux valgus (displacement of the great toe toward the other toes).
- flared lateral soles for stability. (See *Therapeutic shoe modifications*.)

Therapeutic shoe modifications

These illustrations show the modifications in custom shoes that can improve stability and accommodate the foot malformations that affect many patients with diabetes.

High top

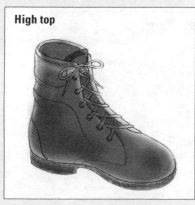

Lateral flare

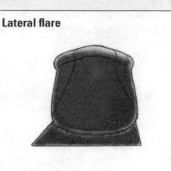

Rocker sole

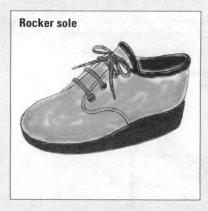

Custom orthotics

Custom orthotics are shoe inserts that serve various functions based on the patient's needs. In general, custom orthotics redistribute pressure, reduce shearing force and friction, and cushion the foot against shocks. If necessary, custom orthotics accommodate the patient's foot deformities as well.

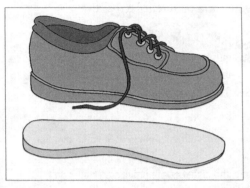

This shoe has a toe box with extra depth and width to accommodate bony deformities, such as claw toes and hallux vagus (displacement of the great toe toward other toes). The shoe can also be modified to allow room for a widened hindfoot/heel. The soft, thick inlay provides comfort and protection.

Walking casts

Walking casts range from total contact casts to splints and walkers.

Cast member

A total contact cast is the gold standard for uninfected neuropathic ulcers on the plantar surface of the foot. Total contact casts are applied by a health care provider such as orthopedic surgeons or podiatrists. Inside the cast, padding is fitted over bony areas of the ankle and leg that are at risk for pressure injuries. The cast is molded to fit snugly to prevent the foot from sliding inside it. This reduces shearing forces over the plantar surface. There are several "kits" available for total contact casts or the casts may be constructed from traditional casting supplies.

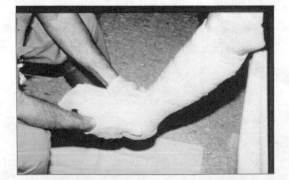

A patient with an infected ulcer is not a candidate for a total contact cast because a cast makes daily assessment, cleaning, and antimicrobial therapy impossible. In addition, inflammation and edema can cause a buildup of pressure within the cast and subsequent tissue damage. In the case of infection, a removable offloading device should be used.

Walk this way

Splints and walkers have cushioned inserts with an outer shell of fiberglass or copolymer. Several splint and walker options are available. One advantage of splints and walkers is that they allow easy inspection of the ulcer. In addition, offloading modifications can be accomplished relatively easily by changing the type of splint or walker in use. However, these devices have disadvantages as well. First and foremost, they don't provide the same degree of pressure and shear relief as a total contact cast. Also, for these therapies to work, the patient must be committed to using the device—a patient can always take a splint off or choose not to use a walker.

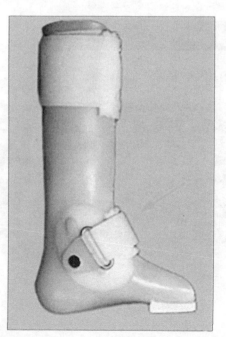

This ankle-foot orthosis is used to relieve pressure from the heel.

Surgical offloading interventions

Surgical offloading procedures include surgical dissection of the wound bed and pressure-inducing bony tissue deformities. Pressure over bony prominences compresses and occludes blood vessels, causing ischemia. Resection (surgical removal) of bony deformities reduces peak plantar pressures. This type of surgery is called *curative surgery* because it removes the pathologic tissue. Examples of curative surgery include exostectomy, digital arthroplasty, bone and joint resections, and partial calcanectomy.

Debridement

Debriding necrotic and nonviable tissue, foreign matter, and microbes from the wound bed expedites wound healing. The most effective method of debridement, surgical debridement, is required in cases of osteomyelitis or when the wound involves a deep abscess or spreading tissue infection. Sharp debridement, which can be performed at the bedside, is an option when surgery isn't necessary or the patient is a poor surgical candidate. Topical proteolytic enzymes can be applied to wound tissue to augment debridement between sessions. (For more information on wound debridement, see Chapter 3.)

Growth factors and cellular tissue products (CTPs) should be considered for the care plan for foot ulcers. (For more information on CTPs, see Chapter 9.)

Matchmaker

Match the three types of ulcers shown here with their names.

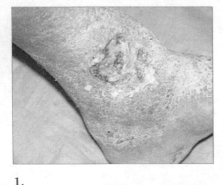

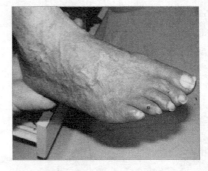

1. _____

2. _____

3. _____

    A.   Arterial ulcer
    B.   Lymphatic ulcer
    C.   Venous ulcer

Answer: 1. C, 2. A, 3. B

Quick quiz

1. Which disorder is the major cause of arterial ulcers?
   A. Atherosclerosis
   B. Diabetes
   C. Venous insufficiency
   D. Lymphedema

Answer: A. Atherosclerosis is the major cause of arterial ulcers.

2. Where is the most common site for a venous ulcer to develop?
   A. Popliteal area
   B. Anterior thigh
   C. Lateral aspect of the foot
   D. Medial aspect of the ankle

Answer: D. Venous ulcers are most common on the medial aspect of the ankle above the malleolus and may extend all the way around the leg.

3. Your patient has venous insufficiency. Their leg edema is best treated by:
   A. compression and leg elevation.
   B. diuretics and compression.
   C. leg elevation and diuretics.
   D. restricting fluid intake and compression.

Answer: A. Compression helps manage edema when the patient is upright. Leg elevation uses gravity to maximize venous return.

4. ABI is:
   A. a guide to venous hypertension.
   B. a value that reflects the amount of blood flow to the ankle.
   C. obtained in a sitting position with the feet flat.
   D. normal if it is above 0.5 mm Hg.

Answer: B. In ABI, the value reflects the ratio of ankle systolic pressure to brachial systolic pressure.

5. The best dressing type for an ischemic ulcer on the toe in a patient who is not revascularized is:
   A. hydrocolloid.
   B. wet to dry.
   C. povidone-iodine.
   D. hydrogel.

Answer: C. An ischemic or arterial ulcer should be kept dry until blood flow to the area is restored.

6. Which sign or symptom is a key indication of progressive arterial insufficiency?
    A. Cyanosis when the foot is in a dependent position
    B. Pain
    C. Edema
    D. Hyperpigmentation of the skin

Answer: B. Pain is the most common presenting symptom in arterial disease with or without an ulcer.

7. Which therapy is the most effective treatment for managing edema?
    A. Hydrotherapy
    B. Compression therapy
    C. Ice therapy
    D. Diuretic therapy

Answer: B. Compression therapy is the most effective way to manage edema.

8. What test is performed first to assess arterial blood flow to the legs in patients with diabetes?
    A. TBI
    B. Doppler ultrasonography
    C. Duplex ultrasonography
    D. ABI

Answer: A. TBI is done for arterial blood flow assessment because ABIs are unreliable in patients with diabetes as their blood vessels are often calcified.

9. The single greatest risk factor for foot ulcers related to diabetes is:
    A. PVD.
    B. peripheral neuropathy.
    C. retinitis pigmentosa.
    D. myopathy.

Answer: B. Peripheral neuropathy is the primary risk factor for foot ulcers related to diabetes.

10. Diabetic ulceration can commonly be found:
    A. around the ankle.
    B. over the sacrum.
    C. on the dorsal surface of the foot.
    D. on the plantar surface of the foot.

Answer: D. Always check the plantar surfaces of the feet for signs of ulcerations. Also check between the toes and on the tips of toes.

11. Which complication commonly results from motor neuropathy?
    A. Charcot neuropathic osteoarthropathy
    B. Diminished sensation
    C. Clawed toes
    D. Poor circulation

Answer: C. Clawed toes commonly result from motor neuropathy, a long-term complication of diabetes.

12. The Semmes–Weinstein monofilament test is used to assess:
    A. blood flow to the feet.
    B. protective sensation of the feet.
    C. pressure on the feet.
    D. temperature of the feet.

Answer: B. During the Semmes–Weinstein monofilament test, the examiner uses a monofilament to assess the patient's protective sensation, or the ability to detect stimuli that may be harmful to the feet.

13. Which statement about the total contact cast is true? Total contact casting is:
    A. a method of redistributing the plantar pressure of the foot.
    B. a special cast just for fractures due to Charcot neuropathic osteoarthropathy.
    C. recommended for use over infected diabetic foot ulcerations.
    D. removable.

Answer: A. The total contact cast is an offloading device that redistributes pressure on the plantar surface of the foot.

Scoring

☆☆☆ If you answered 11 to 13 questions correctly, you've got a reason to grin! You offloaded this quiz in a jiffy.

☆☆ If you answered six to 10 questions correctly, brag to your friends! You zipped through this quiz without decompression.

☆ If you answered fewer than six questions correctly, let out a sigh! Plantar your feet and move onward and upward.

Select references

Beuscher, T. (2022). The importance of shoe selection: Clinical practice alert. *Journal of Wound, Ostomy, Continence Nursing, 49*(1), 87–88. https://doi.org/10.1097/WON.0000000000000838

Bonham, P. A., Brunette, G., Crestodina, L., Droste, L. R., Gonzalez, A., Kelechi, T. J., Ratliff, C. R., & Varnado, M. F. (2021). *Guideline for management of patients with lower-extremity wounds due to diabetes mellitus and/or neuropathic disease* (WOCN Clinical Practice Guideline Series 3). Wound, Ostomy, Continence Nurses Society.

Bowers, S., & Franco, E. (2020). Chronic wounds: Evaluation and management. *American Family Physician, 101*(3), 159–166. https://www.aafp.org/dam/brand/aafp/pubs/afp/issues/2020/0201/p159.pdf

Estelle, E., & Mathioudakis, N. (2018). Update on management of diabetic foot ulcers. *Annals of the New York Academy of Sciences, 1411*(1), 153–165. https://doi.org/10.1111/nyas.13569

Isoherranen, K., Kallio, M., O'Brien, J. J., & Lagus, H. (2020). Clinical characteristics of lower extremity ulcers. *Journal of the European Wound Management Association, 21*(1), 51–58. https://doi.org/10.35279/jewma202011.08

Kelechi, T. J., Brunette, G., Bonham, P. A., Crestodina, L., Droste, L. R., Ratliff, C. R., & Varnado, M. F. (2020). 2019 guideline for management of wounds in patients with lower-extremity venous disease (LEVD): An executive summary. *Journal of Wound, Ostomy, and Continence Nursing, 47*(2), 97–110. https://doi.org/10.1097/WON.0000000000000622

Lane, K. L., Abusamaan, M. S., Voss, B. F., Thurber, E. G., Al-Hajri, N., Gopakumar, S., Le, J. T., Gill, S., Blanck, J., Prichett, L., Hicks, C. W., Sherman, R. L., Abularrag, C. J., & Mathioudakis, N. N. (2020). Glycemic control and diabetic foot ulcer outcomes: A systematic review and meta-analysis of observational studies. *Journal of Diabetes and Its Complications, 34*(10). https://doi.org/10.1016/j.jdiacomp.2020.107638

Laopoulou, F., Kelesi, M., Fasoi, G., Vasilopoulos, G., & Polikandrioti, M. (2020). Perceived social support in individuals with diabetic foot ulcers. *Journal of Wound, Ostomy, and Continence Nursing, 47*(1), 65–71. https://doi.org/10.1097/WON.0000000000000614

Masuda, E., Ozsvath, K., Vossler, J., Woo, K., Kistner, R., Lurie, F., Monahan, D., Brown, W., Labropoulos, N., Dalsin, M., Khilnai, N., Wakefield, T., & Gloviczki, P. (2020). The 2020 appropriate use criteria for chronic lower extremity venous disease of the American Venous Forum, the Society for Vascular Surgery, the American Vein and Lymphatic Society, and the Society of Interventional Radiology. *Journal of Vascular Surgery: Venous and Lymphatic Disorders, 8*(4), 505–525. https://doi.org/10.1016/j.jvsv.2020.02.001

Monteiro-Soares, M., Boyko, E. J., Jeffcoate, W., Mills, J. L., Russell, D., Morback, S., & Game, F. (2020). Diabetic foot ulcer classifications: A critical review. *Diabetes Metabolism Research and Reviews, 36*(Suppl. 1). https://doi.org/10.1002/dmrr.3272

Monteiro-Soares, M., Russell, D., Boyko, E. J., Jeffcoate, W., Mills, J. L., Morback, S., & Game, F. (2020). Guidelines on the classification of diabetic foot ulcers (IWGDF 2019). *Diabetes Metabolism Research and Reviews, 36*(Suppl. 1). https://doi.org/10.1002/dmrr.3273

Murphy, G. A., Woelfel, S. L., & Armstrong, D. G. (2020). What to put on (and what to take off) a wound: Treating a chronic neuropathic ulcer with an autologous homologous skin construct, offloading and common sense. *Oxford Medical Case Reports, 2020*(8), 259–263. https://doi.org/10.1093/omcr/omaa058

Mutasem, A., Al Ayed, M. T., Robert, A. A., & Al Dawish, M. A. (2020). Clinical utility of the ankle-brachial index and toe brachial index in patients with diabetic foot ulcers. *Current Diabetes Review, 16*(3), 270–277. https://doi.org/10.2174/1573399815666190531093238

O'Connor, J., & Varnado, M. F. (2022). Lower extremity neuropathic disease. In L. L. McNichol, C. R. Ratliff, & S. S. Yates (Eds.), *Wound, Ostomy, and Continence Nurses Society core curriculum: Wound management* (2nd ed., pp. 539–584). Wolters Kluwer.

O'Meara, S., Cullum, N., Nelson, E. A., Dumville, J. C. (2012). Compression for venous leg ulcers. *Cochrane Database of Systematic Reviews, 2011*(11), 1–155. https://doi.org/10.1002/14651858.CD000265.pub3

Schecter, M. C., Fayfman, M., Khan, L. S. M. F., Carr, K., Patterson, S., Ziemer, D. C., Umpierrez, G. E., Rajani, R., & Kempker, R. R. (2020). Evaluation of a comprehensive diabetic foot ulcer care quality model. *Journal of Diabetes and Its Complications, 34*(4). https://doi.org/10.1016/j.jdiacomp.2019.107516

Schneider, C., Stratman, S., & Krisner, R. S. (2021). Lower extremity ulcers. *Medical Clinics, 105*(4), 663–679. https://doi.org/10.1016/j.mcna.2021.04.006

Singer, A. J., Tassiopoulos, A., & Kirsner, R. S. (2017). Evaluation and management of lower-extremity ulcers. *The New England Journal of Medicine, 377*(16), 1559–1567. https://doi.org/10.1056/NEJMra1615243

Varaki, E. S., Gargiulo, G. D., Penkala, S., & Breen, P. P. (2018). Peripheral vascular disease assessment in the lower limb: A review of current and emerging non-invasive diagnostic methods. *BioMedical Engineering Online, 17*, 1–27. https://doi.org/10.1186/s12938-018-0494-4

Zakin, E., Abrams, R., & Simpson, D. M. (2019). Diabetic neuropathy. *Seminars in Neurology, 39*(5), 560–569. https://doi.org/10.1055/s-0039-1688978

Chapter 8

Atypical and malignant wounds

Just the facts

In this chapter, you'll learn about:

◆ causes and treatment of atypical wounds

◆ neoplasms

◆ treatment of neoplasms

Chronic wounds are considered atypical when the etiology of the wound is unknown, the location of the wound is different from common chronic wounds, and its appearance varies from common chronic wounds.

Usually, atypical wounds are slow to heal and do not respond to conventional therapies. For a correct diagnosis, a skin or tissue biopsy can determine the cell and tissue morphology, so a definitive treatment may be initiated. Atypical wounds may occur anywhere on the body, but the lower extremities are a common site for vasculitis, pyoderma gangrenosum, calciphylaxis, sickle cell anemia ulcers, and basal or squamous cell carcinomas.

Causes of atypical wounds

Potential causes of atypical wounds are categorized as external, metabolic or autoimmune, inflammatory, infectious, or neoplastic.

External causes
• Bites
• Radiation
• Trauma
• Chemical

Metabolic and autoimmune disorders
• Calciphylaxis
• Thromboangiitis obliterans

• Epidermolysis bullosa
• Sickle cell anemia
• Systemic lupus erythematosus
• Scleroderma

Inflammatory processes
Pyoderma gangrenosum

Infection
Necrotizing fasciitis

Neoplasms
• Basal cell carcinoma
• Kaposi sarcoma
• Lymphoma
• Squamous cell carcinoma
• Melanoma

External causes

Bites from insects and animals, radiation, trauma, and chemicals are external causes of wounds. Wounds from trauma and radiation are discussed in more detail in Chapter 5, "Acute Wounds."

Bites

The bite of a recluse spider usually manifests as a red plaque that can sometimes be identified by two small puncture marks surrounding the erythema. Vesicle formation may occur and then necrosis develops within a couple of days. These generally resolve without further complications. Topical antibiotic creams may also be effective in preventing secondary staphylococcal infection from an open wound.

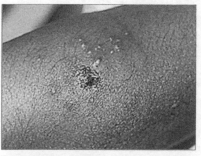

Erythematous lesion with central eschar caused by a spider bite.

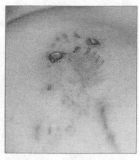

Wounds from several dog bites.

Chemicals

Intravenous extravasation ulcers

Extravasation is the unintentional administration of a vesicant, irritant, or nonvesicant solution into surrounding tissue. This is an example of a chemical wound. Vesicants (chemotherapy agents, certain electrolyte solutions, radiographic contrast media, and vasopressors) are solutions capable of causing tissue injury or destruction for an extended period of time. Irritants and nonvesicants such as alkylating agents, carmustine, or vincristine can also be destructive, but these tend to be excreted more quickly.

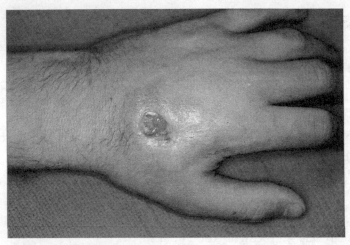

Chronic ulceration from chemotherapy infiltration.

Necrotic drug eruptions

Necrotic drug eruptions can include heparin- and warfarin-induced necrosis. For injectable anticoagulants, the necrosis occurs at the site of infusion or injection; warfarin-induced necrosis commonly occurs on the breasts, buttocks, thighs, and abdomen. The abundance of small dermal blood vessels in fatty tissue may explain why warfarin-induced necrosis is more common in some areas. Drug necrosis is rare but can occur between the first and 10th day of starting anticoagulation after a large initial loading dose has been given. Although the precise cause of the drug reaction is unknown, it is speculated to be related to the protein C, protein S, and antithrombin III anticoagulant cascade that causes an immune response. More research is needed to better understand the pathogenesis of warfarin-induced necrosis.

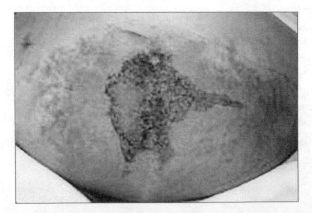

Metabolic and autoimmune disorders

Calciphylaxis

Calciphylaxis, also known as calcific uremic arteriolopathy, is a serious disorder that causes skin ischemia and necrosis and most commonly affects patients in end-stage kidney disease. The pathogenesis is poorly understood. The reduction of arteriolar blood flow is caused by calcification, fibrosis, and thrombus formation. Hyperparathyroidism, deficiencies in inhibitors of vascular calcification, and chronic inflammation have also been implicated.

Ischemic necrosis is a manifestation, and in some cases, pain may precede the actual eruption of the skin lesion. The lesions present as nodules, plaques, nonhealing ulcers, and/or cutaneous necrosis, particularly in areas of high adiposity such as the thigh. Diagnosis is made by clinical appearance, history of comorbidities (i.e., kidney disease), and tissue biopsy to look for classic calciphylaxis morphology.

Thromboangiitis obliterans

Also known as Buerger disease, thromboangiitis obliterans is a rare form of vasculitis that affects the arteries and the veins. It is an inflammatory condition that leads to thrombosis in some superficial veins as well as small and medium-sized arteries. It causes arterial ischemia in distal extremities and superficial thrombophlebitis.

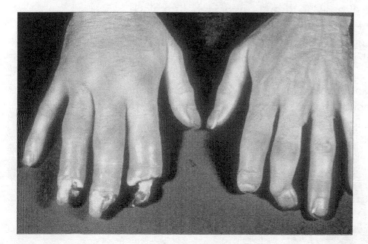

Epidermolysis bullosa

Epidermolysis bullosa (EB) is a heterogeneous group of hereditary, mechanobullous disorders that cause varying degrees of skin and mucosa fragility. Genetic mutations affect skin structural proteins. There are four major types of EB, based on the ultrastructural level of tissue damage in the skin: epidermolysis bullosa simplex (EBS), junctional epidermolysis bullosa (JEB), dystrophic epidermolysis (DEB), and Kindler epidermolysis bullosa (KEB). Depending on the level of blistering and the type of mutation, each of the subtypes of EB is different. There is no specific targeted care for EB, but treatment is generally supportive and includes wound care, infection control, nutritional support, and prevention and treatment of any complications that may occur.

Sickle cell disease

Sickle cell disease is a hemoglobinopathy characterized by the predominance of hemoglobin S. The sickling of red cells is caused by inheritance of homozygosity for hemoglobin S and hemoglobin C or a beta thalassemia. Two observational studies, the Cooperative Study of Sickle Cell Disease in the United States (2019) and the Jamaica Cohort Study (2018) in Jamaica, have provided reliable information on the clinical course of sickle cell anemia in the context of sickle cell ulcers. These studies began in the early 1970s and followed several hundred patients for at least 10 years.

Ulcer formation

Sickled hemoglobin cells lead to abnormal erythrocyte adhesiveness with reflexive vasoconstriction. The intima proliferation of the blood vessel leads to segmental narrowing of medium-sized arteries and degenerative changes of the media, as well as obstruction of the vasa vasorum, all contributing to the vaso-occlusive events that cause sickle cell crisis. The patient is predisposed to thrombosis or embolism blocking the arterial supply to all or part of the affected organ. Patients are plagued by recurrent vaso-occlusive crises with ischemic tissue damage causing pain and eventually organ failure. Patients have described the pain as feeling as if there is broken glass cutting them from inside. Patients may require intravenous pain medication and blood transfusions. The hemolytic anemia produced by the sickled cells causes aplastic crises, megaloblastic anemia, leg ulcers, gallstones, and gout.

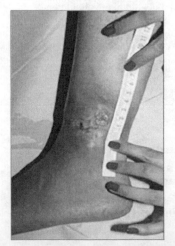

Systemic lupus erythematosus

Systemic lupus erythematosus (SLE) ulcers most commonly occur on the scalp and face and sometimes look like psoriasis. SLE ulcers can be aggravated by sunlight and other ultraviolet light.

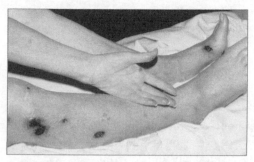

Red, scaly systemic lupus erythematosus ulcer.

Systemic scleroderma

Systemic scleroderma causes hardening of the skin and tissues that support organs and is classified as a connective tissue disease. The word *scleroderma* means thickening of the skin. In this autoimmune disease, fibrosis occurs most commonly on the hands but can also be seen on the face, neck, and upper chest. Acrocyanosis, bluish color of the tissue on the extremities, may occur with scleroderma. When scleroderma is localized to the skin and/or subcutaneous tissue, it is called morphea.

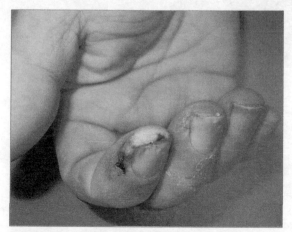

Acrocyanosis and ulcer formation in scleroderma.

Systemic scleroderma is a chronic multisystem disease causing widespread vascular dysfunction and progressive fibrosis of the skin and internal organs. Signs and symptoms of scleroderma are puffy skin that slowly becomes hard and thicker than normal skin, stiff joints because the skin supporting them does not stretch as well, and small white lumps containing calcium in or under the skin on fingers, a condition called calcinosis cutis. Raynaud phenomenon causes the fingers and toes to turn whitish or purplish-blue in response to cold or stress due to lack of blood flow. This may not be visible in people with darker skin tones. Treatment goals usually involve managing the symptoms associated with the skin changes of localized scleroderma while trying to prevent complications as they occur in the normal progression of the disease.

Inflammatory processes

Pyoderma gangrenosum

Pyoderma gangrenosum ulcers are examples of wounds due to an inflammatory process. The ulcerative type occurs most commonly on the legs after injury or trauma. The atypical type of pyoderma gangrenosum occurs on the torso and upper limbs. Often, multiple small pustular or bullous lesions merge into one large ulcer. The ulcers are usually painful, and the disease is characterized by ulcer recurrence and/or exacerbation of lesions, known as pathergy. This phenomenon of pathergy should be acknowledged when considering surgical debridement of these ulcers.

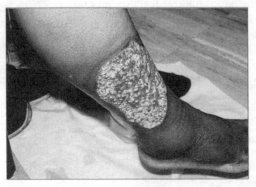

Painful, open ulcer with reddish-purple irregular borders.

Infections

A variety of microorganisms may cause atypical wounds. In particular, beta-hemolytic *Streptococcus pyogenes* can cause necrotizing fasciitis.

Necrotizing fasciitis

Necrotizing fasciitis is a severe, potentially life-threatening type of infection in which bacteria enter the body through a minor wound and release harmful toxins that interfere with the tissue's blood supply.

Extensive tissue damage often occurs under the skin, and a common first symptom is tenderness. Known colloquially as "flesh-eating bacteria," beta-hemolytic *S. pyogenes* is the most common organism to cause necrotizing fasciitis; however, no single organism is responsible for the infection. Frequently, two or more organisms combine and form a synergistic gangrene. Treatment requires extensive debridement of necrotic tissue, usually in an operating room. Management requires a multidisciplinary approach with surgeons, infectious disease physicians, nutritionists, and seasoned wound care specialists experienced in the management of complex wounds.

Classic signs

- Warm skin and a painful bump or spot on the skin
- Typically, a bronze or purple-colored blister forms with a rapidly spreading area of erythema.
- Tissue necrosis progresses with gangrene of the area.

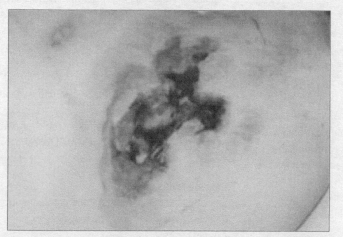

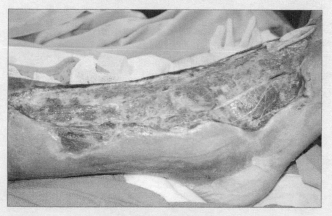

Treatments

Bites
Black widow spider bite
- Immediate medical attention
- Cool compresses
- Elevation, if possible
- Antivenom
- Calcium gluconate
- Antihistamines
- Analgesics
- Local wound care with nonadhesive or low-adhesive dressings to minimize pain

Brown recluse spider bite
- Cool compresses
- Elevation, if possible
- Analgesics
- Systemic corticosteroids
- Aggressive local wound care
- Debridement
- Grafting

Dog bite
- Immediately irrigate the wound with copious amounts of normal saline solution. Don't immerse and soak the wound because this may allow bacteria to float back into the tissue.
- Ask the person about the animal that bit them to determine whether there is a risk of rabies.
- Antibiotics
- Rabies therapy
- Tetanus vaccination
- Local wound care with nonadhesive or low-adhesive dressings to minimize pain
- Topical steroids may be needed to manage intense itch.
- Debridement and grafting if the wound is extensive

Chemical
Intravenous extravasation ulcers
- Immediate cessation of the infusion
- Flushing of the area with normal saline solution within 24 hours
- Local infiltration of the affected area with dilute antidote (varies depending on the drug extravasated)
- Debridement and topical care depending on wound characteristics
- Grafting
- Possible amputation if gangrene results

Necrotic drug eruptions
- Discontinuation of warfarin
- Intravenous heparin
- Debridement

Metabolic and autoimmune disorders
Calciphylaxis
- Requires a multidisciplinary approach involving nephrologists, plastic surgeons, dietitians, and wound care specialists
- Local wound care depending on wound exudate management
- Pain management
- Surgical debridement for infected wounds with excessive drainage
- Nonsurgical debridement for noninfected, dry wounds
- Hyperbaric oxygen therapy (reserved for refractory wounds)

Thromboangiitis obliterans
- Smoking abstinence (cornerstone of treatment)
- Calcium channel blockers such as nifedipine
- Arterial bypass
- Major or minor amputations
- Avoidance of cold temperatures
- Aspirin
- Vasodilators
- Surgical sympathectomy for pain management

Epidermolysis bullosa
- No targeted therapy for EB (more research needed)
- Supported wound care for the protection of frail, blistering bullae
- Prevention and treatment of complications
- Nutritional support

Sickle cell anemia
- Management of venous stasis (leg elevation compression therapy)
- Wound bed management (absorbent dressing for wet wounds and moist dressings for dry wounds)
- Pain management
- Debridement of devitalized tissue
- Application of allograft or engineered skin tissue for refractory ulcers

Systemic lupus erythematosus
- Systemic management of underlying disease
- Corticosteroids (systemic, topical)
- Immunosuppressants (e.g., azathioprine, cyclophosphamide)
- Hyperbaric oxygen therapy
- Local wound care based on wound assessment

Systemic scleroderma
- Systemic management of underlying disease
- Nitrates, such as nitroglycerin, for vasodilation
- Debridement
- Hyperbaric oxygen therapy
- Local wound care—nonocclusive dressings with nonadhesive or low-adhesive surfaces commonly treated like vascular wounds

Inflammatory processes
Pyoderma gangrenosum
- Systemic management of underlying disease
- Corticosteroids (topical, systemic, intralesional)
- Immunosuppressive agents such as cyclosporine (systemic, topical)
- Antimicrobial agents, such as tetracycline and vancomycin
- Antitumor necrosis factor (alpha) medications, such as infliximab and etanercept
- Blood products
- Immunomodulators, such as intravenous immunoglobulin
- Hyperbaric oxygen
- Local wound care with low-adhesive dressings such as with foams, gels, and silicone dressings

Infection
Necrotizing fasciitis
- Frequent surgical debridement
- Broad-spectrum antibiotics
- Grafting or flap
- Aggressive local wound care
- Negative pressure wound therapy
- Local wound care (if extensive, dressing changes may need to be done under anesthesia)
- Consider hyperbaric oxygen therapy to demarcate necrotic tissue quickly.

Neoplasms

Nonmelanoma skin cancers, basal cell carcinomas, and squamous cell carcinomas are the most common types of skin cancers. Kaposi sarcoma, lymphomas, and melanomas are less common, but all can present as atypical wounds. Establishing the diagnosis requires a skin biopsy and is essential to determining the treatment.

Basal cell carcinoma is the most common skin cancer arising from the basal layer of the epidermis.

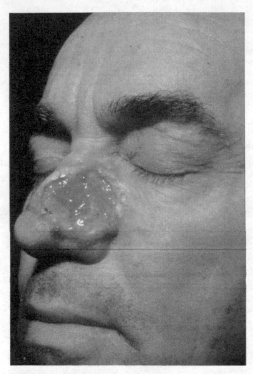

This basal cell carcinoma was untreated. It eventually ulcerated and invaded deeper tissue.

Squamous cell carcinomas originate in the keratinocyte and manifest as malignant, keratinizing, squamous proliferations generated from the epidermis.

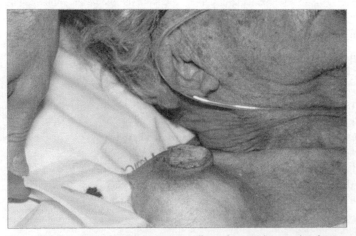

After not being treated, this squamous cell carcinoma ulcerated to form the malignant wound shown here.

Malignant wounds can develop from skin cancer that has not been treated or has recurred.

Lymphomas of the skin are cutaneous proliferation of T or B cells of the type that may cause pruritus, patch-like erythematic rash, or nodular skin lesions. A skin biopsy with immunodiagnostic phenotyping is generally how the diagnosis is made. The goal of treatment is to limit the lymphoma to the cutaneous skin and prevent it from getting to the bloodstream and lymph nodes. The treatment depends on the staging of the disease, ranging from an early stage 1A to 2A, consisting of papules, patches, or plaques with limited if any lymph node involvement. Treatment is a combination of phototherapy, topical steroid creams, topical retinoids, topical imiquimod, local radiation, and photopheresis if there is blood involvement.

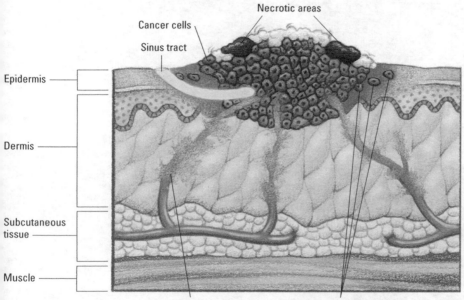

Early recognition of skin rashes, erythematous patches, and ulceration is important for the clinician to identify. Malignant tumors caused by a metastasis of a primary tumor can infiltrate the epidermis of the skin or may occur due to cancer of the skin. These wounds grow rapidly and commonly invade surrounding tissues and organs, sometimes causing sinus tracts and fistulas. Malignant wounds may present as an ulceration or cauliflower-like appearance; are poorly perfused with friable, fragile blood vessels; and contain large amounts of necrotic tissue. The most common locations are the head, neck, chest, and abdomen. Many occur with patients who have lymphoma, leukemia, or untreated skin cancers. Malignant wounds most commonly occur in patients with breast cancer; however, they can also occur in patients with cancer of the head, neck, chest, and abdomen.

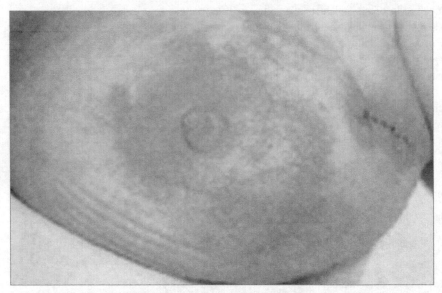

Inflamed carcinoma of the breast.

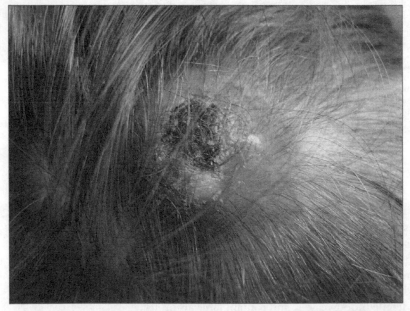

This malignant wound resulted from lymphoma that metastasized to the patient's scalp.

When a primary tumor outgrows its blood supply, it can invade the skin, resulting in a malignant wound.

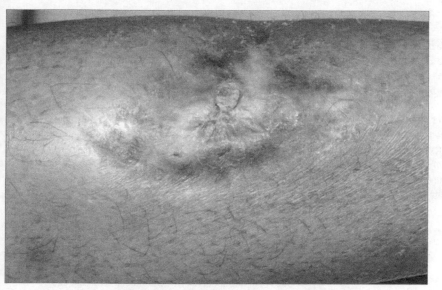

A squamous cell carcinoma resulting from a burn scar.

Chronic wounds or even scar tissue can evolve into a malignant wound. This type of malignant wound is called a Marjolin ulcer.

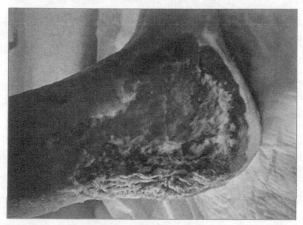

A large, invasive squamous cell carcinoma.

Complications

Problem	Causes	Management strategies
Odor	Nonviable, necrotic tissue and excessive drainage create an ideal environment for bacterial growth. These polymicrobial bacteria are responsible for causing odor. Odor-causing bacteria can be aerobic, such as *Klebsiella*, *Proteus*, *Pseudomonas*, and *Staphylococcus*, or they can be anaerobic such as *Clostridium* and *Bacteroides fragilis*. Odor can cause nausea, vomiting, and loss of appetite for the patient.	• Change dressings and gently irrigate the wound with tap water or normal saline solution at frequent intervals. • Use antimicrobial solutions or wound cleansers as needed. • Apply topical antimicrobials to reduce the amount of bacteria. Consider metronidazole gel or crushed metronidazole tablets, Iodoflex or Iodosorb, or silver-containing products as indicated. • Select from foam, calcium alginate, hydrofiber, composite, and occlusive dressings based on wound characteristics. See Chapter 9 for more information on dressings. • Antiseptic solutions such as acetic acid or sodium hypochlorite can reduce odor but might sting and require dressing changes at a minimum. • Use charcoal dressings, such as Carbonet, CarboFlex, and Actisorb Plus. • Use room deodorizers and odor-masking techniques such as: – Peppermint, lavender, or lemon scents – Mentholatum (e.g., Vicks VapoRub) applied near the patient's or caregiver's nostrils to minimize the perception of odor – A tray of kitty litter, baking soda, or charcoal under the patient's bed to absorb odors – Room ventilation – Pouching system to the wound to contain drainage and help control odors
Bleeding	Malignant cells stimulate angiogenesis. Thrombocytopenia and disseminated intravascular coagulopathy and malnutrition are factors common with cancer, leading to increased vascular permeability and promotion of a loss of protein and fibrinogen. This causes the blood vessels surrounding a malignant wound to become friable and fragile and the blood to have an impaired ability to clot.	• Use nonadherent or low-adhesive dressings (such as silicone dressings) to minimize tissue trauma and reduce the risk of bleeding. • Avoid frequent or unnecessary dressing changes. • Consider using alginate dressings and/or hemostatic agents (e.g., Gelfoam, Surgicel, Spongostan, silver nitrate, Oxycel) for small bleeding areas. • Apply epinephrine-soaked gauze in layers for larger areas. • Assist with surgical intervention (cauterization) or the application of topical epinephrine 1:1,000 to control profuse bleeding. • Administer oral antifibrinolytics (e.g., tranexamic acid, aminocaproic acid) as prescribed to control severe bleeding.

Problem	Causes	Management strategies
Exudate (drainage)	The leakage of fibrinogen and plasma colloids by vessels in the wound causes exudate to form. Bacteria in the wound release enzymes that liquefy tissue, producing additional exudate.	• Use highly absorbent dressings (e.g., calcium alginate, foam, hydrofiber) in wounds with moderate to large amounts of exudate. • Administer topical or systemic antimicrobials as prescribed to reduce bacterial load and exudate. • Use a wound drainage system such as a pouch on wounds with large amounts of exudate. (Avoid using a negative pressure system.) • Protect the surrounding skin from maceration and irritation. • Use a stockinette, tube sleeves, and binders when possible to secure dressings and minimize tape to skin.
Pain	Pressure on nerve endings from edema and the tumor as well as exposure of the dermis to air may cause chronic pain. Dressing changes and other procedures may also worsen pain.	• Assess pain level using a 1–10 pain scale. • Remove old dressings, caring not to pull fragile skin. • Use saline, wound cleansers, and emollients to remove adhesive and debris. • Apply antibacterial products and culture concerning wounds. • Offer local analgesia, prilocaine/lidocaine 2%. • Cetacaine topical anesthetic spray can be used on normal skin to numb the skin prior to a deep injection. • Choose dressings that are absorbent for large, draining wounds and for dry wounds, use nonadherent surfaces, and add moisture to a dry wound bed.
Pruritus (itching)	Edema, bacteria, and tumor all cause cellular inflammation and destruction. This causes the skin to stretch and the peripheral nerves become irritated, commonly resulting in pruritus. Fungal infections may also cause pruritus.	• Emollients, hydrogel sheet dressings, and other topically applied agents can be stored in the refrigerator and then applied to the wound. • Apply menthol creams to the affected area. • Advise the patient to use cool or lukewarm water to bathe or shower rather than hot water. • Advise the patient that antihistamines may only have a limited effect on the pruritus associated with malignant wounds. • Administer oral medications such as gabapentin, doxepin, or mirtazapine as ordered. • Apply topical agents such as tacrolimus and lidocaine before capsaicin (to reduce stinging) and topical cannabinoid agonist agents for temporary relief.

Treatment of neoplasms: Compassionate care

The goal behind any wound management system is to protect the wound and the surrounding areas and to provide an ideal environment for healing. However, because malignant wounds often occur near the end of a patient's life, treatment typically focuses on minimizing complications, controlling symptoms, and offering psychological support rather than on healing. Reducing the size of malignant wounds through radiation and chemotherapy frequently aids in treatment by reducing odor, bleeding, and drainage.

Malignant wounds are a complication of cancer and usually occur in patients with advanced disease. When treatment becomes palliative, not curative, the goals are management of challenging symptoms and improving the quality of life for patients and their families.

Quick quiz

1. When a primary lesion outgrows its blood supply and invades the surrounding skin, which objective is not a primary goal of care?
   A. Diagnosing the wound
   B. Minimizing the complications
   C. Healing the wound
   D. Managing the odor

Answer: C. The goal for any wound management system is to protect the wound and the surrounding tissue and to provide an ideal environment for healing. Because malignant wounds often occur at the end of life, treatment typically focuses on minimizing complications, controlling symptoms, and offering psychological support rather than on healing.

2. Which is the best method to manage a heavily draining wound?
   A. Chilled hydrogel sheets
   B. Silver nitrate application
   C. Alginate and foam dressing
   D. Metronidazole gel and gauze dressing

Answer: C. Alginates absorb drainage and foam absorbs excess drainage and traps it in the dressing.

3. Which potentially life-threatening type of wound infection releases harmful toxins?
   A. Cellulitis
   B. Atypical mycobacteria
   C. Necrotizing fasciitis
   D. Pyoderma gangrenosum

Answer: C. Necrotizing fasciitis is a rapidly progressing skin infection due to a combination of two or more microorganisms that invade the underlying deep fascia, causing necrosis and tissue death.

4. At which site is warfarin unlikely to cause necrosis?
    A.   Site of the infusion or injection
    B.   Breast
    C.   Buttocks
    D.   Umbilicus

Answer: A. Warfarin is only available in pill form and cannot be injected. The abundance of small dermal blood vessels in fatty tissue may explain why warfarin-induced necrosis is more common in the breast, buttocks, and umbilicus.

5. Which skin disorder causes ischemia and tissue necrosis in patients with end-stage kidney disease?
    A.   Calciphylaxis
    B.   Marjolin ulcer
    C.   Necrotizing fasciitis
    D.   Epidermolysis bullosa

Answer: A. Calciphylaxis is a rare, clinically progressive cutaneous necrosis that frequently occurs in patients with end-stage kidney disease. Cutaneous and subcutaneous calcification develops and tissue death can occur.

6. What is the most important reason for accurately recognizing an ulcer as an atypical wound ulcer?
    A.   The wound may be contagious.
    B.   Treatment varies based on the etiology of the wound.
    C.   The standard wound healing therapies will not work.
    D.   Treatment must be billed correctly.

Answer: B. It is critical to recognize the wound etiology when the cause is a process other than pressure, stasis, or neuropathy. A correct diagnosis will ensure the appropriate treatment.

7. Which inflammatory condition most commonly occurs in the hands?
    A.   Necrotizing fasciitis
    B.   Warfarin-induced necrosis
    C.   Thromboangiitis obliterans
    D.   Epidermolysis bullosa

Answer: C. Thromboangiitis obliterans is a rare form of vasculitis that causes thrombosis of the distal arteries and veins, frequently resulting in ischemia in distal extremities.

Scoring

☆☆☆ If you answered all seven questions correctly, congratulations! You are extraordinary with the not-so-ordinary.

☆☆ If you answered five or six questions correctly, nicely done! You have demonstrated you can identify the un-usual.

☆ If you answered fewer than five questions correctly, don't despair! A quick review will reveal a-typical presentation.

Select references

Bauer, C. (2022). Oncology-related skin and wound care. In L. L. McNichol, C. R. Ratliff, & S. S. Yates (Eds.), *Wound, Ostomy, and Continence Nurses Society core curriculum: Wound management* (2nd ed., pp. 668–695). Wolters Kluwer.

Distler, O., & Cozzio, A. (2016). Systemic sclerosis and localized scleroderma—Current concepts and novel targets for therapy. *Seminars in Immunopathology, 38*(1), 87–95. https://doi.org/10.1007/s00281-015-0551-z

Kucisec-Tepes, N. (2013). Atypical wounds. *Journal of Wound Management, 13*(1), 86–87. https://pubmed.ncbi.nlm.nih.gov231938251

National Heart, Lung, and Blood Institute. (2019). *Cooperative study of sickle cell disease (CSSCD).* https://biolincc.nhlbi.nih.gov/studies/csscd/#:~:text=The%20 Cooperative%20Study%20of%20Sickle,and%20mortality%20of%20the%20 disease

Pecone, D., Agarwal, A. G., & Cardones, A. R. (2022). Wounds caused by dermatological conditions. In L. L. McNichol, C. R. Ratliff, & S. S. Yates (Eds.), *Wound, Ostomy, and Continence Nurses Society core curriculum: Wound management* (2nd ed., pp. 652–667). Wolters Kluwer.

Pieper, B. A. (2022). Atypical lower extremity wounds. In L. L. McNichol, C. R. Ratliff, & S. S. Yates (Eds.), *Wound, Ostomy, and Continence Nurses Society core curriculum: Wound management* (2nd ed., pp. 585–602). Wolters Kluwer.

Ratnagobal, S., & Sinha, S. (2013). Pyoderma gangrenosum: Guideline for wound practitioners. *Journal of Wound Care, 22*(2), 68–73. https://doi.org/10.12968/ jowc.2013.22.2.68

Serjeant, G. R., Chin, N., Asnani, M. R., Serjeant, B. E., Mason, K. P., Hambleton, I. R., & Knight-Madden, J. M. (2018). *Causes of death and early life determinants of survival in homozygous sickle cell disease: The Jamaican cohort study from birth.* https://www.ncbi.nlm.nih.gov/pmc/articles/PMC5832208/

Watkins, J. (2016). Diagnosis, treatment and management of epidermolysis bullosa. *British Journal of Nursing, 25*(8), 428–431. https://doi.org/10.12968/bjon .2016.25.8.428

Wolfe, S. (2022). Assessment and management of wound-related infections. In L. L. McNichol, C. R. Ratliff, & S. S. Yates (Eds.), *Wound, Ostomy, and Continence Nurses Society core curriculum: Wound management* (2nd ed., pp. 633–651). Wolters Kluwer.

Young, T. (2017). Caring for patients with malignant and end-of-life wounds. *Wounds UK, 13*, 20–29. https://www.researchgate.net/publication/318092217

Chapter 9

Wound management

Just the facts

In this chapter, you'll learn about:

◆ criteria to use for determining best wound management

◆ types of dressings used in wound care and the features, indications, advantages, and disadvantages of each type

◆ indications, contraindications, and application methods for therapeutic modalities

A look at wound management

Over time, wound care has developed from a practice that focused primarily on care of the injury to a process that also considers the complexities of the patient's general health, possible underlying disease, and specific wound characteristics. As wound care knowledge has increased, so have the number and types of products available to aid healing.

As you read, keep in mind that dressings and adjunct wound care products are tools that can help promote healing, but they aren't the only tools you'll need. Unless concurrent problems, such as malnutrition, oxygenation, circulatory disorders, patient mental illnesses, and knowledge deficits, are also addressed, the healing process stalls. In addition, no dressing or topical agent can compensate for an incomplete assessment. In short, let the findings of a thorough assessment guide your wound care product selection. (See *Tips for selecting wound care products*.)

Tips for selecting wound care products

When planning care, let the big picture guide your choices. Ask yourself these important questions:
• What information did you get from your assessment?
  – Don't forget the cause of the wound and how long it has been present. Identifying causal factors is an important aspect of the wound care.
  – Is there excess exudate as evidenced by saturated dressings and/or maceration around the wound? If so, a more absorbent dressing would be ideal. Always protect the periwound skin unless contraindicated based on the dressing selection.

(continued)

Tips for selecting wound care products *(continued)*

- How large is the wound? Would it be more cost-effective to use an advanced wound care product such as negative pressure wound therapy (NPWT) to facilitate granulation tissue or closure?
- After cleansing, does the wound (not the old dressing) have an unpleasant odor? Do you suspect infection (inflammation in addition to fever, pus, advancing cellulitis, changes in lab work, and/or sudden unexplained increase in pain)? If so, is a culture warranted? For a description of culture technique, see Chapter 3, "Wound Bed Preparation."
- Is there tunneling, undermining, or a cavity that needs to be lightly filled?
- Does the wound need more moisture as evidenced by dry dressings when changed or fibrin slough forming on the wound bed? If so, a hydrogel adds moisture, and transparent films and hydrocolloids maintain moisture.
- Should the wound be debrided? If so, which method is best for the patient? Keep in mind that a wound that is not likely to heal in a timely manner should be kept dry, and the scab (eschar) should be protected and kept dry. Examples include an arterial insufficiency wound on the foot or a wound on a patient in hospice care who is no longer moving or eating.
- Are the wound edges open and secured to subcutaneous tissue or closed (rolled under, scarred, or undermined)? Wound edges must be open and adhered to subcutaneous tissue for complete healing to occur.
- How often does the dressing need to be changed? It usually takes at least 8 hours for a wound to achieve homeostasis after a dressing change. The less often dressing changes are needed, the better. Dressings for noninfected wounds without necrotic tissue should be changed two to three times per week.
- What is the simplest method of closing the wound? Which is most cost-effective?
- Is the patient in a health care facility or at home?
  - If the patient is in a health care facility, which companies have contracts to supply wound care products to your facility? Learn about these products first. It's good for everyone if money can be saved while the job still gets done!
  - If the patient is at home, can they afford the supplies they need? Simple and affordable aren't necessarily synonymous. If not, is financial assistance available? Who provides wound care at home? If the patient can't perform this important task, can family members or friends help? Is home health care an option? If so, is the patient eligible?

Evidence-based practice dictates these wound care principles:
- Cleanse the wound before each dressing change. Determine the need for sterile supplies based on whether the wound is acute or chronic. Normal saline, tap water, wound cleanser, or an antimicrobial may be necessary depending on the wound.
- Debride wounds with conservative, sharp, surgical, autolytic, biologic, or enzymatic methods as necrotic tissue impedes wound healing.
- Provide moist wound healing: Select the primary dressing based on the appearance of the majority of the wound bed.
- Consult a certified wound care nurse.

All the rage

Keep in mind that new products arrive almost daily, and others are updated or improved regularly. Because the quality of the care that you provide depends on your level of knowledge, it is imperative that you stay up to date by periodically reviewing the available products. However, that does not always mean that newer is better! Newer is often more expensive and may not add to your ability to accomplish your goals for the wound (e.g., add moisture, control bacteria).

Wound dressings

As medical research has afforded a better understanding of wounds and the healing process, manufacturers have developed new materials and sophisticated dressing options that promote better healing. Gauze may be used when daily dressing changes are necessary because the wound is infected or being debrided. Otherwise, advanced wound dressings are more effective in terms of both healing and cost because they result in less frequent dressing changes and protect the wound much better.

Moisture level, likelihood of tissue trauma caused by adherence, infection control, and wound dimensions are just some of the factors that affect wound dressing selection. The level of moisture in the wound bed is critical to the success or failure of healing. Consequently, one fundamental way to classify dressings is by their effect on wound moisture. Ask yourself if the dressing adds, absorbs, or does not affect wound moisture. (See *Dressing for the occasion*.)

Dressing for the occasion

Some dressings absorb moisture from a wound bed; some add moisture to it. Others help maintain the existing moisture level. Use this chart to quickly determine the category of dressing appropriate for your patient.

Absorbs moisture	Neutral (maintains existing moisture level)	Adds moisture
• Alginates	• Composite dressings	• Gels (amorphous, sheet, impregnated hydrogel gauze)
• Gauze	• Transparent films	• Medical-grade honey
• Foams	• Cellular tissue products	
• Polymer dressings	• Collagen dressings	
• Super-absorbent pads	• Contact layers	
• Cellulose (hydrofibers)	• Hydrocolloids	
• NPWT		
• Cadexomer iodine		

Gauze but not forgotten

World War II initiated the use of gauze as a dressing; it is absorbent like facial tissue but unable to absorb more than minimal fluid, and it cannot retain fluid at all. Also keep in mind that bacteria can penetrate 17 layers of gauze, so it can't help protect the wound from infection or protect others from cross-contamination. Even on closed incisions, a dressing that is occlusive and absorptive and can remain in place for 24 to 48 hours is better. When using gauze in an open wound, monitor whether it is drying out between dressing changes because a dry cell (desiccation) is a dead cell! If gauze is not staying moist with saline, use hydrogel to make sure it stays moist. When filling dead space with moistened gauze, always "fluff" the gauze before placing it in the wound.

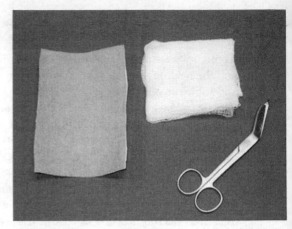

Alginate and hydrofiber dressings

Alginate dressings are made from seaweed, and hydrofiber dressings are made of cellulose. Both dressings are nonwoven and very absorptive. They are available as soft, sterile pads or ropes. These dressings absorb excessive exudate and may be used on infected wounds. As they absorb exudate, many turn into a gel that keeps the wound bed moist and promotes healing. These nonadhesive and nonocclusive dressings also promote autolysis by drawing wound fluid into the wound bed that contains natural enzymes. However, if you notice they are not very moist when removed, a different type of dressing may be necessary.

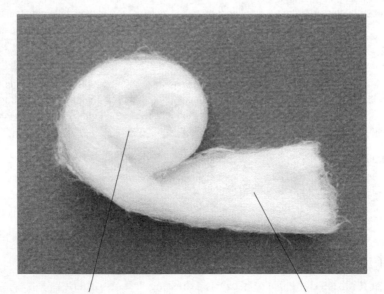

Very soft, nonwoven fibers turn into a biodegradable gel as they absorb exudate.

Fibers encourage hemostasis in minimally bleeding wounds.

Examples of alginate dressings include:
- AlgiSite M
- KALTOSTAT

- Maxorb CMC/Alginate
- Sorbsan
- Melgisorb
- NU-SORB
  Examples of hydrofiber dressings include:
- Aquacel
- Durafiber
- Opticell

When they're used

Use alginate and hydrofiber dressings only on wounds with moderate to heavy drainage and in wound tunnels with drainage. If using this type of dressing in tunnels, make sure it remains intact and does not leave particles behind.

What's the advantage?

Alginate and hydrofiber dressings are beneficial because they:
- hold up to 20 times their own weight in fluid.
- may be cut to fit wound dimensions.
- may be layered for more absorption.
- come in ropes for deep wound filling.

What to consider

Alginate and hydrofiber dressings:
- require secondary dressings.
- shouldn't be used on dry eschar or wounds with light drainage.
- may dehydrate the wound bed of a dryer wound and cause desiccation (cell death due to drying).

Antimicrobial dressings

Antimicrobial dressings protect against bacterial overload—an improvement on topical antibiotics, which are sensitizers—that is, chemicals that frequently cause allergies. Use of antimicrobial dressings can help us protect the wound from infection, so we can use antibiotics to treat infection as advised by the Centers for Disease Control and Prevention (CDC). Active ingredients, such as silver, cadexomer iodine, sodium hypochlorite, methylene blue/gentian violet, hypochloric acid, and polyhexamethylene biguanide (PHMB), provide antimicrobial effects. Most dressing categories include antimicrobial options. That means we can consider both moisture balance and bacterial balance when choosing a dressing.

Examples of antimicrobial dressings include:
- Acticoat (a line of many different dressing materials with nano-crystalline silver)

- Durafiber Ag, AquacelAG, OpticellAG+ (cellulose hydrofiber with silver)
- Iodosorb Gel and Iodoflex Pads (with cadexomer iodine)
- SilvaSorb, Arglaes (hydrogel with silver)
- Hydrofera Blue (absorbent dressings with methylene blue and gentian violet)
- AMD gauze, Telfa, foam (with PHMB)
- Amerigel hydrogel (with Oakin, an antimicrobial oak extract)
- Sorbion Sachet, Cutimed Siltec (absorbent dressings that attract and bond bacteria)
- Prontosan hydrogel (with PHMB)
- Anasept hydrogel (with sodium hypochlorite)
- Medihoney, TheraHoney, ManukaMed (Medical-grade honey wound care products encourage osmotic flow of fluid. Honey contains glucose oxidase, an enzyme that converts glucose to hydrogen peroxide, which may contribute to some of its antibacterial properties, and there are indications that honey has independent antibacterial properties as well as antifungal properties.)

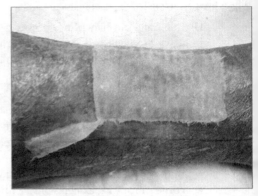

- MultiDex gel or powder (Hyperosmolar sugar like maltodextrin kills germs.)
- Xcel Antimicrobial (a cellulose dressing that can absorb or donate moisture; contains PHMB)

When they're used

Use antimicrobial dressings as primary or secondary dressings on wounds that are at high risk for infection, are infected, or are nonhealing.

What's the advantage?

Antimicrobial dressings:
- decrease numbers of bacteria (called *bioburden*).
- help control odor because they reduce bacteria that cause the odor.
- work against a variety of microorganisms.

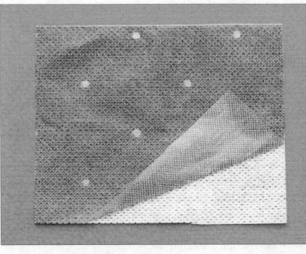

What to consider

Along with antimicrobial dressings, the patient may still require systemic antibiotic therapy for a clinically infected wound. In addition, some antimicrobial dressings may:

- produce a hypersensitivity reaction in patients sensitive to such product ingredients as silver or iodine.
- occasionally sting when applied.
- contribute to the development of resistant organisms if overused.
- emit their own chemical odors.

Collagen dressings

Collagen dressings function like a scaffold to give wound cells a structure on which to grow. They are harvested from various animals and contain protein fibers but no cells. Because of this, rejection is not an issue, but allergies still can occur. We must also be sensitive to the recipient's beliefs and inform them of the animal source. Different religions have rules that some people may practice about avoiding any intake of materials from certain animals.

Examples of collagen dressings include:

- BCG Matrix
- Promogran
- Promogran Prisma
- Oasis
- Stimulen
- HYCOL
- BioPad
- Puracol
- Endoform

When they're used

Use collagen dressings for healthy partial- and full-thickness injuries, skin grafting donor sites, and second-degree burns that seem a bit slow to progress to healing.

What's the advantage?

The biggest advantage of collagen dressings is that they may shorten healing times as they provide a scaffold for cells to use for healing.

Collagen dressings encourage wound healing by stimulating the deposit of collagen fibers necessary for the growth of tissue and blood vessels.

These highly absorbent dressings also maintain a moist wound environment.

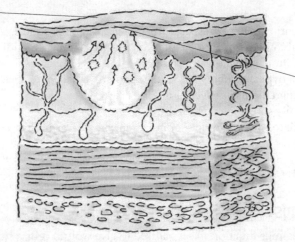

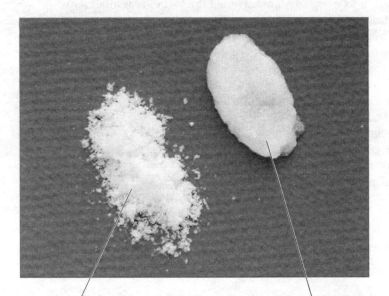

Some bovine collagen is processed into fine particles, as shown here. These particles can then be shaken into a wound bed.

Mixing with moist exudate in the wound, the particles gel as they absorb many times their weight in excess fluid.

What to consider

Collagen dressings:

- are made with bovine, porcine, or avian collagen.
- may cause allergic reactions to the animal protein.
- mostly require secondary dressings.
- should only be used after wound is free of bacteria and necrotic tissue.

Composite dressings

Composite dressings are hybrid dressings that combine two or more types of dressings into one. For example, a three-layer composite dressing can include a bottom layer of a meshed semiadherent or nonadherent material (allows excess exudate to travel through to the next layer while keeping the wound bed slightly moist and protected from other things sticking to it); a middle layer (composed of an absorptive material which pulls excess exudate away and holds it); a top or cover layer (protects the wound from bacterial invasion and keeps exudate from leaking out).

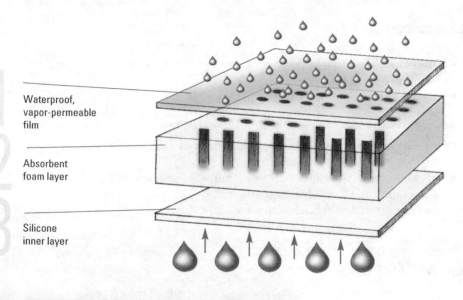

1 Waterproof, vapor-permeable film

2 Absorbent foam layer

3 Silicone inner layer

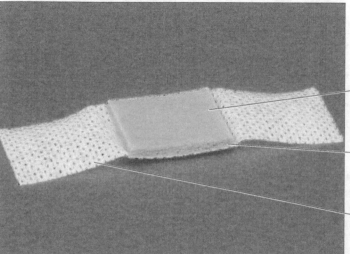

A thin, transparent, semipermeable film allows the exchange of gas and water vapor while blocking bacteria.

A highly absorbent foam-type matrix slowly releases ingredients that clean and moisturize the wound.

The adhesive backing consists of a breathable cloth.

Examples of composite dressings include:
- Alldress
- Compdress Island Dressing
- COVADERM Plus
- COVRSITE
- MPM Multi-Layered Dressing
- TELFA PLUS Island Dressing

When they're used

Use composite dressings as primary or secondary dressings on wounds with minimal to moderate drainage. They can also be used to protect peripheral and central intravenous (IV) lines.

What's the advantage?

Composite dressings are:
- all-in-one dressings that come in various combinations to suit each patient's wound care needs.
- available in multiple sizes and shapes.

What to consider

Composite dressings can't be used on third-degree burns. In addition, they:
- may not absorb drainage or provide a moist wound bed (depending on the product selected).
- can't be cut to fit without losing some of the dressing's integrity.

Contact layer dressings

Contact layer dressings are single-layer dressings made of woven or perforated material suitable for direct contact with the wound's surface. These nonadherent contact layers prevent other dressings from sticking to the surface of the wound.

Examples of contact layer dressings include:
- Mesh dressings: Mepitel, Versatel, Restore Contact Layer Flex, Adaptic Touch, Silflex, Acticoat Flex
- Other contact layers: Conformant 2 Wound Veil, Telfa Clear, Profore Wound Contact Layer, Dermanet, Drynet

When they're used

Use contact layer dressings to let drainage flow to a secondary dressing while preventing that dressing from adhering to the wound. The mesh type can be used under a NPWT dressing to prevent the granulation tissue from becoming embedded in the foam or gauze.

What's the advantage?

Contact layer dressings:
- decrease the pain and tissue trauma experienced during dressing changes.
- can be used with topical medications, fillers, and gauze dressings.
- that are mesh type should overlap the wound edges because the dressing will keep the wound bed moist and at the same time keep the skin edges dry.
- are often available already attached to a foam or other absorptive dressing to catch any exudate.

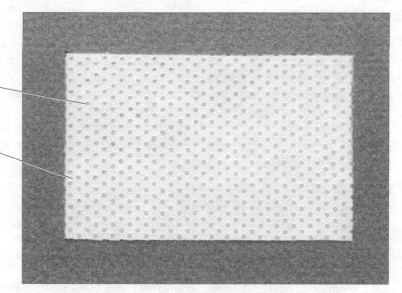

Holes allow drainage to pass through to a secondary dressing.

During dressing changes, the contact layer remains in place to protect the wound from trauma.

What to consider

Contact layer dressings require a secondary dressing and are contraindicated for use on third-degree burns. They are often made of silicone because of silicone's nonallergenic and nonstick properties. Silicone-based adhesives minimize pain during removal because of the interactive properties of silicone with the oils of the epidermis. Silicone adhesives will adhere as the dressing warms to body temperature after application and will begin to self-release as the oils of the epidermis build, facilitating easier removal.

Foam dressings

Foam dressings are absorbent spongelike dressings that may include an adhesive or silicone border. They provide a moist healing environment and thermal insulation along with a bit of padding to protect the wound.

Examples of foam dressings include:

- Allevyn
- CarraSmart
- Hydrosorb
- Cutimed Siltec
- Lyofoam
- Mepilex
- OptiFoam
- PolyTube Tube-Site Dressing
- Tielle Plus

When they're used

Use foam dressings as primary or secondary dressings on wounds with minimal to heavy drainage and around tubes such as percutaneous gastrostomy tubes. For heavy drainage, consider placing an absorbent primary layer covered by a foam dressing or choose one of the foams that includes super-absorbent materials. For delicate skin or wound tissue, consider a foam dressing with a silicone layer.

What's the advantage?

Foam dressings may be used in combination with other products. Those with an adhesive or silicone border don't require a secondary dressing. In addition, foam dressings can:

- be used on infected wounds if changed daily or longer if they contain an antimicrobial.
- manage heavier drainage because they wick moisture from the wound and allow evaporation (those without a cover).
- be used around tubes (such as a tracheostomy) because they don't fray like gauze.

What to consider

Without an adhesive border, foam dressings may require a secondary dressing, tape, wrap, or net. In addition, they:

- may have an adhesive border that may stick to the skin or wound base.
- may cause maceration if not changed regularly (those without silicone attached to protect skin).
- aren't recommended for nondraining wounds.

Additionally, PolyMem is a polymeric membrane dressing (PMD) and is slightly different than a traditional foam dressing. PMDs incorporate features of foams, films, and hydrocolloids.

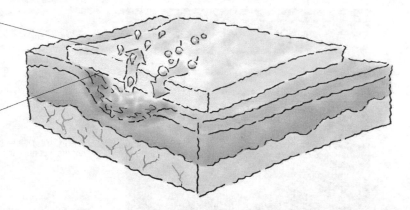

Foam outer layer
- Provides comfort
- Allows water to evaporate
- Permits the free flow of oxygen and other gases

Inner contact layer
- Wicks drainage away from wound
- Allows trauma-free removal because of low adherence to wound surface

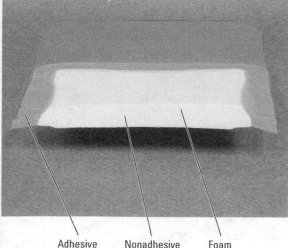

This foam dressing has an adhesive border to secure the dressing over the wound bed.

Adhesive border	Nonadhesive contact layer	Foam

Adhesive foam dressing.

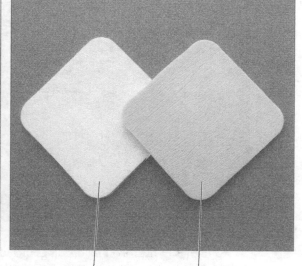

Nonadhesive contact layer	Top layer of semipermeable film

Nonadhesive foam dressing.

Hydrocolloid dressings

Hydrocolloid dressings are adherent, moldable wafers made of a carbohydrate-based material. Most have a waterproof backing. They're impermeable to oxygen, water, and water vapor, and most provide minimal absorption. These dressings turn to gel as they absorb moisture, help maintain a moist wound bed, and promote autolytic debridement.

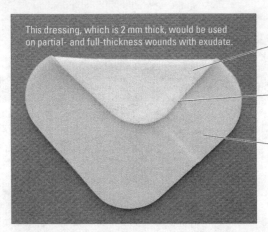

This dressing, which is 2 mm thick, would be used on partial- and full-thickness wounds with exudate.

The exterior surface protects the wound from outside contaminants.

The hydrocolloid layer turns to gel as hydrocolloids absorb moisture.

The adhesive layer adheres to the surrounding skin, but not the wound; adherence decreases as gel forms.

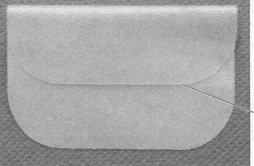

Thin hydrocolloid dressings are used on partial-thickness and shallow full-thickness wounds with minimal exudate and to protect areas at risk for skin breakdown.

The hydrocolloid interior of this dressing is less than 1 mm thick.

Examples of hydrocolloid dressings include:
- Band-Aid Advanced Healing Bandages (available over the counter)
- DuoDERM CGF
- Restore Cx Wound Care Dressing
- 3M Tegasorb Hydrocolloid
- Comfeel Hydrocolloid
- FlexiCol

When they're used

Use hydrocolloid dressings on partial-thickness wounds with minimal drainage in order to maintain the natural wound fluids. For wounds with necrotic tissue or slough that are draining minimally, these dressings can aid in effective autolytic debridement by keeping the wound bed moist at all times so our natural enzymes can do their job. Hydrocolloid dressings can also serve as secondary dressings and can be used as skin protection under medical devices, braces, or cast edges to prevent friction and pressure.

What's the advantage?

Hydrocolloid dressings are beneficial because they:

- maintain moisture by stopping evaporation and becoming gelatinous as they absorb drainage.
- may require changing only two to three times each week.
- can be easily removed from the wound base if it is moist.
- are available in contoured forms for use on specific sites.

What to consider

Hydrocolloid dressings shouldn't be used on burns or infected or wet wounds. Be sure to watch the skin at the edges for maceration. In addition, they:

- may have an odor when removed that occurs when exudate gels the material.
- can cause periwound skin stripping when removed, especially if changed too often.
- can cause maceration or hypergranulation (also called "proud flesh").
- may be warmed prior to or after placement to maximize adhesion.

Hydrogel dressings

Hydrogel dressings are water-, oil-, or glycerin-based dressings that add moisture to dry wounds and don't adhere to the wound bed. They provide limited absorption (some are 96% water themselves) and are available as tubes of gel (amorphous) or in flexible sheets, impregnated gauze, or impregnated gauze strips. Hydrogel dressings promote autolytic debridement by keeping the wound bed moist.

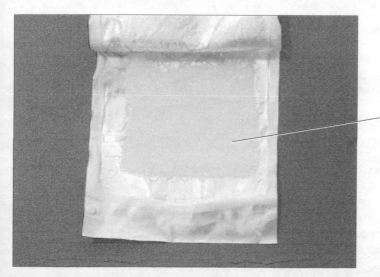

Hydrogel-impregnated gauze
- Hydrates wounds
- Softens necrotic tissue
- Cools and soothes burning wounds (such as skin tears and dermal wounds)

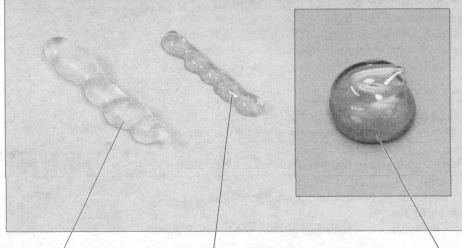

Amorphous hydrogels are gels packaged in tubes. Depending on the components in the gel, amorphous hydrogels have a number of uses.

Plain hydrogel
- Creates a moist wound environment
- Promotes autolytic debridement

20% sodium chloride gel
- Increases the level of sodium in the wound bed
- Has an enhanced ability to soften and remove necrotic tissue

Hydrogel with additives (such as alginate)
- Absorbs low to moderate amounts of drainage

Examples of amorphous hydrogel dressings include:
- Aquasorb Hydrogel
- Carrasyn Gel with Acemannan Hydrogel
- CURASOL Gel
- Intrasite Gel
- Normlgel (gelled saline)
- SAF-Gel
- Skintegrity Gel
- Solosite Gel
- MediHoney, TheraHoney, ManukaMed (honey dressings from the Manuka flower)
- MultiDex Gel (hypertonic sugar)
- Spandgel

Examples of sheet hydrogels include:
- AquaClear
- DermaGel, Elastogel (glycerin-based sheets)
- TOE-AID Toe and Nail Dressing
- Spandgel Sheets

An example of an impregnated gauze strip hydrogel is Curity Packing Strip gauze. Even though products like this are called packing strips, remember dead space is *gently* filled. The wound should not be stuffed with dressing material.

When they're used

Use hydrogel dressings on dry wounds and wounds with minimal drainage to add moisture or on wounds with necrotic tissue or slough to moisten them enough to allow autolytic debridement.

What's the advantage?

Hydrogel dressings come in sheets, impregnated gauze pads and strip gauze, and as amorphous gel. They add moisture to dry or minimally draining wounds. When applied, they may provide cooling that soothes and eases pain.

What to consider

Amorphous gel hydrogel dressings require a secondary dressing. For shallow wounds, composite dressings may be used as many have a nonadherent layer that does not absorb the gel. When filling dead space in a deep wound, follow the package directions for amorphous gel. Gauze that has been moistened with normal saline and fluffed should be used as a filler so that the gel is not absorbed into the gauze. Sterile gels are more expensive but useful if there is bone, tendon, or organ exposed in the wound. In addition, amorphous gels:

- can macerate the surrounding skin if it is not protected.
- may necessitate daily dressing changes.
- vary in viscosity among brands and according to the product's base (water, oil, or glycerin).

Super-absorptive dressings

Super-absorptive dressings have highly absorbent material, such as cellulose, polymer, or polyacrylate beads. Various forms are available, including gels, pads, and pillows.

Examples of specialty absorptive dressings include:

- 3M Tegaderm Superabsorber
- Exudry
- Cutisorb Ultra
- Sofsorb
- TENDERSORB WET-PRUF Abdominal Pads
- Xtrasorb
- Eclypse Border
- OptiLock
- Sorbion Sachet
- LeukoMed

When they're used

Use super-absorptive dressings on infected or noninfected wounds with moderate to heavy drainage.

What's the advantage?

Super-absorptive dressings:
- are highly absorbent (holding up to 33% more moisture than alginates).
- typically require less frequent changes.
- are available in a variety of forms.

What to consider

Some absorptive dressings can't be used on burns or on wounds with little or no drainage.

Transparent film dressings

Transparent film dressings are clear, adherent, nonabsorptive, polyurethane dressings. They're semipermeable to oxygen and water vapor but not to water itself. Transparency allows visual inspection of the wound while the dressing is in place. Transparent film dressings maintain a moist wound environment and promote autolysis in dry wounds. Because they are waterproof, these dressings are also used to protect IV sites and other invasive tubes.

To avoid skin stripping when these are removed, always use a skin protectant on the periwound skin. Several techniques for removal include: using an adhesive remover or any oil and rubbing it along the edge you are removing; loosening the opposite corners of the dressing and pulling it parallel to the skin, stretching the dressing (this loosens

Backing is removed before application, leaving a clear, membranelike dressing.

Film allows the exchange of water vapor and oxygen while being impermeable to fluids and bacteria.

Transparent film allows visual inspection of the wound while the dressing is in place.

the adhesive bond without tearing skin); and placing a hydrocolloid or pectin wafer frame around the edges of the wound and placing the clear film dressing on that (when removing the clear film, use an adhesive remover or oil and it will slip right off the wafer).

Examples of transparent film dressings include:

- BIOCLUSIVE Transparent Dressing
- BlisterFilm
- ClearSite Transparent Membrane
- OpSite FLEXIGRID
- 3M NexCare Waterproof Bandages (available over the counter)
- 3M Tegaderm Transparent Dressing

When they're used

Use transparent film dressings as the primary dressing on partial-thickness wounds with minimal exudate and on wounds with eschar (dry, leathery, black necrotic tissue) to promote autolysis. Transparent film may also be used as a secondary dressing over a hydrogel to promote autolysis, but do not use transparent film over medicated ointments or enzymes as the occlusive dressing can potentiate the effects of the ointment. Transparent films can also be used as a secondary dressing to secure a wound filler.

What's the advantage?

Transparent film dressings:

- are very flexible.
- allow you to see the wound without removing the dressing.
- are adherent but won't stick to a moist wound.
- aren't bulky.

What to consider

Transparent film dressings don't absorb drainage, making them appropriate only for partial-thickness wounds or shallow, full-thickness wounds with minimal exudate. They can, of course, be combined with an absorptive pad. These dressings do not stick to moist skin, such as in some areas of the body where perspiration is more common. In addition, the adhesive can strip skin around the wound if the dressing is removed incorrectly. Skin integrity is especially important to remember when dressings are applied to fragile skin, for example, the skin of very young and older individuals. (See Chapter 4 for more information on medical adhesive-related skin injuries.)

Wound fillers

Wound fillers are specialized dressings used to fill deeper wounds and tunnels. They're made of various materials and come in many forms, including acrylate strands, granules, powders, bags of polymer, and gels. Wound fillers can add moisture to the wound bed or absorb drainage, depending on the product. Other dressing types may be used as wound fillers, such as alginates, hydrofibers, and gel-impregnated gauze.

Examples of special wound fillers include:
- Bard Absorption Dressing
- Flexigel Strands
- Cutimed Cavity
- PolyMem WIC Cavity Filler and Rope Wound Filler
- TenderWet Cavity

When they're used

Use wound fillers as primary dressings on infected or noninfected wounds with minimal to heavy drainage that require dead space to be filled.

What's the advantage?

Wound fillers come in several forms with different absorption abilities. These dressings would be cost-effective to use (rather than gauze) in a noninfected wound without necrotic tissue so that the dressing can be left in place for 2 to 5 days. This may be cost-effective because the highest cost of a dressing change is often the staff time spent doing it, not the cost of the dressing material. Because it is also known to be better for healing to change dressings less often (in a clean, noninfected wound), this is great for the patient as well.

What to consider

Wound fillers can't be used on third-degree burns. For highly exudating wounds, consider NPWT if appropriate. Also, the wormlike appearance of some wound filler products can alarm some patients.

See Appendix 6 to quickly compare dressings, their actions, indications for use, contraindications, and application tips.

Additional therapeutic modalities

Therapeutic modalities promote wound healing by:
- physically or mechanically debriding particulate and bacterial necrosis.
- killing microorganisms or controlling bioburden (microorganism number).
- reducing or controlling edema and wound fluids.
- increasing blood flow and tissue oxygenation.
- enhancing immune and/or connective tissue cell function.
- providing scaffolding for tissue growth.

Cellular, acellular, and matrix-like products (CAMPs)

In 2022 a consensus panel of 11 experts convened to discuss cellular and/or tissue-based products (CTPs) and best practice for their use. The panel defined CAMPs as "A broad category of biomaterials, synthetic materials or biosynthetic matrices that support repair or re-generation of injured tissues through various mechanisms of action" (Wu et al., 2023, S4). This consensus document is suggested by the panel to be used in conjunction with the 2019 consensus document, Implementing TIMERS (Atkin et al., 2019).

Growth factors

Growth factors are an important form of biotherapy because of the key role they play in the healing process—stimulating cell proliferation.

Getting the factors straight

Wound healing is a complex process that the body undertakes to replace or repair injured tissue. If various growth factors aren't syn-thesized, secreted, and removed from tissues with correct timing, the wound healing process can stall. This leaves the wound bed in a chronic state of confusion, unable to heal.

The master factor

In the past decade, growth factors have been studied to determine exactly how they function in healing and how they may be used in the treatment of chronic wounds. (See *Understanding growth factors*.) Particular focus has been placed on platelet-derived growth fac-tor (PDGF), which some experts call the *master factor*. Although the specific growth factor or other mechanism that initiates wound heal-ing isn't known, PDGF is known to play a central role by attracting fibroblasts (components of granulation tissue) and inducing them to divide. This is central to wound healing because fibroblasts are re-sponsible for collagen formation.

Understanding growth factors

Key growth factors that play an important role in wound healing include:

Type	Description
Transforming growth factor beta (TGF-β)	Controls movement of cells to sites of inflammation and stimulates extracellular matrix (ECM) formation
Basic fibroblast growth factor (bFGF)	Stimulates angiogenesis (the development of blood vessels)
Vascular endothelial growth factor (VEGF)	Stimulates angiogenesis
Insulin-like growth factor (IGF)	Increases collagen synthesis
Epidermal growth factor (EGF)	Stimulates epidermal regeneration

Trials and tribulations

The key growth factors PDGF, TGF-β, bFGF, and EGF have been through or are currently undergoing testing in clinical trials. At this time, the only synthetic growth factor approved for use in wound care is becaplermin (Regranex Gel 0.01%), which has a biologic activity similar to that of endogenous PDGF. Becaplermin is indicated only for the treatment of lower extremity diabetic neuropathic ulcers and has been shown to increase wound closure in these ulcers by 43% when compared to placebo gel.

Penny-sized potency

Becaplermin is used to treat lower extremity neuropathic ulcers that have adequate blood flow and involve tissues at or below the subcutaneous level. It can be applied to wounds using a sterile applicator, such as a swab, a tongue blade, or saline-moistened gauze. Per the manufacturer recommendations, the applied amount of becaplermin depends on the size of the ulcer, it should be recalculated at a weekly or biweekly rate, and a penny-size thickness should be applied over the ulcer. The wound can then be dressed with a saline-moistened gauze. Keep in mind that becaplermin is contraindicated for necrotic and infected wounds, in patients with poor blood supply to the legs, or on known neoplasms at the application site.

Acellular matrix dressings

Acellular matrix dressings contain nonliving products derived from allogeneic, xenographic, synthetic, or biosynthetic materials. An antigen–antibody reaction does not occur as there are no living cells. These ECM dressings provide the scaffold that the nonhealing wound needs to support the attachment and migration of fibroblasts, keratinocytes, and endothelial cells.

Cellular and/or tissue–based wound products

CTPs include more than just protein fibers. They include living or preserved animal or human tissue. Using these products would not be the same as an autograft (skin taken from the same person at a site remote to the wound) but they would have definite advantages over other dressings. Because of this, they are coded differently by Medicare and other insurance companies.

Advanced therapies are considered after the wound has not progressed with traditional wound therapies and the cause of the wound, optimized systemic support, and patient-related factors have been addressed. They should only be used after the wound is free of bacteria and necrotic tissue. CTPs are available refrigerated, frozen, and dried, depending on the manufacturer. Again, check with your facility to identify which CTPs are available.

Product	What it replaces	What it's made from	What it's used for
Cellular products, living skin equivalent			
Apligraf (cultured in vitro)	Epidermis and dermis	Type 1 collagen Human fibroblasts Human keratinocytes	Venous ulcers Neuropathic ulcers
Grafix (noncultured intact tissues)	ECM	Growth factors and cells of the ECM	Acute and chronic wounds including burns and neuropathic foot ulcers
Acellular products, nonviable cells			
Oasis	ECM	Porcine small intestinal submucosa	Neuropathic ulcers, venous ulcers, partial- and full-thickness wounds, pressure injuries, surgical wounds (donor sites/grafts, post-Mohs surgery, post-laser surgery, podiatric, wound dehiscence)
EpiFix	Epithelial cells, basement membrane, avascular connective tissue	Dehydrated human amniotic membrane epithelial tissue	Acute and chronic wounds (e.g., neuropathic foot ulcers, burns)
DermACELL	ECM components, growth factors, cytokines, matrikines	Acellular human skin	Neuropathic foot ulcers, chronic nonhealing wounds (second- and third-degree burns, breast reconstruction, dehiscence)

Ultrasound

Low-frequency ultrasound (mechanical pressure waves delivered at 20 to 30 kHz, which are above the range of human hearing) is used in treatments for patients with both open and closed wounds because of its nonthermal and thermal effects. Ultrasound appears to have optimal effects when used during the inflammatory phase of wound healing. It speeds the wound's progress through the healing phases. It has also been shown to be effective in the proliferative phase of wound healing by increasing collagen extensibility, circulation, pain threshold enzymatic activity, cell membrane permeability, and nerve conduction velocity.

Cavitation sensation

Ultrasound can be used for more than visualization; it has therapeutic properties as well. Nonthermal effects of ultrasound include acoustic cavitation and microstreaming.

- In acoustic cavitation, gaseous microbubbles are made to expand and contract rhythmically in the tissues being treated. These microbubbles are thought to stimulate biologic phenomena such as the activation of ionic channels in cellular membranes.
- Microstreaming is another nonthermal effect that results from cavitation. Cavitation causes fluids close to the microbubbles to stream by, thus stimulating the cells in close proximity. In this way, ultrasound increases calcium conductance in fibroblasts, which is important because collagen secretion is a calcium-dependent process.

Gets the blood flowing

Ultrasound's thermal effects include increased blood flow to tissue, which results in increased tissue healing. Ultrasound also increases white blood cell (WBC) migration and promotes a more orderly arrangement of collagen in both open and closed wounds.

This might be a job for ultrasound

Ultrasound is indicated to:
- encourage debridement of necrotic tissue (via cavitation and microstreaming).
- increase wound healing.
- enhance blood flow and oxygen transport.
- decrease pain.
- increase collagen elasticity.
- decrease inflammation.
  Contraindications for ultrasound include:
- active profuse bleeding.
- malignant tissue.
- acute infections.
- deep vein thrombosis.
- ischemic areas.
- plastic implants or implanted electronic devices.
- irradiated areas.
- treatment over the gonads, spinal cord, eyes, or a pregnant person's uterus.

Electrical stimulation

Electrical stimulation (E-stim) can help healing by changing the positive and negative polarity in the wound. As is true in the heart, negative and positive charges are an important signal for healing. Wound tissue naturally has a positive charge, while epithelium has a negative charge. When the wound is filled in, this helps the skin grow toward the wound tissue since opposite charges attract. This characteristic is often lost in chronic wounds and when it can be reestablished, the wound may respond by healing. The therapy is not Food and Drug Administration (FDA) approved for wounds at this time so prior authorization is recommended. E-stim should be provided by a physical therapist who has expertise in this modality.

E-stim is used to enhance healing of recalcitrant wounds, especially chronic pressure injuries. It is delivered through a device that has conductive electrodes, which are applied either within the wound itself or to the periwound skin.

Zap it!

E-stim can be used to:
- promote wound healing.
- orient cells.
- promote cellular migration.
- enhance blood flow.
- increase protein synthesis and wound bed formation.
- destroy microorganisms.
- increase angiogenesis.
- increase tissue oxygenation.
- reduce wound bioburden or microbial content.
- reduce pain (wound and diabetic neuropathic pain).

Lack of stimulation

Contraindications for E-stim include:
- malignant tissue.
- untreated osteomyelitis.
- treatment over the pericardial area or areas related to control of cardiac and respiratory function (e.g., neck or thorax).
- treatment over some implanted electronic devices (e.g., a pacemaker).

Hyperbaric oxygen

Hyperbaric oxygen (HBO) therapy is the delivery of 100% oxygen through a sealed chamber at pressures greater than atmospheric pressure via a total-body chamber, such as that used for decompression therapy for divers. Another delivery method involves a smaller chamber used just for the limbs.

In demand

HBO delivered by a whole-body chamber increases the amount of dissolved oxygen in the blood available for wound healing. This increased availability of oxygen in the blood can be used by cells, such as neutrophils, that employ oxygen-dependent processes.

(The processes by which neutrophils destroy microorganisms are oxygen based, as is cellular metabolism in general.) In addition, the increased availability of oxygen for tissues apparently relieves relative hypoxia in wounded tissues.

HBO a go!

Evidence supports systemic HBO treatment for patients with non-healing wounds, such as neuropathic ulcers and venous and arterial insufficiency ulcers. Patients with venous ulcers who don't improve with traditional therapies may benefit when compression therapy is paired with systemic HBO treatment. Another possible use for HBO is in treating patients with neuropathic foot ulcers. HBO increases nitric oxide production in the wound. Nitric oxide is a unique free radical important in vasodilation and neurotransmission, which play major roles in diabetic wound healing. Keep in mind, patient selection for HBO therapy is usually based on the measurement of oxygen tension around the wound using transcutaneous oxygen pressure ($TcPO_2$). An in-chamber $TcPO_2$ higher than 200 mm Hg with the patient breathing 100% oxygen is the best indicator of success or failure.

HBO is contraindicated for patients taking certain medications, such as bleomycin, disulfiram, cisplatin, mafenide, and doxorubicin, or patients who are experiencing pneumothorax.

Topical HBO

Topical HBO, also known as topical oxygen therapy (TOT), provides a supply of oxygen through an airtight chamber or soft-sided "bag" that is sealed around a wound present on the trunk or limb of the body. This method does not rely on systemic circulation but may increase the oxygen levels in plasma flowing to the wound itself.

When it's used
- When conventional methods do not produce improvement in wound healing
- With other wound healing strategies

What to consider
A total assessment of the wound, the length of time the wound has been present (if it is chronic), and other modalities used must be taken into consideration before contemplating the use of topical HBO.

What's the advantage?
HBO therapy is a painless treatment that may provide the necessary oxygen to tissues in order to maximize healing potential.

Medical leech therapy

Leech therapy, or *hirudotherapy*, was approved in 2004 by the FDA as a medical device for use after reconstructive or plastic surgery.

When it's used

- Medicinal leeches may be used when a surgical flap or wound is not healing due to venous congestion. It provides temporary relief of the pressure from the excess blood collection.
- They are also used by surgeons following reattachment of digits, ears, limbs, and penile replantation.

What's the advantage?

It is difficult to attach veins to serve new tissue, so leech therapy keeps the pressure out of the tissue until it can drain old blood naturally when it develops veins to do so. When leeches attach, they usually feed between 20 and 60 minutes, each removing about 5 to 15 mL of blood. Leeches detach spontaneously and the wound created continues to exude blood for approximately 6 hours, releasing up to an additional 50 mL of blood. Medical leeches are raised in farms under sterile conditions and are destroyed once used.

What to consider

- Be sure to have a protocol in place prior to ordering medical leeches. They must be stored and fed properly.
- The health care provider order should include the number of leeches to be used, the area of the body to be treated, and the duration and frequency of the therapy.
- Complete a thorough medication history as certain medications, supplements, and vitamins can increase a patient's risk of bleeding or suppress the patient's immune response. Nonsteroidal antiinflammatory medications, steroids, ginseng, and ginkgo biloba are a few examples of potential contraindications.
- A neurovascular assessment of the area to be treated to detect any signs of arterial insufficiency is important.
- Smoking and caffeine ingestion before therapy is contraindicated to reduce vasoconstriction.
- The staff and patient must also be well prepared in order to address the *ick* factor of using something from the animal kingdom on the wound.
- A protocol is available at www.leechesusa.com.

Negative pressure wound therapy

NPWT, considered an advanced therapeutic modality, can be used when a wound fails to heal in a timely manner or has a large amount of exudate. It is also used often over a flap or graft to ensure a better "take" and reduce local edema and over closed incisions to ensure that edges stay closed and any edema is removed from within. Systems consist of either a foam or gauze dressing matched or cut to the size of the wound, suction tubing, and a vacuum pump with or without a canister for exudate. One end of the suction tubing is placed over the dressing or attached via a special connector to the top of the dressing and the other end connects to the vacuum pump with or without a canister. The dressing is sealed securely in place with adhesive drape that extends 1¼ to 2 in (3 to 5 cm) over adjacent skin all around the dressing.

When turned on, the pump reduces air pressure beneath the dressing, drawing off exudate and reducing edema in surrounding tissues. This process reduces bacterial colonization, promotes granulation tissue development, increases the rate of cell mitosis, and spurs the migration of epithelial cells within the wound. Special training is required to operate this device. (See *Understanding NPWT*.)

Understanding NPWT

NPWT encourages healing by applying localized subatmospheric pressure at the site of the wound. This reduces edema and bacterial colonization and stimulates the formation of granulation tissue. This illustration shows the components of an NPWT device.

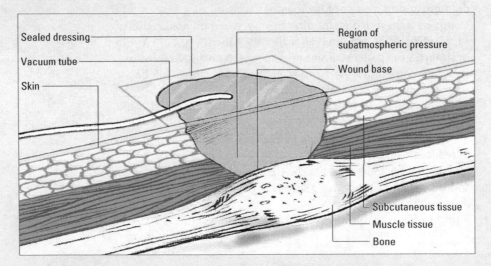

Mini-me

There are now several versions available of most brands of NPWT devices. There are regular-sized pumps for handling large wounds or those with heavy exudate. There are smaller, portable versions that run on batteries and have smaller canisters. There are also very small versions that are single-use devices, and many of these are disposed of after 1 week. One of the "mini-me" versions uses no batteries; the suction is produced via a spring inside. Some versions have no containers for exudate but instead come with dressings capable of holding small amounts (30 to 60 mL) of exudate as a gel.

Examples of NPWT

This field continues to evolve. The following examples are not the only options a provider may have for NPWT as other products may enter the market.

Traditional
- Vacuum-assisted closure (VAC) (several versions and sizes available, 3M)
- Invia (Medela)
- Renasys (Smith+ Nephew)
- SVED (Cardinal Health)
- Engenex (ConvaTec)

Disposable
- PICO (Smith+ Nephew)
- SNAP (3M)
- Prevena (3M)

When it's used

NPWT is useful in managing slow-healing acute, subacute, or chronic exudative wounds with cavities. It is ideal for pressure injuries or surgical wounds with depths greater than 1 cm. It is also used for short periods over flap grafts and newly closed incisions to reduce edema in the tissue and keep edges approximated.

What's the advantage?

NPWT devices:
- clean deeply and can manage small to large amounts of drainage.
- can manage multiple wounds when dressings are cut to bridge two or more wounds (or when a Y-connector connects two wounds to one unit).
- have rechargeable batteries and are small enough to fit in a pouch that can be worn at the waist or over the shoulder; others require no battery.

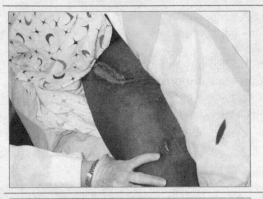

Thigh wounds to be treated with NPWT using the bridging technique

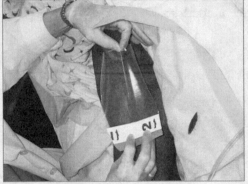

Drape placed between wounds for the foam bridge to protect intact skin from suction

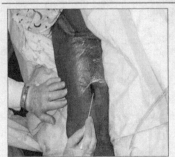

Foam gently filled into the lower wound

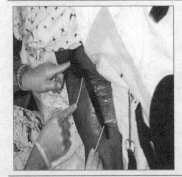

Foam gently filled into the upper wound and "bridge" foam placed on the drape so that each end touches the wound foam

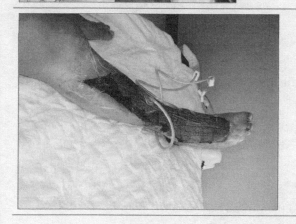

Drape placed over the entire foam dressing; suction will be applied to the middle of the dressing after cutting a hole in the drape and using a larger, round piece of foam to fit the suction pad.

Wounds on anterior and posterior leg; each wound has its own suction catheter as the wounds are large. Only one machine is used with a Y-connector for the suction tubings.

What to consider

NPWT is contraindicated for use with untreated osteomyelitis, malignancies, and wounds with excessive necrotic tissue or unexplored fistulas. In addition:

- the foam or gauze dressing must not extend out onto bare skin or the skin will be damaged. The skin may be protected with plastic drape or a hydrocolloid.
- it is important to cushion any suction tubing or connectors to prevent a device-associated pressure injury. One method is to use hydrocolloid under the edges with solid ostomy seals around the tubing to help get an airtight seal. A method called *bridging* requires the skin to be covered from the wound to a *neutral* place on the body (e.g., away from a bony prominence) and then placing a strip of foam on top of that, then draping to seal it.
- incorrect use of the NPWT device, such as improperly setting the pressure, can result in damage to the wound or skin, so it is essential to have education about the device being used.

NPWT with instillation

NPWT may also be used with instillation of a topical solution with removal during the negative pressure cycle. This is meant to provide wound cleansing between dressing changes. The instillation fluid may be normal saline or an antimicrobial solution.

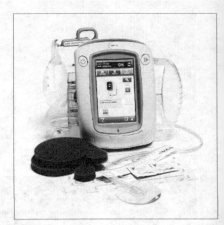

When it's used

- traumatic wounds
- surgical wounds
- diabetic wounds
- venous wounds
- pressure injuries
- infected wounds
- full-thickness burns after excision
- after evacuation of a hematoma once hemostasis has occurred

What's the advantage?

Instillation aids in cleansing of the wound surface, washing away devitalized tissue, and lessening bacterial load. Solutions used must be compatible with the NPWT products used.

What to consider

The history and condition of the patient and the wound bed remain primary considerations when using this dressing technique. The solution, amount of time the solution is in contact with the wound (dwell time), the number of times a day it is done, and the negative pressure setting are ordered by the provider.

This MIST is a must

In MIST therapy, ultrasound energy is transferred directly to the wound through a sterile saline mist. MIST enhances wound healing and decreases bacterial and necrotic debris in tissue by:

- enhancing fibroblast migration rates (shown in the laboratory).
- increasing collagen levels (shown in an animal wound model).
- decreasing bacterial numbers (shown in the laboratory and a patient case study) and disruption of biofilm.
- enhancing blood flow through vasodilation and increased angiogenesis.
- reducing sustained inflammation and matrix metallopeptidase.

Noncontact normothermic wound therapy

Noncontact normothermic wound therapy increases the temperature of the wound bed, thereby promoting increased blood flow in the area of the wound. The dressing in this system has a dome that contains a special electronic warming card. Once in place, the card heats to 100.4°F (38°C), bathing the wound in radiant heat. The closely sealed wound covering promotes a moist environment in the wound bed. This system is designed to remain in place for 72 hours.

When it's used

As ordered, use the noncontact normothermic wound therapy on acute or chronic, full- or partial-thickness wounds, regardless of etiology, that have failed to heal with traditional therapies, including wounds with compromised blood flow, such as some arterial or diabetic foot ulcers.

What's the advantage?

Noncontact normothermic wound therapy:
- can absorb a small to moderate amount of drainage in the wound covering.
- doesn't disturb the wound when removed.
- can be used on infected wounds.

What to consider

Noncontact normothermic wound therapy is contraindicated for use on third-degree burns. In addition, it requires specific dressings and thorough patient teaching related to dressing changes and heat management.

The only noncontact normothermic wound therapy system on the market is the Warm-Up Therapy System.

Therapeutic light

In therapeutic light modalities, light or its energy is used to aid in wound healing. The modalities include ultraviolet (UV) treatment and laser therapy.

UV treatment

Although not a form of light, UV energy or radiation is commonly categorized as therapeutic light. UV energy lies between x-rays and visible light on the electromagnetic spectrum. It has been used for more than 100 years for the treatment of slow-healing and infected wounds. In a systematic review of literature regarding UV light as an adjunctive treatment, Inkaran et al. (2021) found that most studies supported improved healing outcomes.

Strike up the bands

UV radiation is typically divided into three spectral bands: UVA, UVB, and UVC. These bands differ in their biologic effects and their depth of penetration through the skin layers.

The utility of UVC has been demonstrated in various wound types. It is primarily used for treatment in patients with infected wounds. An added benefit of UVC is that it kills a broad spectrum of microorganisms with low exposure times and isn't likely to generate resistant microorganisms.

UV utility

Indications for UV treatment include:
- chronic, slow-healing wounds.
- infected or heavily contaminated wounds.
- necrotic wounds.
  Contraindications for UV treatment include certain chronic disease states, such as:
- diabetes.
- pulmonary tuberculosis.
- hyperthyroidism.

Application of UVC radiation

Primarily used to treat patients with infected wounds, UVC radiation kills a broad spectrum of microorganisms with low exposure times. Here's how it's used.

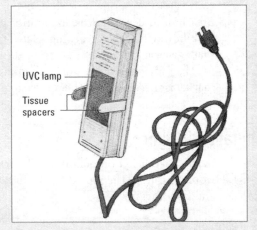

UVC lamp

Tissue spacers

Cover-up

First, the skin around the wound is protected with a thick application of UV-impenetrable ointment, such as zinc oxide or petroleum. Other skin areas are covered with clean sheets. The eyes of the patient and the person administering the therapy must be covered with UV protective glasses.

Turn-on

The UVC lamp is placed 1 in (2.5 cm) from the surface and then turned on for 30 to 60 seconds. This is done once daily for about 1 week or until the infection has cleared. Fungal infections may require a slightly longer treatment time (90 seconds).

Space-out

Tissue spacers, as shown later, may be added to maintain the appropriate distance of the lamp from the wound.

- systemic lupus erythematosus.
- cardiac disease.
- kidney disease.
- hepatic disease.
- acute eczema.
- herpes simplex.

Laser therapy

The word "laser" comes from an acronym for "light amplification by simulated emission of radiation." Lasers can be divided into two groups:

- Cold lasers, also known as *low-level laser therapy* (LLLT), include the helium neon (red laser) and the gallium arsenide, gallium aluminum, and gallium aluminum-arsenide lasers. Resulting tissue changes are attributed to the biologic effects of radiation.
- Hot lasers encompass the carbon dioxide laser and other lasers used for surgical dissection.

In wound healing, cold lasers (LLLT) assist wound closure by promoting cell proliferation and migration and nerve regeneration. The treatment consists of either placing the laser probe directly over selected treatment points for a specific time according to the dosage required or using a gridlike pattern and continuously moving the probe over this grid for a specific treatment time. Success of LLLT and its respective effects are dependent on wavelength, power, dose, and time of application. In a 2014 literature review by Silva Dias Andrade et al., LLLT was shown to promote major physiologic effects when applied to the skin, such as reduction of inflammation, angiogenesis, epithelial and fibroblast proliferation, collagen synthesis and deposition, and wound contracture. It was also determined that doses of 3 to 6 J/cm^2 and wavelengths between 623.8 and 1,000 nm are most effective in the wound healing process.

Laser tag

Indications for LLLT include:

- slow-healing wounds.
- nerve regeneration.
- pain relief.
  Contraindications for LLLT include treatments over:
- the eye.
- a hemorrhage.
- a malignancy.
- a pregnant person's uterus.
- photosensitive skin.

Quick quiz

1. What type of dressing is most appropriate for a patient with a dry wound?
   A. Super-absorptive pad
   B. Amorphous hydrogel
   C. Alginate
   D. Foam

Answer: B. A dry wound needs added moisture to promote wound healing, so an amorphous hydrogel dressing should be used.

2. Which dressing type is most absorbent?
   A. Hydrocolloid
   B. Foam
   C. Nonadherent contact layer
   D. Alginate/hydrofiber

Answer: D. Although foams also have some absorptive capacity, alginate dressings are the most absorbent.

3. You smell an unpleasant odor as you remove your patient's dressing. Which type of dressing may cause this finding?
   A. Alginate
   B. Hydrocolloid
   C. Composite
   D. Foam

Answer: B. Hydrocolloid dressings absorb minimal drainage and turn to gel. This gel can have an unpleasant odor when exposed during dressing changes.

4. Which wound care device uses negative air pressure to deep clean a wound?
   A. NPWT
   B. Warm-Up Therapy System
   C. Alpha-Stim
   D. MIST therapy

Answer: A. NPWT generates negative pressure that draws off exudate, bacteria, and excessive moisture.

5. Which growth factor is marketed as Regranex?
   A. TGF-β
   B. PDGF
   C. IGF
   D. VEGF

Answer: B. Becaplermin (Regranex Gel 0.01%) is the only genetically engineered growth factor substance approved by the FDA for use in wound care. It has a biologic activity similar to that of PDGF produced by the body.

6. What type of UV light is used for infected wounds?
    A. UVA
    B. UVB
    C. UVC
    D. UVD

Answer: C. UVC is primarily used for the treatment of infected wounds because it kills a broad range of microorganisms with short exposure times. Also, it isn't likely to generate resistant microorganisms.

7. What's the maximum recommended impact pressure for pulsatile lavage?
    A. 5 psi
    B. 10 psi
    C. 15 psi
    D. 20 psi

Answer: C. Unless there's a specific order for a higher-impact pressure or a provider is present to supervise, impact pressure shouldn't exceed 15 psi.

8. Which type of therapy increases the amount of dissolved oxygen in the blood?
    A. Ultrasound
    B. Electrical stimulation
    C. Laser
    D. HBO

Answer: D. By increasing the amount of dissolved oxygen in the blood, HBO therapy increases the availability of oxygen to wounded tissues, which improves healing.

9. Which condition is contraindicated for the use of electrical stimulation?
    A. Untreated osteomyelitis
    B. Chronic pressure injuries
    C. Decreased tissue oxygenation
    D. Decreased blood flow

Answer: A. Electrical stimulation is contraindicated for a patient with untreated osteomyelitis.

10. Which type of growth factor increases collagen synthesis during wound healing?
    A. VEGF
    B. IGF
    C. EGF
    D. bFGF

Answer: B. IGF plays an important role in wound healing by increasing collagen synthesis.

Scoring

☆☆☆   If you answered all 10 questions correctly, shout it out! Your
knowledge of wound care products is second to none.

☆☆   If you answered eight questions correctly, we'd like to shake your
hand! You've obviously absorbed all the material on wound care
products.

☆   If you answered fewer than five questions correctly, that's OK! We'll
count this one as warm-up therapy.

Select references

Atkin, L., Bućko, Z., Conde Montero, E., Cutting, K., Moffatt, C., Probst, A.,
Romanelli, M., Schultz, G. S., & Tettelbach, W. (2019). Implementing
TIMERS: The race against hard-to-heal wounds. *Journal of Wound Care,*
28(Suppl 3a), S1–S49. https://doi.org/10.

Bates, A. N., & Ercolano, E. (2021). Development and implementation of a simple
wound care guideline for minor skin lesions: A quality improvement project.
Journal of Wound, Ostomy, and Continence Nursing, 48(4), 285–291. https://
doi.org/10.1097/WON.0000000000000778

Benskin, B. L. (2018). Evidence for polymeric membrane dressings as a unique dressing
subcategory, using pressure ulcers as an example. *Advances in Skin & Wound*
Care, 7(12), 419–426. https://doi.org/10.1089/wound.2018.0822

Bishop, A. (2019). Hyperbaric oxygen therapy for problem wounds: An update. *Wounds*
UK, 15(4), 26–31. https://www.wounds-uk.com/resources/details/hyperbaric-
oxygen-therapy-problem-wounds-update

Chen, R., Salisbury, A., & Percival, S. L. (2020). A comparative study on the cellular
viability and debridement efficiency of antimicrobial-based wound dressings.
International Wound Journal, 17(1), 73–82. https://doi.org/10.1111/iwj.13234

Crumley, C. (2022). Topical wound therapy products with ionic silver. *Journal*
of Wound, Ostomy and Continence Nursing, 49(4), 308–313. https://doi
.org/10.1097/WON.0000000000000884

Golledge, J., & Singh, T. P. (2019). Systematic review or meta-analysis: Systematic
review and meta-analysis of clinical trials examining the effect of hyperbaric
oxygen therapy in people with diabetes-related lower limb ulcers. *Diabetic*
Medicine, 36(7), 813–826. https://doi.org/10.1111/dme.13975

Grigatti, A., & Gefen, A. (2022). What makes a hydrogel-based dressing advantageous
for the prevention of medical device-related pressure ulcers. *International*
Wound Journal, 19(3), 515–530. https://doi.org/10.1111/iwj.13650

Inkaran, J., Tenn, A., Martyniuk, A., Farrokhyar, F., & Cenic, A. (2021). Does UV light as
an adjunct to conventional treatment improve healing and reduce infection
in wounds? A systematic review. *Advances in Skin & Wound Care, 34*(4), 1–6.
https://doi.org/10.1097/01.ASW.0000734384.52295.92

Jaszarowski, K., & Murphree, R. (2021). Wound cleansing and dressing selection. In
L. L. McNichol, C. R. Ratliff, & S. S. Yates (Eds.), *Wound, Ostomy and Conti-*
nence Nurses Society core curriculum: Wound management (2nd ed., pp. 156–170).
Wolters Kluwer.

Kim, P. J., Attinger, C. E., Constantine, T., Crist, B. D., Faust, E., Hirche, C. R., Lavery, L., Messina, V. J., Ohura, N., Punch, L. J., Wirth, G. A., Younis, I., & Téot, L. (2020). Negative pressure wound therapy with instillation: International consensus guidelines update. *International Wound Journal*, *17*(1), 174–186. https://doi.org/10.1111/iwj.13254

Landau, Z., & Schattner, A. (2001). Topical hyperbaric oxygen and low energy laser therapy for chronic diabetic foot ulcers resistant to conventional treatment. *The Yale Journal of Biology and Medicine*, *74*(2), 95–100.

Murdoch, J., Robinson, M., Rossato, M., Ryrie, M., Robinson, M., & Searle, R., & Murdoch, J. (2021). Use of NPWT as part of a Hospital @ Home wound management service. *Journal of Community Nursing*, *35*(4), 50–57. https://www.jcn.co.uk/journals/issue/08-2021/article/use-npwt-part-hospital-home-wound-management-service

Nguyen, J. K., Huang, A., Siegel, D. M., & Jagdeo, J. (2020). Variability in wound care recommendations following dermatologic procedures. *Dermatologic Surgery*, *46*(2), 186–191. https://doi.org/10.1097/DSS.0000000000001952

Rastogi, A., Bhansali, A., & Ramachandran, S. (2019). Efficacy and safety of low-frequency, noncontact airborne ultrasound therapy (Glybetac) for neuropathic diabetic foot ulcers: A randomized, double-blind, sham-control study. *The International Journal of Lower Extremity Wounds*, *18*(1), 81–88. https://doi.org/10.1177/1534734619832738

Silva Dias Andrade, F. S., Oliveira Clark, R. M., & Ferreira, M. L. (2014). Effects of low-level laser therapy on wound healing. *Revista do Colégio Brasileiro de Cirurgiões*, *41*(02), 129–133. https://doi.org/10.1590/S0100-69912014000200010

Snyder, D., Sullivan, N., Margolis, D., & Schoelles, K. (2020). *Skin substitutes for treating chronic wounds*. Agency for Healthcare Research and Quality (US). https://pubmed.ncbi.nlm.nih.gov/32101391/

Szweda, P., Gorczyca, G., & Tylingo, R. (2018). Comparison of antimicrobial activity of selected, commercially available wound dressing materials. *Journal of Wound Care*, *27*(5), 320–326. https://doi.org/10.12968/jowc.2018.27.5.320

Thanigaimani, S., Singh, T., & Golledge, J. (2021). Topical oxygen therapy for diabetes-related foot ulcers: A systematic review and meta-analysis. *Diabetic Medicine*, *38*(8), e14585. https://doi.org/10.1111/dme.14585

Tottoli, E. M., Dorati, R., Genta, I., Chiesa, E., Pisani, S., & Conti, B. (2020). Skin wound healing process and new emerging technologies for skin wound care and regeneration. *Pharmaceutics*, *12*(8), 735. https://doi.org/10.3390/pharmaceutics12080735

van Rijswijk, L., & Gray, M. (2012). Evidence, research, and clinical practice: A patient-centered framework for progress in wound care. *Journal of Wound, Ostomy, and Continence Nursing*, *39*(1), 35–44. https://doi.org/10.1097/WON.0b013e3182383f31

Webber, L., Cornish, W., Cummins, A., & Henshaw, F. R. (2022). Portable negative pressure wound therapy (NPWT) is an effective therapy for hard-to-heal-wounds in the community: A case series. *Wound Practice & Research*, *30*(2), 108–111. https://doi.org/10.33235/wpr.30.2.108-111

Wu, S., Carter, M., Cole, W., Crombie, R., Kapp, D. I., Kim, P., Milne, C., Molnar, J., Niezgoda, J., Woo, K., Zabel, D., & Hamm, R. (2023). Best practice for wound repair and regeneration: Use of cellular, acellular and matrix-like products (CAMPs). *Journal of Wound Care*, *32*(4 SUPPL B), S1–S32.

Chapter 10

Pediatric skin and wound care fundamentals

Just the facts

In this chapter, you'll learn about:

◆ how skin changes in the pediatric years

◆ common pediatric wounds and skin conditions

◆ what to consider when creating a plan of care for children

◆ dressings for pediatric wound care

A look at the skin

Anatomy and physiology

In a short period of time, children's skin goes through many changes. From infancy to adolescence, the child's skin is constantly changing. The fundamentals of the skin's structure remain unchanged but the function of the skin changes. In the first year of life, the skin is more permeable to products because of its structure. The skin may appear translucent depending on the amount of brown fat or the gestational age at birth. Infants born prior to 40 weeks of gestation have under-developed skin structures. When full term, the infant's skin is well developed with a functioning stratum corneum; however, it is still susceptible to skin damage and toxicity.

For the infant born prior to 40 weeks, the stratum corneum develops after birth by exposure to air and the environment. The development of the stratum corneum for the premature infant takes a couple of weeks to up to a month depending on the level of prematurity. The collagen structure is immature and develops over time, affecting the skin's permeability and tensile strength. A premature baby is more susceptible to skin tears and toxicity than the term infant. However, all infants are susceptible to skin damage from adhesives, moisture, friction, and pressure.

The layered look

A patient's level of skin maturation determines how the practitioner selects products for skin integrity and wound healing. Regardless of age, all children should have dressings that minimize pain and maximize time between dressing changes. Similar to adults, wounds can take up to 3 hours to reach the body temperature after a dressing change. During this time, the wound is no longer in an active healing phase. Caloric requirements for children are higher than those of adults given their rapid growth and metabolism; frequent dressing changes will further compound the caloric needs. For children with wounds, the caloric requirements are increased, and for toddlers who are picky eaters, meeting caloric requirements can be a challenge. Therefore, it is imperative to maximize time between dressing changes and use products that promote wound healing to optimize the healing environment.

Common pediatric skin or wound conditions

Eczema

Eczema is a broad term encompassing seven categories of inflammatory conditions that result in erythematous dry, scaly patches of skin. The lack of filaggrin is a potential genetic component of eczema, while inflammatory triggers is another component. Atopic dermatitis is another term for eczema, a common condition in childhood that may follow the child into adulthood.

Itchiness over the dry patchy skin is the most common symptom. Minimizing exposure to allergen triggers such as certain foods, fabrics, and chemicals can help control flare-ups. A daily routine can keep the skin moisturized with pH-balanced cleansing products, moisturizers that are both humectant and emollient, and only using fragrances or skin products that are hypoallergenic. Patches of eczema are common over areas of flexion and extension such as the elbow or knees and are prone to infections from itching. Blistering may also occur.

Allergic dermatitis

Allergic dermatitis can occur at any time in childhood. The itchy area may present as a rash or hives and be extremely uncomfortable. The allergen exposure may be systemic (e.g., from being ingested) or localized (e.g., from direct contact with the skin). Allergic dermatitis is managed both topically and systemically with steroids to control the inflammatory response.

Incontinence-associated dermatitis

Incontinence-associated dermatitis is common in children who are incontinent. Zinc-based clear barrier creams are an effective way to prevent perineal skin irritation related to moisture and chemical irritants associated with stool and urine. For rashes that appear or persist despite the use of barrier cream, the clinician should evaluate for satellite lesions. In the presence of erythema, irritated skin that has maculopapular lesions and/or satellite lesions may require an additional imidazole-based antifungal ointment.

Epidermolysis bullosa

Epidermolysis bullosa is a rare and devastating skin condition that results in blistering of the skin with minimal friction. There are four types of epidermolysis bullosa, with the most severe form affecting the mucosal membranes. Life expectancy for children diagnosed with epidermolysis bullosa depends on the form. With the mildest form, life expectancy is about 50 years, and with the most severe form, life expectancy is generally the first year of life or shorter (Has et al., 2020). The blisters that form open up and are difficult to heal. The goal of care is to prevent new blisters from forming and promote fast healing. Protecting high-friction areas with soft foam with or without silicone adhesion, moisturizer, and dressings with antimicrobials are components of the plan of care.

What to consider when creating the plan of care

A good plan of care for wound healing in pediatrics meets the patient where they are in their life and supports emotional and physical development. Recommending dressings that do not require intrusive dressing changes supports the child and their progression of developmental milestones. This also limits the risk for regression. Regression can occur in different forms. For example, a child who is toilet-trained may regress and begin to be incontinent. An older child who is independent in activities of daily living may want help; a formerly social adolescent may regress to isolation. It is the clinician's responsibility to develop a plan of care that avoids the risk for regression. The child should be able to participate in their daily activities with their dressing in place.

The clinician needs to understand how the child spends most of their day and what it looks like. It is important to engage the child and caregiver in the plan of care. Educating the primary caregiver is another important element for ensuring wound healing. It is important to avoid restricting the child's activity and movement with the dressing as much as possible. The dressing should not cause pain, and the plan should require minimal systemic narcotics as much as possible.

The plan of care for dressing changes should include age-appropriate distraction and engagement of the child. Engaging the child by creating a comfortable environment for dressing changes facilitates a healing environment.

Dressing selection dos and don'ts

The choice of dressings depends on the child, the type of wound, and the goal for healing. See Chapter 9, "Wound Management," for more on dressings.
• DO use dressings that promote cell growth and migration by providing a moist environment without drying out the wound bed.
• DO use silicone technology and avoid aggressive adhesive tapes; this helps with avoiding pain and anxiety with dressing changes.
• DO consider medical-grade honey, which has proven effective on pediatric wounds.
• DO NOT use silver dressings that donate silver to the wound; these can lead to silver toxicity. Nondonating silver dressings are safe to use in children.
• DO NOT use aggressive adhesives.

Negative pressure therapy is a safe and effective method for promoting healing of wounds in pediatric patients. For children in the acute care setting under close supervision by the wound care team, the negative pressure dressing is often changed twice a week to minimize anxiety and pain associated with the dressing change and to promote undisturbed healing. During this time, the child is closely monitored by the multidisciplinary team for any changes in condition warranting the removal of the dressing such as signs of infection, including sudden increase in inflammatory markers, fever, pain, and periwound erythema.

Maintaining skin integrity

Throughout all stages of life, maintaining skin integrity requires evidence-based practice. Pediatric skin functions best when the pH is kept between 4 and 7 with a pH-balanced cleanser. Using a moisturizer that acts as both a humectant and emollient will help bring moisture to the epidermis and maintain it. A product that is nonallergenic or hypoallergenic and safe for use in infants is dimethicone 6%. For incontinent children, using a zinc-based clear moisture cream with each diaper change can prevent moisture maceration and candida, otherwise referred to as diaper rash. When diaper rash does not respond to this first-line care, the clinician may consider treating the candida infection with miconazole 2%. Moisture maceration and prevention within skin folds and under trach ties or neck folds is easily managed with moisture-wicking fabric that contains nondonating silver, which is safe for use in children (Singh, 2016).

Pressure injury prevention across the age spectrum

Implementing a bundled approach to pressure injury (PI) prevention in pediatrics is an effective way to maintain skin integrity. Over the last decade, global PI prevalence has been reduced from 5.88% to as low as 0.2% with a bundled approach to prevention (Singh et al., 2018). A bundled approach includes a validated skin risk assessment tool managing moisture, support surface, mobility, skin integrity, and appropriate devices.

Pressure injury prevention bundles

Risk factors	Mitigating risk factors
Validated risk assessment tools	• Acute care: On admission and daily, after any change in condition • Home or long-term care: On admission, monthly, and with any change in condition
Moisture (skin's natural tensile strength is fostered by using pH-balanced cleansers and humectant- and emollient-based moisturizers)	• Hypoallergenic moisturizers containing dimethicone foster the skin's natural ability to withstand friction and shear forces. • Gently cleanse daily and apply moisturizer to foster skin's tensile strength and promote skin's natural ability to protect itself.
Incontinence	Clear or zinc-based barrier creams and ointments
Fungal	Creams from imidazole category such as 2% miconazole
Perspiration	Moisture-wicking fabric (safe to use in the neonatal population but safety not validated in the premature infant <32 weeks)
Immobility	Select a support surface to envelop and disperse pressure over the body, especially the bony prominences. Pressure redistribution with support surfaces is available for overhead warmers, isolettes, and cribs: • Fluidized positioners • Use these to change pressure points when repositioning is not possible (make small indents in the fluidized positioner to remove pressure from an ear or occiput). • Fluidized positioners can help minimize physiologic startles in the premature infant (promotes comfort, a sense of security, and a proper position).
Pressure, shear, microclimate	Five-layered bordered foam in the appropriate size to cover a bony prominence or other at-risk skin area

Risk factors	Mitigating risk factors
Devices	• When possible change resting pressure points or resting position every 2–4 hours. • Five-layer foam cut to fit and placed directly under the device (absorbs perspiration and disperses skin pressure)
Face masks	Use two different masks (there are different pressure points with each type). Change every 4 hours. Place five-layer thin foam between face mask and skin interface.
Pulse oximeter probe	Apply transparent film over the probe before placement. Change position every 4 hours. Avoid cohesive elastic dressing over oximeter probe.

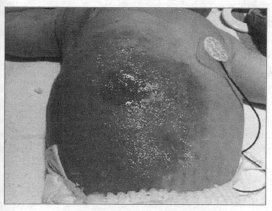

Abdominal candida surrounding an emergent ileostomy site. This can be prevented by containing drainage and protecting surrounding skin with barrier ointments.

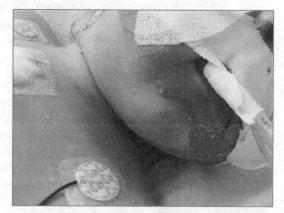

Facial candida from saliva from the mouth. This can be prevented by applying liquid skin protector around the mouth prior to applying tape.

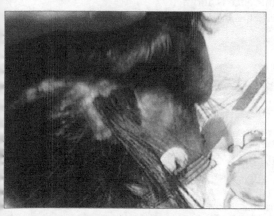

Occipital pressure injury (caused by a blanket roll) may be prevented by using the fluidized positioner to assist with maintaining different head positions.

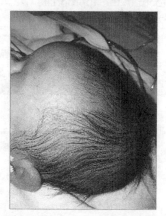

Area of irritation on the forehead caused by an electro-encephalogram lead. Use a liquid skin protector before applying any adhesives to fragile skin.

An effective support surface or positioner will envelop and disperse pressure over bony prominences. Fluidized air positioning aids can help minimize physiologic startles in the premature infant, promoting comfort and a sense of security while providing proper positioning.

Bundled interventions can include a different combination of approaches. The skin's natural tensile strength is supported by using pH-balanced cleansers and humectant emollient-based moisturizers. Hypoallergenic moisturizers that contain dimethicone foster the skin's natural ability to withstand friction and shear forces. Daily gentle cleansing and application of moisturizer help skin's tensile strength and promote its natural ability to protect itself.

Areas of the skin that are under devices are at greatest risk for skin breakdown. Changing pressure points or resting position of devices every 2 to 4 hours as tolerated can prevent skin breakdown. Using two different face masks with pediatric patients requiring nonintubation respiratory support is an effective way to safely provide respiratory support without causing skin breakdown. Thin foam cut to fit directly under the device in resting position on the skin will further promote skin integrity by absorbing intertriginous moisture or small beads of sweat. For devices with resting positions that cannot be changed, a small piece of thin foam placed under the nonmovable device, such as the plastic components of the arterial line or bumper portion of the gastric tube, is an effective way to maintain skin integrity. Some devices are essential, and the resting position can be changed every 2 to 4 hours; however, while in direct contact with the skin, the device may inadvertently cause skin damage. In extremely premature infants and very sick neonates, the pulse oximeter probe may result in skin damage that may be prevented by placing transparent film over the probe prior to placing it on the patient. The five-layered bordered foam in the appropriate size to cover a bony prominence is another component of a bundle to effectively address microclimate, friction, and pressure.

Quick quiz

1. What is one approach to preventing pediatric PIs that has been demonstrated to be effective and is evidence based?
    A. Using hydrocolloids over bony prominences
    B. Turning pediatric patients every 2 hours
    C. This remains a challenge without an effective method beyond using pillows.
    D. Using a bundled approach addressing risk assessment, support surface, moisture, and nutrition

Answer: D. Studies show that no one intervention alone prevents PIs but interventions addressing the different risk factors for skin injury implemented at the same time as a bundle have a greater impact in maintaining skin integrity.

2.   The wound care nurse at a large acute care facility has been asked to help on the pediatric unit. Which is an effective approach to managing acute wounds in pediatrics?
    A.   Using the same policies that are used for adults
    B.   Identifying the nurse's limitations and telling the pediatric unit to consult with a pediatric specialist
    C.   Understanding a comprehensive approach should be taken to account for developmental stage, age, mobility, and type of wound
    D.   Knowing pediatric patients may try to remove dressings so strong adhesives should be used

Answer: C. Developing a patient-centered plan of care for pediatric wound care requires integration of the child's developmental stage, age, mobility, activity, and home life, as well as implementing the principles of wound care.

3.   A 9-year-old patient with a long-term history of eczema is admitted to your facility for cellulitis. You have been consulted to recommend a dressing. What is your approach in recommending a dressing?
    A.   Use a standard dressing consisting of gauze and tape.
    B.   Use a standard dressing consisting of bordered foam.
    C.   Meet with the patient and caregiver for an assessment before suggesting a dressing.
    D.   It does not matter since eczema and cellulitis are difficult to treat.

Answer: C. Prior to developing a plan of care, the wound care clinician should meet with the child and family to understand the needs of the patient and then develop a plan of care.

4.   You meet an adolescent patient who is engaged in their own care and wants to learn about their condition. They have not met anyone other than their primary care provider yet in the facility where you work. What should you do next?
    A.   Tell the patient you will discuss the care plan with their caregiver.
    B.   Quickly examine the affected area, recommend a dressing, and move to your next patient.
    C.   Sit down and ask the patient to tell you more about what they want to learn and ask about their existing skin care routine.
    D.   Tell the patient you will call their primary care provider to explain.

Answer: C. Engaging with an adolescent who is asking questions fosters a therapeutic relationship.

5. The caregiver of a patient with eczema tells you they normally buy whatever body wash and moisturizer is on sale. As a wound care specialist, you recognize this could be an issue because:
   A. sale items are never reliable.
   B. only expensive body wash and skin care products are reliable.
   C. pH-balanced, hypoallergenic products are recommended for optimal skin care for eczema.
   D. only prescription-strength products work for eczema.

Answer: C. Optimizing skin pH, minimizing allergen exposure, and maximizing a balance of moisture are priorities in the management of eczema.

6. Common skin conditions in pediatrics include:
   A. lower extremity wounds.
   B. traumatic wounds from falls and accidents.
   C. skin issues related to poor hygiene.
   D. eczema, epidermolysis bullosa, and dermatitis.

Answer: D. Eczema, epidermolysis bullosa, and dermatitis are more common in the pediatric population than lower extremity wounds, traumatic wounds from falls and accidents, and skin issues related to poor hygiene.

Scoring

☆☆☆ If you answered all six questions correctly, congratulations! You have knowledge across the age spectrum.

☆☆ If you answered four or five questions correctly, good job! Your learning is growing across the spectrum but there's more to go.

☆ If you answered fewer than four questions correctly, don't worry! After a review you will know more than before.

Select references

Baharestani, M. M. (2007). Use of negative pressure wound therapy in the treatment of neonatal and pediatric wounds: A retrospective examination of clinical outcomes. *Ostomy Wound Management, 53*(6), 75–85. https://www.hmpgloballearningnetwork.com/site/wmp/content/use-negative-pressure-wound-therapy-treatment-neonatal-and-pediatric-wounds-a-retrospective-

de Jesus, L. E., Martins, A. B., Oliveira, P. B., Gomes, F., Leve, T., & Dekermacher, S. (2018). Negative pressure wound therapy in pediatric surgery: How and when to use. *Journal of Pediatric Surgery, 53*(4), 585–591. https://doi.org/10.1016/j.jpedsurg.2017.11.048

Delmore, B., VanGilder, C., Koloms, K., & Ayello, E. A. (2020). Pressure injuries in the pediatric population: Analysis of the 2008–2018 International Pressure Ulcer Prevalence Survey data. *Advances in Skin & Wound Care, 33*(6), 301–306. https://doi.org/10.1097/01.ASW.0000661812.22329.f9

Harper, J., & Oranje, A. P. (2019). *Harper's textbook of pediatric dermatology* (4th ed.). John Wiley & Sons Ltd.

Has, C., Bauer, J. W., Bodemer, C., Bolling, M. C., Bruckner-Tuderman, L., Diem, A., Fine, J. D., Heagerty, A., Hovnanian, A., Marinkovich, M. P., Martinez, A. E., McGrath, J. A., Moss, C., Murrell, D. F., Palisson, F., Schwieger-Briel, A., Sprecher, E., Tamai, K., Uitto, J., … Mellerio, J. E. (2020). Consensus reclassification of inherited epidermolysis bullosa and other disorders with skin fragility. *British Journal of Dermatology, 183*(4), 614–627. https://doi.org/10.1111/bjd.18921

Paller, A. S., & Mancini, A. J. (2020). *Paller and Mancini—Hurwitz clinical pediatric dermatology E-book: A textbook of skin disorders of childhood and adolescence.* Elsevier Health Sciences.

Rowe, A. D., McCarty, K., & Huett, A. (2018). Implementation of a nurse driven pathway to reduce incidence of hospital acquired pressure injuries in the pediatric intensive care setting. *Journal of Pediatric Nursing, 41*, 104–109. https://doi.org/10.1016/j.pedn.2018.03.001

Singh, C. D. (2016). Use of a moisture wicking fabric for prevention of skin damage around drains and parenteral access lines. *Journal of Wound, Ostomy, and Continence Nursing, 43*(5), 551–553. https://doi.org/10.1097/WON.0000000000000249

Singh, C. D., Anderson, C., White, E., & Shoqirat, N. (2018). The impact of pediatric pressure injury prevention bundle on pediatric pressure injury rates: A secondary analysis. *Journal of Wound, Ostomy and Continence Nursing, 45*(3), 209–212. https://doi.org/10.1097/WON.0000000000000439

Singh, C. D., & Shoqirat, N. (2019). Pressure redistribution crib mattress: A quality improvement project. *Journal of Wound, Ostomy, and Continence Nursing, 46*(1), 62–64. https://doi.org/10.1097/WON.0000000000000500

Appendices and index

Bates–Jensen Wound Assessment Tool
Instructions for use

General guidelines

Fill out the rating sheet to assess a wound's status after reading the definitions and methods of assessment described later. Evaluate once a week and whenever a change occurs in the wound. Rate according to each item by picking the response that best describes the wound and entering that score in the item score column for the appropriate date. When you have rated the wound on all items, determine the total score by adding together the 13 item scores. The HIGHER the total score, the more severe the wound status. Plot the total score on the wound status continuum to determine progress. If the wound has healed/resolved, score items 1, 2, 3, and 4 as = 0.

Specific instructions

1. **Size:** Use ruler to measure the longest and widest aspect of the wound surface in centimeters; multiply length × width. Score as = 0 if wound healed/resolved.

2. **Depth:** Pick the depth and thickness most appropriate to the wound using these additional descriptions; score as = 0 if wound healed/resolved:
   1 = Tissues damaged but no break in skin surface
   2 = Superficial, abrasion, blister, or shallow crater. Even with and/or elevated above skin surface (e.g., hyperplasia)
   3 = Deep crater with or without undermining of adjacent tissue
   4 = Visualization of tissue layers not possible due to necrosis
   5 = Supporting structures include tendon, joint capsule

3. **Edges:** Score as = 0 if wound healed/resolved. Use this guide:
Indistinct, diffuse	=	Unable to clearly distinguish wound outline
Attached	=	Even or flush with wound base, <u>no</u> sides or walls present; flat
Not attached	=	Sides or walls <u>are</u> present; floor or base of wound is deeper than edge

Rolled under, thickened	=	Soft to firm and flexible to touch
Hyperkeratosis	=	Callous-like tissue formation around wound and at edges
Fibrotic, scarred	=	Hard, rigid to touch

4. **Undermining:** Score as = 0 if wound healed/resolved. Assess by inserting a cotton-tipped applicator under the wound edge; advance it as far as it will go without using undue force; raise the tip of the applicator so it may be seen or felt on the surface of the skin; mark the surface with a pen; and measure the distance from the mark on the skin to the edge of the wound. Continue process around the wound. Then use a transparent metric measuring guide with concentric circles divided into four (25%) pie-shaped quadrants to help determine percent of wound involved.

5. **Necrotic tissue type:** Pick the type of necrotic tissue that is <u>predominant</u> in the wound according to color, consistency, and adherence using this guide:

White/gray nonviable tissue	=	May appear prior to wound opening; skin surface is white or gray
Nonadherent, yellow slough	=	Thin, mucinous substance; scattered throughout wound bed; easily separated from wound tissue
Loosely adherent, yellow slough	=	Thick, stringy, clumps of debris; attached to wound tissue
Adherent, soft, black eschar	=	Soggy tissue; strongly attached to tissue in center or base of wound
Firmly adherent, hard/black eschar	=	Firm, crusty tissue; strongly attached to wound base <u>and</u> edges (like a hard scab)

6. **Necrotic tissue amount:** Use a transparent metric measuring guide with concentric circles divided into four (25%) pie-shaped quadrants to help determine percent of wound involved.

7. **Exudate type:** Some dressings interact with wound drainage to produce a gel or trap liquid. Before assessing exudate type, gently cleanse wound with normal saline or water. Pick the exudate type that is <u>predominant</u> in the wound according to color and consistency, using this guide:

Bloody	=	Thin, bright red
Serosanguineous	=	Thin, watery pale red to pink
Serous	=	Thin, watery, clear

Purulent   =   Thin or thick, opaque tan to yellow or green; may have offensive odor

8. **Exudate amount:** Use a transparent metric measuring guide with concentric circles divided into four (25%) pie-shaped quadrants to determine percent of dressing involved with exudate. Use this guide:

None   =   Wound tissues dry

Scant   =   Wound tissues moist; no measurable exudate

Small   =   Wound tissues wet; moisture evenly distributed in wound; drainage involves ≤25% dressing

Moderate   =   Wound tissues saturated; drainage may or may not be evenly distributed in wound; drainage involves >25% to ≤75% dressing

Large   =   Wound tissues bathed in fluid; drainage freely expressed; may or may not be evenly distributed in wound; drainage involves >75% of dressing

9. **Skin color surrounding wound:** Assess tissues within 4 cm of wound edge. Dark-skinned persons show the colors "bright red" and "dark red" as a deepening of normal ethnic skin color or a purple hue. As healing occurs in dark-skinned persons, the new skin is pink and may never darken.

10. **Peripheral tissue edema and induration:** Assess tissues within 4 cm of wound edge. Nonpitting edema appears as skin that is shiny and taut. Identify pitting edema by firmly pressing a finger down into the tissues and waiting for 5 seconds; on release of pressure, tissues fail to resume previous position and an indentation appears. Induration is abnormal firmness of tissues with margins. Assess by gently pinching the tissues. Induration results in an inability to pinch the tissues. Use a transparent metric measuring guide to determine how far edema or induration extends beyond wound.

11. **Granulation tissue:** Granulation tissue is the growth of small blood vessels and connective tissue to fill in full-thickness wounds. Tissue is healthy when bright, beefy red, shiny, and granular with a velvety appearance. Poor vascular supply appears as pale pink or blanched to dull, dusky red color.

12. **Epithelialization:** Epithelialization is the process of epidermal resurfacing and appears as pink or red skin. In partial-thickness wounds, it can occur throughout the wound bed as well as from the wound edges. In full-thickness wounds, it occurs from the edges only. Use a transparent metric measuring guide with concentric circles divided into four (25%) pie-shaped quadrants to help determine percent of wound involved and to measure the distance the epithelial tissue extends into the wound.

Bates–Jensen Wound Assessment Tool

NAME

Complete the rating sheet to assess wound status. Evaluate each item by picking the response that best describes the wound and entering the score in the item score column for the appropriate date. If the wound has healed/resolved, score items 1, 2, 3, and 4 as = 0.

Location: Anatomic site. Circle, identify right (R) or left (L) and use "X" to mark site on body diagrams:

_____	Sacrum and coccyx	_____	Lateral ankle
_____	Trochanter	_____	Medial ankle
_____	Ischial tuberosity	_____	Heel
_____	Buttock	_____	Other site:_____.

Shape: Overall wound pattern; assess by observing perimeter and depth.

Circle and <u>date</u> appropriate description:

_____	Irregular	_____	Linear or elongated
_____	Round/oval	_____	Bowl/boat
_____	Square/rectangle	_____	Butterfly Other Shape

Item	Assessment	Date score	Date score	Date score
1. Size*	*0 = Healed, resolved wound 1 = Length × width <4 cm² 2 = Length × width 4.0–< 16 cm² 3 = Length × width 16.1–< 36 cm² 4 = Length × width 36.1–<80 cm² 5 = Length × width >80 cm²			
2. Depth*	*0 = Healed, resolved wound 1 = Nonblanchable erythema on intact skin 2 = Partial-thickness skin loss involving epidermis and/or dermis 3 = Full-thickness skin loss involving damage or necrosis of subcutaneous tissue; may extend down to but not through underlying fascia; and/or mixed partial and full thickness and/or tissue layers obscured by granulation tissue 4 = Obscured by necrosis 5 = Full-thickness skin loss with extensive destruction, tissue necrosis, or damage to muscle, bone, or supporting structures			
3. Edges*	*0 = Healed, resolved wound 1 = Indistinct, diffuse, none clearly visible 2 = Distinct, outline clearly visible, attached, even with wound base 3 = Well-defined, not attached to wound base 4 = Well-defined, not attached to base, rolled under, thickened 5 = Well-defined, fibrotic, scarred, or hyperkeratotic			

Item	Assessment	Date score	Date score	Date score
4. Undermining*	*0 = Healed, resolved wound 1 = None present 2 = Undermining <2 cm in any area 3 = Undermining 2–4 cm involving <50% wound margins 4 = Undermining 2–4 cm involving >50% wound margins 5 = Undermining >4 cm or tunneling in any area			
5. Necrotic Tissue Type	1 = None visible 2 = White/gray nonviable tissue and/or nonadherent yellow slough 3 = Loosely adherent yellow slough 4 = Adherent, soft, black eschar 5 = Firmly adherent, hard, black eschar			
6. Necrotic Tissue Amount	1 = None visible 2 = <25% of wound bed covered 3 = 25% to 50% of wound covered 4 = >50% and <75% of wound covered 5 = 75% to 100% of wound covered			
7. Exudate Type	1 = None 2 = Bloody 3 = Serosanguineous: thin, watery, pale red/pink 4 = Serous: thin, watery, clear 5 = Purulent: thin or thick, opaque, tan/yellow, with or without odor			
8. Exudate Amount	1 = None, dry wound 2 = Scant, wound moist but no observable exudate 3 = Small 4 = Moderate 5 = Large			
9. Skin Color Surrounding Wound	1 = Pink or normal for ethnic group 2 = Bright red and/or blanches to touch 3 = White or gray pallor or hypopigmented 4 = Dark red or purple and/or nonblanchable 5 = Black or hyperpigmented			
10. Peripheral Tissue Edema	1 = No swelling or edema 2 = Nonpitting edema extends <4 cm around wound 3 = Nonpitting edema extends >4 cm around wound 4 = Pitting edema extends <4 cm around wound 5 = Crepitus and/or pitting edema extends >4 cm around wound			

Item	Assessment	Date score	Date score	Date score
11. Peripheral Tissue Induration	1 = None present 2 = Induration, <2 cm around wound 3 = Induration 2–4 cm extending <50% around wound 4 = Induration 2–4 cm extending >50% around wound 5 = Induration >4 cm in any area around wound			
12. Granulation Tissue	1 = Skin intact or partial-thickness wound 2 = Bright, beefy red; 75% to 100% of wound filled and/or tissue overgrowth 3 = Bright, beefy red; <75% and >25% of wound filled 4 = Pink and/or dull, dusky red and/or fills ≤25% of wound 5 = No granulation tissue present			
13. Epithelialization	1 = 100% wound covered, surface intact 2 = 75% to <100% wound covered and/or epithelial tissue extends >0.5 cm into wound bed 3 = 50% to <75% wound covered and/or epithelial tissue extends to >0.5 cm into wound bed 4 = 25% to <50% wound covered 5 = <25% wound covered			
	TOTAL SCORE			
	SIGNATURE			

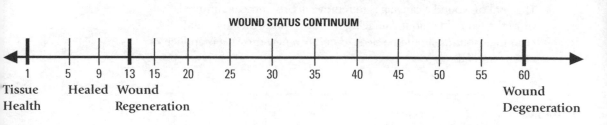

WOUND STATUS CONTINUUM

1   5   9   13   15   20   25   30   35   40   45   50   55   60

Tissue   Healed   Wound   Wound
Health   Regeneration   Degeneration

Plot the total score on the Wound Status Continuum by putting an "**X**" on the line and the date beneath the line. Plot multiple scores with their dates to see at a glance regeneration or degeneration of the wound.

Wound bed preparation

Before doing any procedures, always:
- confirm the patient's identity using two patient identifiers according to your facility's policy.
- medicate patient as needed.
- provide privacy and explain the procedure to the patient to allay their fears and promote cooperation.
- position the patient in a way that maximizes their comfort while allowing easy access to the wound site.
- review the wound care orders.
- assemble the equipment at the patient's bedside and inspect supplies for expiration dates.
- use clean or sterile technique, depending on your facility's policy.
- loosen lids on cleaning solutions and medications for easy removal.
- attach an impervious plastic trash bag to the overbed table to hold used dressings and refuse.
- use personal protective equipment as needed.
- wash hands.
- use standard precautions.

Cleaning the wound

The goal of wound cleansing is to remove debris and contaminants from the wound without damaging healthy tissue. After an initial cleaning, wounds should be cleaned before a new dressing is applied and as needed.

What you need

- Impervious plastic trash bag
- Linen saver pad
- Two pairs of clean or sterile gloves (depending on facility policy)
- Personal protective equipment if indicated
- Prescribed cleanser, such as sterile normal saline solution, wound cleanser, sterile water
- Clean or sterile container (depending on facility policy)
- Materials as needed for wound care
- Skin protectant wipe (skin sealant) or other protective skin barrier

Step by step

1. **Remove the soiled dressing.**
   Put on clean gloves. Roll or lift an edge of the dressing, and then gently remove it while supporting the surrounding skin. When possible, remove the dressing in the direction of hair growth.

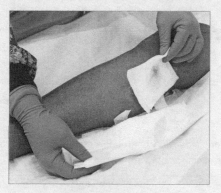

2. **Inspect the dressing and wound.**
   Note the color, amount, and odor of drainage and necrotic debris.

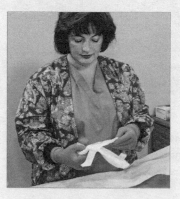

3. **Clean the wound.**
   When cleaning a wound, move from the least contaminated area to the most contaminated area. Also, be sure to use a clean gauze pad for each wipe.

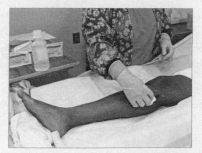

(continued)

Step by step *(continued)*

- For a linear-shaped wound, such as an incision, gently wipe from top to bottom in one motion, starting directly over the wound and moving outward.

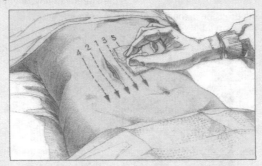

- For an open wound, such as a pressure injury or around a drain, gently wipe in concentric circles, again starting directly over the wound/drain and moving outward.

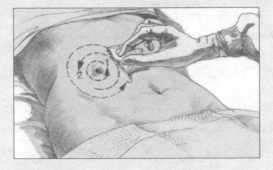

4. **Dry the wound.**
   Using the same procedure as for cleaning a wound, dry the wound using dry gauze pads. Pat dry; do not rub.
5. **Reassess the condition of the skin and wound.**
   Note the character of the clean wound bed and surrounding skin.

Wound irrigation

Irrigation cleans tissues and flushes cell debris and drainage from an open wound. It also helps prevent premature surface healing over an abscess pocket or infected tract. After irrigation, lightly fill open wounds to absorb additional drainage and fill dead space.

What you need

- Impervious plastic trash bag
- Linen saver pad
- Emesis basin

- Two pairs of clean or sterile gloves (depending on facility policy)
- Personal protective equipment if indicated
- Prescribed irrigant, such as sterile normal saline solution or sterile water, or other prescribed solution
- 35-mL piston syringe with 19G needle or catheter and clean or sterile container or commercial wound irrigation set
- Skin protectant wipe (skin sealant) or other protective skin barrier
- Materials as needed for wound care

Getting ready

Mark any container with the date it was opened. Don't use any solution that has been open longer than 24 hours. As needed, dilute the prescribed irrigant to the correct proportions with sterile water or normal saline solution. Some facilities may have the pharmacy prepare this for you. Be sure to check your facility policy. Allow the solution to reach room temperature or warm it to 90°F to 95°F (32.2°C to 35°C).

Step by step

1. **Prepare the solution and equipment.**
   Fill the irrigating device with irrigating solution.
2. **Irrigate the entire wound thoroughly.**
   Use a face shield or mask and goggles in case of a splash. Gently instill a slow, steady stream of solution into the wound. Make sure the solution flows from the clean area to the dirty area of the wound to prevent contamination of clean tissue. To prevent tissue damage, don't force the needle or angiocatheter into the wound. Irrigate until you've administered the prescribed amount of solution or until the solution returns clear. Note the amount of solution administered. Keep the patient positioned to allow complete wound drainage. Devices used to irrigate a wound should provide gentle, low-pressure irrigation and may include a bulb syringe or a 35-mL piston syringe with an 18G needle or angiocatheter.

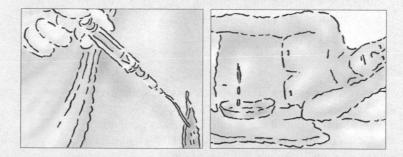

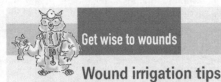

Wound irrigation tips

How can you avoid mess or spillage when irrigating a wound in a hard-to-reach location? Here are some tips you can follow.

Limb wounds

You can soak an arm or a leg wound in a large vessel of warm irrigating fluid, such as water, normal saline solution, or an appropriate antiseptic. Remember that this method is contraindicated in patients with cellulitis, unstable coagulation studies, or deep vein thrombosis.

If possible, rinse the wound several times and carefully dispose of the contaminated liquid in the appropriate location.

Trunk or thigh wounds

Because they're difficult to irrigate, trunk or thigh wounds require some ingenuity. One method uses an ostomy irrigation pouch applied over the wound. (Run warm solution through an infusion set and collect it in a drainage bag.)

You can also use a large syringe for irrigation. Where possible, direct the flow at right angles to the wound and allow the fluid to drain by gravity. Doing so requires careful positioning of the patient, either in bed or on a chair. The patient may need analgesia during the treatment.

If irrigation isn't possible, you'll have to swab the wound clean, which is time-consuming. Swab away exudate before using antiseptic or saline solution to clean the wound (taking care not to push loose debris into the wound).

Positioned for success

- Make sure to explain to the patient what you will be doing.
- Ask the patient to tell you if they experience any discomfort or pain during the procedure.
- Keep the patient positioned to allow further wound drainage into the basin.
- Clean the area around the wound with normal saline solution and pat dry with gauze; wipe intact surrounding skin with a skin protectant wipe and allow it to dry.

Practice pointers

- Try to coordinate wound irrigation with the wound care specialist or health care provider visit so that they can inspect the wound.
- Irrigate with a bulb syringe if the wound is small or not particularly deep or if a piston syringe is unavailable. However, use a bulb syringe cautiously because this type of syringe doesn't deliver enough pressure to adequately clean the wound.

Collecting a wound culture

Heavily colonized and infected wounds (those with heavy bacterial or fungal overgrowth) are unable to properly heal. Cultures can help determine the involved organism and guide treatment. One common wound culture collection method is the surface swab technique (see Levine technique below). Other methods, including syringe aspiration and punch tissue biopsy, are performed by health care providers. Remember, the surface swab technique obtains bacteria colonized only on the wound's surface. For a more accurate culture, needle aspiration of fluid or punch tissue biopsy should be used.

What you need

- Clean gloves
- Normal saline solution
- Sterile gauze pads
- Sterile culture tube with transport medium (or commercial collection kit for aerobic culture)
- Special anaerobic culture tube containing carbon dioxide or nitrogen
- Clean or sterile dressings for the wound
- Laboratory request form
- Patient labels

Step by step culture using Levine method

When obtaining a wound culture, follow standard precautions and maintain sterile technique throughout each of these steps.

1. **Inspect and cleanse.**
   - Cleanse wound with normal saline solution.
   - Remove/debride nonviable tissue, and blot with sterile gauze.
   - Wait 2 to 5 minutes.
2. **Swab**
   - Identify a healthy area of wound about 1 cm² (*do not culture exudate, pus, eschar, or heavily fibrous tissue*).
   - Moisten the swab with nonpreserved normal saline solution if the wound bed is dry.
   - Rotate the end of a sterile applicator over a 1-cm² area for 5 seconds (technique suggests alginate-tipped applicator). Apply sufficient pressure to swab to cause tissue fluid to be expressed.

(continued)

Step by step culture using Levine method *(continued)*

3. **Place the swab in the appropriate culture medium.**
   - When the tip of the swab is saturated, break the tip using sterile technique into a collection device designed for quantitative cultures.
   - If the wound is open and has viable tissue, immediately place the swab in an aerobic culture tube. If the wound has necrotic tissue or sinus tracts, obtain both an aerobic and an anaerobic culture.
4. **Label the culture tube.**
   Follow the facility policy. Include the patient's name, the date and time, the source location of the specimen, and your name or initials. You may be asked about any antibiotics the patient is taking. Immediately send the tube to the laboratory.

Collecting an anaerobic specimen

Because most anaerobes die when exposed to oxygen, they must be transported in tubes filled with carbon dioxide or nitrogen. Before specimen collection, the small inner tube containing the swab is held in place with a rubber stopper.

After collecting the specimen, quickly replace the swab in the inner tube and depress the plunger to separate the inner tube from the stopper. The swab is forced into the larger tube, exposing the specimen to a carbon dioxide–rich environment.

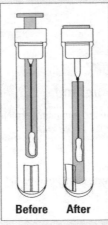

Before   After

Appendix 3

Pressure injury prevention algorithm

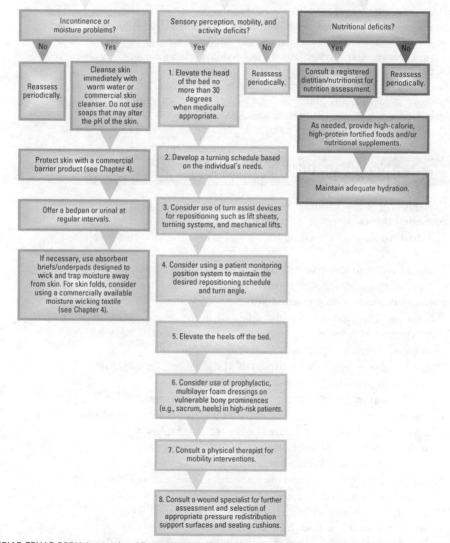

Assess for pressure injury risk using a validated risk assessment scale.

Incontinence or moisture problems?

No → Reassess periodically.

Yes → Cleanse skin immediately with warm water or commercial skin cleanser. Do not use soaps that may alter the pH of the skin.

Protect skin with a commercial barrier product (see Chapter 4).

Offer a bedpan or urinal at regular intervals.

If necessary, use absorbent briefs/underpads designed to wick and trap moisture away from skin. For skin folds, consider using a commercially available moisture wicking textile (see Chapter 4).

Sensory perception, mobility, and activity deficits?

Yes:
1. Elevate the head of the bed no more than 30 degrees when medically appropriate.
2. Develop a turning schedule based on the individual's needs.
3. Consider use of turn assist devices for repositioning such as lift sheets, turning systems, and mechanical lifts.
4. Consider using a patient monitoring position system to maintain the desired repositioning schedule and turn angle.
5. Elevate the heels off the bed.
6. Consider use of prophylactic, multilayer foam dressings on vulnerable bony prominences (e.g., sacrum, heels) in high-risk patients.
7. Consult a physical therapist for mobility interventions.
8. Consult a wound specialist for further assessment and selection of appropriate pressure redistribution support surfaces and seating cushions.

No → Reassess periodically.

Nutritional deficits?

Yes → Consult a registered dietitian/nutritionist for nutrition assessment.

As needed, provide high-calorie, high-protein fortified foods and/or nutritional supplements.

Maintain adequate hydration.

No → Reassess periodically.

Data from 2019 NPIAP, EPUAP, PPPIA International Pressure Injury Clinical Practice Guidelines and Munoz, N., Posthauer, M. E., Cereda, E., Schols, J., & Haesler, E. (2020). The role of nutrition for pressure injury prevention and healing: The 2019 international clinical practice guideline recommendations. *Advances in Skin & Wound Care, 33,* 123–136.

Prevention and treatment of pressure injuries: Nutrition guidelines for adults

Sources: Haesler, E. (Ed.). (2019). *European Pressure Ulcer Advisory Panel, National Pressure Injury Advisory Panel and Pan Pacific Pressure Injury Alliance. Prevention and treatment of pressure ulcers/injuries: Clinical practice guideline.* European Pressure Ulcer Advisory Panel, National Pressure Injury Advisory Panel and Pan Pacific Pressure Injury Alliance. Cambridge Media. Munoz, N., Posthauer, M. E., Cereda, E., Schols, J., & Haesler, E. (2020). The role of nutrition for pressure injury prevention and healing: The 2019 international clinical practice guideline recommendations. *Advances in Skin & Wound Care, 33*(3), 123–136. https://doi.org/10.1097/01.ASW.0000653144.90739.ad

Prevention of pressure injuries

1. Consider the impact of impaired nutritional status on the risk of pressure injuries.
2. Conduct nutritional screening for individuals at risk of a pressure injury.
3. Conduct a comprehensive nutrition assessment for adults at risk of a pressure injury who are screened to be at risk for malnutrition and for all adults with pressure injuries.
4. Develop and implement an individualized nutrition care plan for individuals at risk for pressure injury who are malnourished or who are at risk of malnutrition.
5. Optimize energy intake for individuals at risk of pressure injuries who are malnourished or at risk of malnutrition.
6. Offer high-calorie, high-protein fortified foods and/or nutritional supplements in addition to the usual diet for adults who are at risk of developing pressure injuries and who are also malnourished or at risk of malnutrition if nutritional requirements cannot be achieved with normal dietary intake.
7. Adjust protein intake for individuals at risk of pressure injuries who are malnourished or at risk of malnutrition.
8. Discuss the benefits and harms of enteral or parenteral feeding to support overall health in light of preferences and goals of care with individuals at risk of pressure injuries who cannot meet their nutritional requirements through oral intake despite nutritional interventions.

9. Provide and encourage adequate water/fluid intake for hydration for an individual at risk for pressure injury when compatible with goals of care.

Treatment of pressure injuries

1. Develop and implement an individualized nutrition care plan for individuals with pressure injuries who are malnourished or who are at risk of malnutrition.
2. Provide 30 to 35 kcal/kg body weight/day for adults with pressure injuries who are malnourished or at risk of malnutrition.
3. Provide 1.25 to 1.5 g protein/kg body weight/day for adults with a pressure injury who are malnourished or at risk of malnutrition.
4. Offer high-calorie, high-protein nutritional supplements in addition to the usual diet for adults with pressure injuries who are malnourished or at risk of malnutrition if nutritional requirements cannot be achieved by normal dietary intake.
5. Provide high-calorie, high-protein, arginine, zinc, and antioxidant oral nutritional supplements or enteral formula for adults with stage 2 or greater pressure injuries who are malnourished or at risk of malnutrition.
6. Discuss the benefits and harms of enteral or parenteral feeding to support pressure injury treatment in light of preferences and goals of care for individuals with pressure injuries who cannot meet their nutritional requirements through oral intake despite nutritional interventions.
7. Provide and encourage adequate water/fluid intake for hydration for an individual with a pressure injury when compatible with goals of care and clinical condition.

Pressure Ulcer Scale for Healing (PUSH)

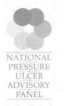

NATIONAL
PRESSURE
ULCER
ADVISORY
PANEL

Pressure Ulcer Scale for Healing (PUSH)
PUSH Tool 3.0

Patient Name_____ Patient ID# _____

Ulcer Location _____ Date _____

Directions:

Observe and measure the pressure ulcer. Categorize the ulcer with respect to surface area, exudate, and type of wound tissue. Record a sub-score for each of these ulcer characteristics. Add the sub-scores to obtain the total score. A comparison of total scores measured over time provides an indication of the improvement or deterioration in pressure ulcer healing.

	0	1	2	3	4	5	Sub-score
LENGTH X WIDTH	0	< 0.3	0.3 – 0.6	0.7 – 1.0	1.1 – 2.0	2.1 – 3.0	
	6	7	8	9	10		
(in cm²)		3.1 – 4.0	4.1 – 8.0	8.1 – 12.0	12.1 – 24.0	> 24.0	
EXUDATE AMOUNT	0	1	2	3			Sub-score
	None	Light	Moderate	Heavy			
TISSUE TYPE	0	1	2	3	4		Sub-score
	Closed	Epithelial Tissue	Granulation Tissue	Slough	Necrotic Tissue		
							TOTAL SCORE

Length x Width: Measure the greatest length (head to toe) and the greatest width (side to side) using a centimeter ruler. Multiply these two measurements (length x width) to obtain an estimate of surface area in square centimeters (cm²). Caveat: Do not guess! Always use a centimeter ruler and always use the same method each time the ulcer is measured.

Exudate Amount: Estimate the amount of exudate (drainage) present after removal of the dressing and before applying any topical agent to the ulcer. Estimate the exudate (drainage) as none, light, moderate, or heavy.

Tissue Type: This refers to the types of tissue that are present in the wound (ulcer) bed. Score as a "4" if there is any necrotic tissue present. Score as a "3" if there is any amount of slough present and necrotic tissue is absent. Score as a "2" if the wound is clean and contains granulation tissue. A superficial wound that is reepithelializing is scored as a "1". When the wound is closed, score as a "0".

- 4 – **Necrotic Tissue (Eschar):** black, brown, or tan tissue that adheres firmly to the wound bed or ulcer edges and may be either firmer or softer than surrounding skin.
- 3 – **Slough:** yellow or white tissue that adheres to the ulcer bed in strings or thick clumps, or is mucinous.
- 2 – **Granulation Tissue:** pink or beefy red tissue with a shiny, moist, granular appearance.
- 1 – **Epithelial Tissue:** for superficial ulcers, new pink or shiny tissue (skin) that grows in from the edges or as islands on the ulcer surface.
- 0 – **Closed/Resurfaced:** the wound is completely covered with epithelium (new skin).

www.npuap.org
11F

PUSH Tool Version 3.0: 9/15/98
©National Pressure Ulcer Advisory Panel

Wound care dressing review

The following companies have products that are listed in the accompanying chart. **This chart is not intended to be an all-inclusive list of or about products available in each classification or from each company.**

This chart contains dressing classifications with some actions, indications, contraindications, and application tips for the classifications.

- Coloplast—Comfeel®, Biatain®, Triad™ Hydrophilic Wound Dressing (https://www.coloplast.us/about-us/coloplast_samples/ostomy_stoma_supplies_catheters_incontinence_samples/?utm_campaign=CP_US_EN_AW_Text_NA_NA_Brand_Exact&gclid=EAIaIQobChMIwrahmeD58QIVgYvICh2y_QhyEAAYASAAEgKaN_D_BwE&gclsrc=aw.ds)
- Convatec—DuoDERM®, AQUACEL® hydrofiber and foam with and without silver; KALTOSTAT® (https://www.convatec.com/advanced-wound-care/skin-care/)
- Covidien—Kendall™/COVIDIEN™ brands—Kerlix, Excilon, AMD™ gauze options, Telfa; Xeroform®, Curasorb (Medtronic now owns this line; https://www.medtronic.com/covidien/en-us/products.html)
- Integra LifeSciences Corp.—MEDIHONEY™, TCC-EZ cast® (https://www.integralife.com/outpatient-clinic-private-office/category/wound-reconstruction-care-outpatient-clinic-private-office)
- Ferris—PolyMem® (www.polymem.com)
- Hollister—Restore® hydrogel, calcium alginate, alginate silver, hydrocolloid (https://www.hollister.com/en/products/wound-care-products)
- MANUKAMED®—MANUKApli, etc. (https://shop.manukamed.com/)
- Medline—Optifoam, Opticell, TheraHoney products (https://www.medline.com/category/Advanced-Wound-Care/Z05-CA01_17)
- Mölnlycke—Mepilex®, Mepitel®, Lyofoam®, Melgisorb®, Mepore® film, Normlgel®, and additional products (https://www.molnlycke.us/)
- Organogenesis Inc.—Apligraf®, Dermagraft®, PuraPly® AM (https://organogenesis.com/advanced-wound-care/)
- Smith & Nephew—Allevyn, IntraSite, SoloSite, OpSite; AlgiSite, Acticoat, Iodosorb, Iodoflex, FlexiGel, Oasis®, Collagenase Santyl® enzyme ointment, Grafix, Stravix (https://www.smith-nephew.com/professional/products/advanced-wound-management/)
- 3M—Tegasorb, Tegaderm, 3M No Sting Cavilon Skin Spray, VAC (https://www.3m.com/3M/en_US/medical-us/skin-and-wound-care/)

Dressing classifications	Actions	Indications	Contraindications	Application tips
Gauze "Gauze" dressings were traditionally woven cotton, nonfilled sponges that may be loosely (Kerlix™) woven or a fine mesh. 2×2 and 4×4 are most common sizes. Gauze now available with antimicrobial properties.	*Kerlix and woven gauze* • Absorbs exudate and allows fluid to transfer to secondary dressing; nonselective debridement of wound bed; fills dead space of wound, sinus tract, or undermining edges • Gauze dressings will (1) debride (ordered as a wet to dry); *this is nonselective debridement and **not recommended**!* (2) absorb some exudate and transfer to secondary dressing.	• Gauze dressings are used on all wound stages. • Most effective on full thickness but need to be changed frequently to maintain moisture. When filling dead space always open and "fluff" the gauze pad.	Moisten with NSS if used as filler in dry wounds.	• Fine mesh gauze to ↓ damage to wound bed on removal (do not use cotton-filled sponges as "debris" can be left in wound) • Fill lightly to avoid compromised blood flow or delay wound closure. • Protect surrounding skin with a skin protector when moist gauze is used or wound is draining. • Change Q4–8 hrs depending on purpose, amount of drainage. • For draining wound, use cotton gauze to "wick" drainage into secondary dressing (such as an ABD).
Noncotton, nonwoven Synthetic gauze is now available in several combinations, polyester and/or rayon.	• Absorbent but does not transfer drainage to secondary dressing as well as cotton gauze • Less adherent—not for debriding • Good for cleaning and prepping			

Dressing classifications	Actions	Indications	Contraindications	Application tips
Alginate and Hydrofiber Dressings (Kaltostat™, SORBSAN®, AlgiSite, SeaSorb, Curasorb™) [Aquacel; Maxorb® Extra CMS/Alginate]	• Absorb moderate to heavy amounts of exudate while maintaining a moist wound bed. • Alginates are derived from seaweed and absorb many times their own weight.	• Wounds with large amounts of exudate that need to be lightly filled • Wounds with necrosis and exudate • Select wounds with sinus tracts and undermining edges depending on ability to *remove all of the dressing material* at each dressing change • Full thickness • Clean or dirty	• Wounds with minimal exudate • Wounds covered with dry eschar	• Absorptive dressings require a secondary or cover dressing. • Change when strikethrough to outer dressing occurs. • Dressings come in ropes or sheets. • Alginates may change to a tan color—assess wound *after* cleansing. • Copolymer starches should be thoroughly rinsed from wound bed before assessment and reapplication.
Antimicrobials Silver Cadexomer iodine Covidien Kendall gauze with AMD™ Honey (TheraHoney; MANUKApli)	• Kill bacteria and reduce bioburden while remaining noncytotoxic for wound healing and cell proliferation • Cadexomer iodine disrupts biofilm.	• Infected wounds • Wounds suspected to have bioburden	• Allergy to product components • Allergy to honey, not bees	• See manufacturer directions. • Use only medical-grade honey.
CAMPs (Cellular, Acellular, and Matrix-Like Products) Apligraf®, Epifix, OASIS® Ultra and Wound Matrix, Grafix, Stravix	Tissues deliver multiple growth factors to wound depending on product.	Nonhealing wounds that have failed conservative therapeutic modalities over a 4-week period	• Allergy to tissue used (bovine, porcine) • Do not use on clinically infected wounds.	See manufacturer directions for additional indications for use and contraindications.
Collagen Dressings PROMOGRAN PRISMA® (matrix of 55% collagen, 44% oxidized regenerated cellulose [ORC] and 1% ORC/silver); PROMOGRAN® 55% collagen, 45% ORC; Puracol® Plus; Puracol® Plus Ag+	Provides collagen matrix to wound bed to accelerate wound healing	To "jump start" a wound that is not healing by providing a collagen matrix for wound to continue healing	• Dry, eschar-covered wounds • Third-degree burns • Not most effective on necrotic wounds • If bovine product, check for allergy to bovine	• Select dressing based on wound bed. • Use cover dressings as needed for absorbency, protection, etc. • Remove by rinsing wound with sterile normal saline and reapplying dressing material.

Dressing classifications	Actions	Indications	Contraindications	Application tips
Contact Layer Mepitel®, Restore TRIACT **Xeroform, Adaptic™**	Silicone dressings Xeroform, Adaptic™ discussed below	• Helps prevent dressing adherence • Helps protect regenerating tissue and minimizes patient pain and trauma during dressing changes • Exudate easily passes through to the secondary absorbent dressing. • Can be cut to wound size without unraveling and shredding.	Heavily exudating wounds unless you are using the dressing as a wound contact layer under negative pressure wound therapy, etc.	Consider applying a skin protection preparation on periwound skin.
Nonadherent dressings Telfa™, Xeroform, Adaptic™	• Telfa is a gauze dressing with minimal absorptive capability and a nonstick surface. • Adaptic™ is knitted cellulose acetate fabric and impregnated with a specially formulated petrolatum emulsion. • Xeroform is a sterile, nonadherent gauze dressing with bacteriostatic action and contains 3% bismuth tribromophenate in a special petrolatum blend on fine mesh gauze.	Telfa™ can be used over ointments, creams, and gels as minimal product absorption into the dressing occurs.	Telfa™ should not be used as a wound contact layer.	Consider applying a skin protection preparation on periwound skin.

Enzymatic Agents Collagenase Santyl®	• Degrade damaged tissues while causing little injury to healthy tissue
	• Ointment selectively targets the collagen strands that hold microscopic cellular debris in place, helping break the cycle of inflammation.
		Necrotic tissue in wound bed	Adverse reactions of periulcer area such as burning, stinging, bleeding, transient dermatitis	• Score (cross-hatch) hard eschar or soften by autolysis before applying enzyme to ↑ penetration.
				• MEND
				  Moisture: Apply damp NSS dressing over ointment and then cover with secondary dressing.
				  Edge-to-edge application on wound
				  Nickel thick application
				  Daily dressing change

Dressing classifications	Actions	Indications	Contraindications	Application tips
Foam (ALLEVYN, Biatain®, Mepilex, Optifoam®)	• Absorbs exudate and traps it within dressing and off wound bed. • Permits moist environment without maceration	• Assists with autolytic debridement of moist wound bed • Maintains moist wound bed • Absorbs moderate to heavy exudate • Insulates wound surface • Provides nontraumatic removal • Partial thickness • Full thickness if dead space is lightly filled (space may be filled with selected foam products) • May be used as a secondary dressing for additional absorption • Clean or dirty	• Wounds with no exudates (*some foams are not as hydrophilic as others and may be used with drier wounds*) • Wounds with dry eschar • Wounds with undermining edges or sinus tracts unless areas are lightly filled	• Foam needs to be secured if it is nonadhesive (tape, gauze wrap, mesh net wrap, elastic bandage). • Use skin protectant around wound to protect from drainage. – Check manufacturer's directions • Change when drainage strikes through to outer edges of foam (or top of foam depending on product) Q2–5 days.
Polymeric Membrane Dressings (PolyMem®)	• PolyMem's Quadra-Foam contains a mild, nontoxic cleansing agent activated by moisture that is gradually released into the wound bed. • Gently expands to fill and conform to the wound • Wicks away up to 10 times its weight in exudates • Keeps the wound bed moist and soothes traumatized tissues, reducing wound pain and providing comfort at the wound site. The moisturizer also keeps the dressing pad from adhering to the wound so it is removed with virtually no pain.	• Assists with autolytic debridement of moist wound bed • Maintains moist wound bed • Absorbs moderate to heavy exudate • Insulates wound surface • Provides nontraumatic removal • Partial thickness • Full thickness if dead space is lightly filled	• Wounds with no exudates (*some foams are not as hydrophilic as others and may be used with drier wounds*) • Wounds with dry eschar • Wounds with undermining edges or sinus tracts unless areas are lightly filled	Foam needs to be secured if it is nonadhesive (tape, gauze wrap, mesh net wrap, elastic bandage).

Dressing classifications	Actions	Indications	Contraindications	Application tips
Hydrocolloid (DuoDERM®, Restore®, Tegasorb™, RepliCare™, Comfeel)	• Contains hydroactive particles • Occlusive • May be adhesive with a tape border • May react with wound exudate to form gel-like covering to maintain moist wound environment	• Assists with autolytic debridement by keeping wound bed moist • Absorbs light to moderate wound drainage • Insulates wound and because of occlusion provides some protection against secondary infection. Used for autolysis • Partial thickness • Shallow full thickness (think ear) • Noninfected wounds	• Highly exudating wounds • Clinically infected wounds • Wounds with sinus tracts or undermining edges unless this "dead space" is lightly filled	• 2–4 cm of intact skin around wound allows for better seal. • May use skin protector around wound to defat area and protect skin from adhesive if fragile skin • Shave or clip excessive hair to ↓ bacterial invasion of wound and ↑ adhesion. • Picture frame edges with tape if dressing is not prepackaged with this feature. • Change Q3 days or when dressing is no longer occlusive, leaking, or wrinkled. • Exudate is usually yellowish and odorous—assess wound **after** cleaning. • Does not require secondary dressing • Occlusive so stool and urine do not contaminate wound unless dressing is not intact
Hydrogel *Hydrogel sheet dressing* (Vigilon®, FLEXIGEL; Derma-Gel®)	• Maintain a moist wound surface as they are composed of mostly water • Nonadherent • Minimal absorption • Autolytic debridement because of eschar hydration • Acts like second layer of skin and decreases pain	• Promotes autolytic debridement • Provides comfort to wound • Partial thickness—Cut to fit wound as moist dressing can macerate intact skin around the wound • Clean or dirty • Consider for skin tears or radiation areas (with radiologist permission).	Moderate to heavily exudating wounds	• Secondary dressings are needed. – Consider non-adherent dressing, tubular dressings, mesh dressings to avoid adhesives. • Change dressings when strikethrough occurs; may be once or twice a day to every other day

Dressing classifications	Actions	Indications	Contraindications	Application tips
Amorphous wound gel (IntraSite™, Carrasyn V™, SoloSite, Normlgel®, DuoDERM® gel, Restore™, Curafil™; Skintegrity®)	• Gels have different hydrophilic properties and therefore have different wound hydrating capacities—check product info. • Promotes granulation and reepithelialization • Hydrates eschar	• Maintain a moist wound surface • Create a moist wound surface by hydrating • Support autolytic debridement • Clean or dirty • Partial thickness or full thickness (remember to lightly fill the dead space) • Partial thickness? Consider using non-adherent gauze to decrease amount of wound gel absorbed by secondary dressing.	• Moderate to heavily exudating wounds • Full thickness if NSS moist, fluffed gauze not used to lightly fill "dead space"	• Gel dressings do not adhere to wound bed and do not destroy fragile tissue while they are maintaining moist environment • Secondary dressings are needed.

Gel-impregnated strip gauze (Restore™ hydrogel-impregnated gauze, Curafil™ hydrogel-impregnated gauze strip)

Transparent, Polyurethane Adhesive Film (OpSite®, Tegaderm™)	• Semipermeable membrane that permits water vapor and oxygen to pass between wound bed and environment but keeps bacteria from coming in because of dressing pore size • Maintains moist wound environment to enhance resurfacing of the wound • Occlusion reduces local wound pain. • Autolytic debridement enhanced by moist, warm environment • Does not require secondary dressing	• Indicated for nondraining wounds. Supports autolytic debridement of dry eschar and fibrin slough • Maintains moist, non-adherent surface next to wound • Protects blisters and superficial wounds • Wound can be monitored through transparent dressing. • Partial thickness • Do not use on infected wounds. • May be used as secondary dressing for selected wounds	• Exudating wounds. Clinically infected wounds • Wounds with sinus tracts or undermining edges unless this "dead space" is lightly filled	• 2–4 cm of intact skin around wound allows for better seal. • Use skin protector around wound to defat area and protect skin from adhesive. • Shave or clip excessive hair to ↓ bacterial invasion of wound and ↑ adhesion. • Change when dressing is leaking or no longer intact or Q3–5 days. • Exudate is usually cloudy and foul smelling until wound is cleansed.

Filling dead space

Filling dead space in a wound prevents surface healing before deep healing. The type of material used depends on the size of the wound and the amount of exudate. If using gauze, consider using roll gauze as you will not leave a piece behind on removal! Cotton mesh gauze used to be the standard. Today, you have more options. See Chapter 9 for more on dressing options.

Step by step

As you follow these steps, be sure to observe standard precautions.

1. **Make sure the material is moist.**
   Use a slight amount of sterile normal saline solution if needed (draining wounds do not usually need added moisture).
2. **Fill the dead space.**
   Use sterile forceps, gloves, and/or cotton-tipped applicators as needed.
   - If using moistened gauze, fluff the moist sterile pad or strip to unclump it.
   - Loosely but thoroughly fill the dead space in the wound. Note that "packing" the wound too tightly can create pressure damage on the granulating cells.
   - Cover all the wound surfaces and edges.
   - Regardless of dressing used, keep dressing in the wound bed because moist dressings can macerate intact tissue.

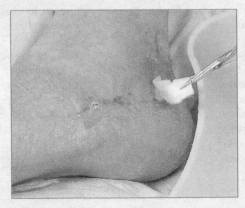
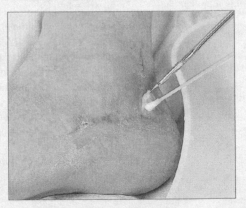

Index

Note: i refers to an illustration; t refers to a table.

Note: i refers to an illustration; t refers to a table.

Note: i refers to an illustration; t refers to a table.

Note: i refers to an illustration; t refers to a table.

Note: i refers to an illustration; t refers to a table.